Medigraph (T.M.)
Manual

Medigraph ^(T.M.) Manual

GEORGE E. PALEY, M.D. and HERBERT C. ROSENTHAL
in collaboration with GRAPHICS INSTITUTE, INC.

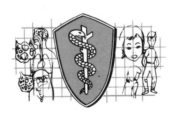

H. S. STUTTMAN CO., Inc.   New York, N.Y. 10016

Publishers

INTRODUCTION

E ARLY RECOGNITION of any illness is the most important single factor in
its treatment and cure. This statement applies equally to minor and
annoying ailments such as some skin disorders, to the major takers of
human life such as heart disease and cancer, as well as to such growing
problems as infectious diseases and drug addiction.

Being aware of the importance of early recognition, the medical profession is abandoning its classic position of telling the patient as little as
possible and entering an era in which doctors endeavor to provide their
patients with authoritative information about the *causes, symptoms, possible complications* and *prevention* of disease.

Thus, signs of disease which are deceptively mild or unnoticed by the
uninformed person may alert the informed patient to seek early treatment.
When disease does strike without warning, knowledge can overcome fear.
The physician will diagnose, prescribe, and follow through with treatment.
The demands on the doctor's time are such, however, that frequently he
cannot stop to explain fully the cause of the illness, the further symptoms
that may develop, and the outlook for complete or partial cure. The informed individual, be he patient or close relative, can derive much comfort
in the possession of authoritative knowledge about the illness, its usual
course and the treatment the physician may choose to combat it.

To convey this knowledge with authority and clarity required the combined efforts of a physician qualified as a specialist in Internal Medicine
and a graphic visualizer with a talent for simplifying technical subjects. The
MEDIGRAPH MANUAL is the result of such collaboration plus staff work by
medical writers, designers and illustrators. Test use of the MEDIGRAPH
illustrations by doctors and patients have demonstrated their unique ability
to explain, inform, and instruct.

The scope of the volume is wide, ranging from the common diseases
of childhood to the ailments of old age, and covering in between the frequent and the rare disorders that afflict persons of all ages.

The text is so organized that the reader can quickly find the information he seeks. The pertinent facts for each disease are immediately at hand,
with text and illustration side by side, eliminating the necessity for leafing

through the volume or consulting an index for various aspects of the same illness. When it is helpful for purposes of conveying a clear understanding of a disease and its action upon the patient, the organ or organs principally affected are illustrated in their position in the body as a whole. Separate drawings show how a specific part is affected, from the hair follicles and pores involved in a case of acne to the intricate involvement of the spine in a slipped disc or of the heart in various types of heart disease. A full color atlas of male and female anatomy, printed on transparent acetate overlays, accurately illustrates each body system and the comparative size and position of each organ shown on the MEDIGRAPH illustrations.

The discussion of each disease begins with a brief summary of its *causes* and how it affects the organ or body system involved. The affected organ and its role in the normal body are described. If the disorder is a functional one, the abnormal changes in the organ and its function are outlined; if the disease is caused by an outside influence such as the presence of bacteria or the absence of some vital nutritive substance, these factors are clearly explained.

There follows a specific description of *symptoms* by which the disease can be recognized, and these symptoms are meticulously illustrated in the accompanying MEDIGRAPH illustrations. If the disease first manifests itself in a rash, for instance, the MEDIGRAPH chart shows the specific type and form of rash that may be noted and follows the stages from its first appearance to its decline as the disease is overcome by treatment. If pain is the first warning sign, the site of its occurrence is shown in the MEDIGRAPH illustration. Many diseases have well-defined stages through which they progress from onset to disappearance, and these stages sometimes affect various parts or organs of the body; each of these is clearly illustrated in the MEDIGRAPH pictures for each disease.

The third section of text on each disease describes the *complications* that may arise, and these, too, are shown in the MEDIGRAPH illustration on the opposite page.

The final section gives advice on *prevention* of the disease, if possible, or the lessening of its impact on the patient if the illness is unavoidable. Forms of treatment that are available to the physician are described, including newly developed methods of surgery, chemotherapy, and others, along with the favorable or unfavorable outlook for recovery. Specific instructions are given for avoiding preventable diseases and advice is provided for the individual whose family is prone to certain diseases.

The MEDIGRAPH illustrations and text cover a broad range of medical conditions that occur with some frequency in doctors' practices throughout the world. They are the distillation of eight years of research, planning and reader testing. It will be gratifying to see a continuation of the evidence that widespread reference to this MEDIGRAPH MANUAL will help the doctor more easily explain to the patient the nature of his illness, and enable doctor and patient to work together to speed the patient's recovery.

H. S. STUTTMAN CO., INC.
Publishers

Contents

Acne 12

Acromegaly and Giantism 14

Addison's Disease 16

Alcoholism 18

Amebiasis and Amebic Dysentery 20

Aneurysms 22

Anthracosis (Coal Miner's Pneumoconiosis) and Asbestosis 24

Anthrax 26

Appendicitis and Peritonitis 28

Arteriosclerosis 30

Peripheral Arteriosclerosis 32

Rheumatoid Arthritis 34

Bell's Palsy 36

Beriberi 38

Botulism 40

Brain Tumors 42

Bronchial Adenoma 44

Bronchial Asthma 46

Bronchiectasis 48

Bronchitis 50

Buerger's Disease 52

Bursitis 54

Breast Cancer 56

Cancers of the Cervix and Uterus 58

Cancer of the Colon and Rectum 60

Lung Cancer 62

Cancer of the Pancreas 64

Skin Cancer 66

Cancer of the Stomach 68

Carbuncles, Furuncles (Boils) and Folliculitis 70

Cataracts 72

Celiac Disease 74

Cerebral Palsy 76
Chagas' Disease 78
Chickenpox 80
Cholera 82
Cirrhosis of the Liver 84
Cold Sores 86
Ulcerative Colitis 88
Conjunctivitis 90
Contact Dermatitis and Drug Reactions 92
Coronary Artery Disease 94
Cretinism and Myxedema 96
Cushing's Syndrome 98
Deviated Septum 100
Diabetes 102
Diphtheria 104
Drug Abuse: Amphetamines 106
Drug Abuse: Barbiturates 108
Drug Abuse: Cocaine 110
Drug Abuse: Heroin 112
Drug Abuse: LSD 114
Drug Abuse: Marijuana and Hashish 116
Drug Abuse: Mescaline and Peyote 118
Drug Abuse: Sniffing of Glue, Solvents, Aerosols, Anesthetics 120
Eclampsia and Preeclampsia 122
Ectopic Pregnancy 124
Emphysema 126
Encephalitis 128
Subacute Bacterial Endocarditis 130
Epilepsy 132
Diseases of the Esophagus 134
Fibroid Tumor 136
Fibromyositis 138
Flu and Grippe 140
Fractures and Dislocations 142
Fungus Infections of the Skin 144
Gallstones 146
Gastritis 148
German Measles 150
Glaucoma 152
Gonorrhea 154
Gout 156
Hansen's Disease 158
Hay Fever 160
Congenital Heart Disease 162
Hypertensive Heart Disease 164

Pulmonary Heart Disease 166
Rheumatic Heart Disease 168
Thyroid Heart Disease 170
Heart Failure 172
Heat Stroke 174
Hemophilia 176
Hemorrhoids (Piles) and Fissures 178
Hepatitis 180
Hiatus (Diaphragmatic) Hernia 182
Inguinal and Other Abdominal Hernias 184
High Blood Pressure 186
Histoplasmosis 188
Hives 190
Hodgkin's Disease 192
Hookworm 194
Hydrocele and Varicocele 196
Hyperparathyroidism 198
Hyperthyroidism 200
Hypoglycemia 202
Hypogonadism and Simmonds' Disease 204
Ileitis 206
Impetigo 208
Intestinal Obstruction 210
Iritis 212
Kidney and Urinary Tract Stones 214
Lead Poisoning 216
Leptospirosis 218
Leukemia 220
Leukoplakia 222
Lice and Scabies 224
Lung Abscess 226
Lupus Erythematosus 228
Malaria 230
Mastoiditis 232
Measles 234
Ménière's Disease (and Labyrinthitis) 236
Meningitis 238
Menopause 240
Mercury Poisoning 242
Migraine Headaches 244
Infectious Mononucleosis 246
Multiple Sclerosis 248
Mumps 250
Myasthenia Gravis 252
Nephritis 254

Neuritis 256
Neurocirculatory Asthenia 258
Orchitis 260
Osteoarthritis 262
Osteomyelitis 264
Ovarian Infection 266
Pancreatitis 268
Parkinson's Disease 270
Pellagra 272
Pericarditis 274
Pernicious Anemia 276
Phlebitis 278
Pilonidal Cyst 280
Pinworm 282
Pityriasis Rosea 284
Pleurisy 286
Pneumonia 288
Poliomyelitis 290
Prostate Gland Enlargement   Cancer of the Prostate 292
Psoriasis 294
Rabies 296
Raynaud's Disease 298
Rheumatic Fever 300
Rickets 302
Rocky Mountain Spotted Fever 304
Roundworm 306
Scarlet Fever 308
Schistosomiasis 310
Scleroderma 312
Scurvy 314
Seborrheic Dermatitis 316
Shingles 318
Sickle Cell Anemia 320
Silicosis 322
Sinusitis 324
Slipped Disc 326
Smallpox 328
Snake Bites 330
Sprains and Strains 332
Sterility 334
Stroke 336
Styes 338
Syphilis 340
Tapeworm 342
Tay-Sachs Disease 344

Tetanus 346

Acute Tonsillitis 348

Toxoplasmosis 350

Trench Mouth 352

Trichinosis 354

Trichomonas 356

Pulmonary Tuberculosis 358

Typhoid Fever 360

Ulcers of the Digestive Tract 362

Undescended Testicles 364

Urinary Tract Tumors and Infections 366

Varicose Veins 368

Vitamin A Deficiency 370

Warts 372

Wens, Milium and Lipoma 374

Whiplash Injury of the Neck 376

Whooping Cough 378

Yellow Fever 380

Index 382

The Human Body in Anatomical Transparencies 385

the disease and its causes   Acne is a chronic disease of the oil glands of the skin which results in formations of blackheads, pustules, cysts, and depressed scars over the face and back primarily. The cause is unknown, but it occurs most usually during adolescence when the oil glands mature and produce larger amounts of oil. The disease ranges from mild to severe. It can last, off and on, from 2 to 20 years. If it is not treated, it can permanently scar the patient.

symptoms   The areas affected appear extremely oily—usually the forehead, chin, and portions around the nose. Many blackheads appear along with some pussy lesions which open easily and dry without scarring after discharging their contents. Squeezing usually drives as much oil back deeper into the skin as it removes, and simply enlarges the inflamed area. Deeper lesions heal more slowly and these frequently leave pitted scars. In severe cases where there are a great many lesions, they can run together and cause abscesses which heal in time but leave behind large areas of disfiguring scar tissue.

complications   There can be secondary infections. Also, a patient can be very distressed and disturbed when unsightly scar tissue remains.

prevention (or lessening of impact)   The acne-prone person can do little to prevent this disease, but he can do a number of things to modify its course and minimize scarring. He should avoid chocolate, iodized salt, fats, fried foods, dairy products, shellfish, mayonnaise, peanut butter, and alcoholic beverages. Personal hygiene should be emphasized—including washing frequently and bathing with anti-bacterial soap. Sun baths can be beneficial and certainly help cosmetically. Very often the doctor will prescribe a program of diet and medication.

Acne

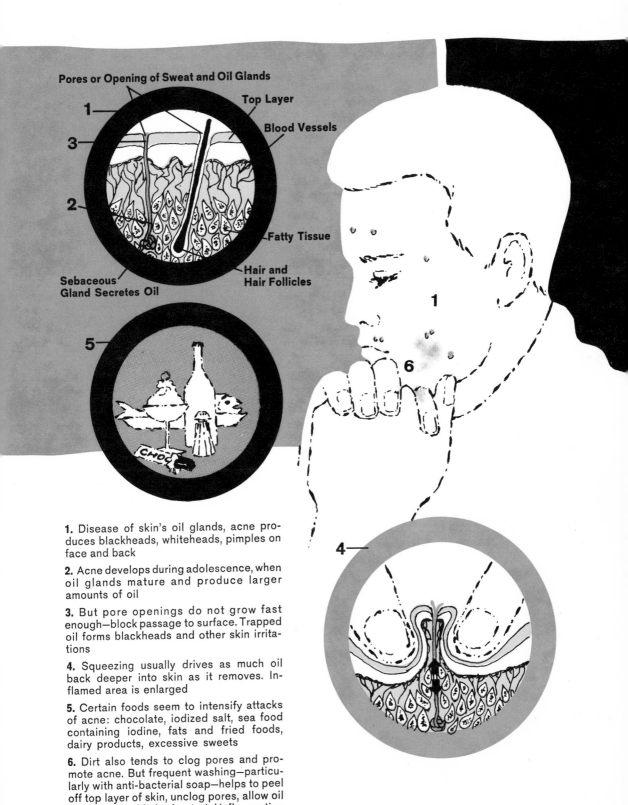

Pores or Opening of Sweat and Oil Glands

1

3

2

Top Layer

Blood Vessels

Fatty Tissue

Hair and
Hair Follicles

Sebaceous
Gland Secretes Oil

5

CHOC

1

6

4

1. Disease of skin's oil glands, acne produces blackheads, whiteheads, pimples on face and back

2. Acne develops during adolescence, when oil glands mature and produce larger amounts of oil

3. But pore openings do not grow fast enough—block passage to surface. Trapped oil forms blackheads and other skin irritations

4. Squeezing usually drives as much oil back deeper into skin as it removes. Inflamed area is enlarged

5. Certain foods seem to intensify attacks of acne: chocolate, iodized salt, sea food containing iodine, fats and fried foods, dairy products, excessive sweets

6. Dirt also tends to clog pores and promote acne. But frequent washing—particularly with anti-bacterial soap—helps to peel off top layer of skin, unclog pores, allow oil to emerge, and fights bacterial inflammation

Acromegaly and Giantism
(Diseases of Overactive Pituitary Gland)

the disease and its causes   These two conditions are brought about by the excessive production of growth hormones by the pituitary gland. The cause of the overproduction of these hormones is usually a small, benign, slow-growing tumor in the pituitary gland.
Both conditions are relatively rare, and both sexes are affected.

symptoms   GIANTISM   When the tumor causes hormone overproduction during the normal growth years, all the organs and the long bones keep growing, resulting at first in a well-proportioned giant. However, if the disease goes undetected and untreated, the giantism can progress to a point where the patient becomes dangerously weakened.
ACROMEGALY   When the tumor causes hormone overproduction *after* the normal growth years, excessive growth occurs in areas other than the long bones. These areas include the soft tissues—such as the lips, tongue, ears, and nose—and the bony structures, causing a protruding lower jaw, spade-like hands, enlarged feet, and a hunched back. Often men become impotent and women cease to menstruate. Headaches, visual impairment, and even blindness sometimes result. The thyroid gland may become involved. Diabetes is not an unusual development. This form of the disease, which appears most often in the third decade, can develop over a period of ten or more years. In occasional cases it runs a rapid course and may end fatally because of heart involvement or inability to resist infection. The disease may stop of its own accord at any point, and the patient may live a comfortable life for many years.

complications   Complications arise when the progress of the disease results in the involvement of other organ systems or the development of other glandular abnormalities. Heart failure, hyperthyroidism, diabetes, and diabetic coma are not unusual.

prevention (or lessening of impact)   When the presence of a tumor is established, it must be destroyed by X ray treatment or surgery. Associated glandular abnormalities are treated with specific replacement hormones. Treatment which controls the disease cannot undo any bodily changes which have already taken place, but it can stop further progression.
There is no way of knowing who will be affected or how this disease can be prevented.

Acromegaly and Giantism

(Diseases of Overactive Pituitary Gland)

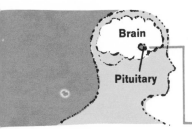

Brain

Pituitary

Tumor of anterior pituitary gland results in overproduction of hormones controlling growth

If tumor becomes active . . .

after normal growth years . . .

Acromegaly

With growth no longer possible in long bones, excessive growth slowly takes place in other areas:

1. Soft tissues—lips, tongue, ears, nose

2. Bony structure—protruding lower jaw, spade-like hands, enlarged feet, hunched back

3. Disturbance of sexual functions—impotence in men, ceasing of menstruation in women

4. Other possible complications—diabetes, visual disturbances and blindness, loss of strength

before normal growth years . . .

Giantism

1. Long bone growth continues, resulting in well proportioned giant 7-8 feet tall

2. However, if not arrested, gigantism may progress to stage of increasing weakness and death

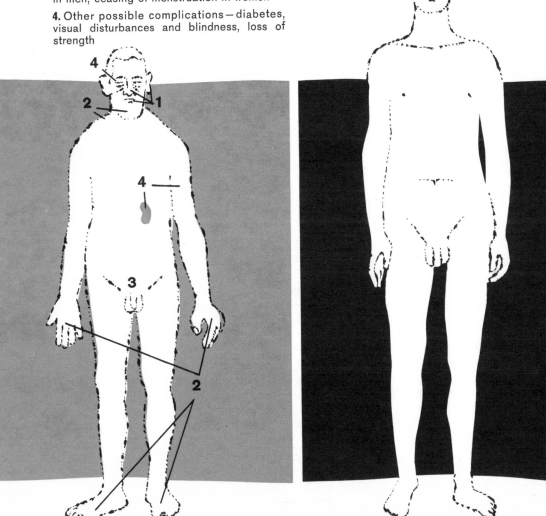

the disease and its causes   The adrenal cortex, which is the outer sheath of the adrenal gland at the upper end of the kidney, secretes over 30 steroid hormones. The proper function of this gland is essential for life. Any condition that interferes with its secretions is potentially serious. Therefore, early recognition of Addison's disease and prompt treatment of it are of the greatest importance.

Addison's disease, or underactivity of the adrenal cortex, is rare. It can develop at any age, although it is found most often in middle life, and occurs equally in both sexes. The course of the disease is slow, but as it develops it can reduce the normal operations of both adrenal glands. In time, the patient suffers from a chronic adrenal insufficiency—lacking the hormones normally produced by the adrenal cortex. While tuberculosis accounts for about 70% of the cases, tumors affecting both glands, and certain bacterial infections, are also implicated. The disease may also be the end result of a condition in which the pituitary gland is not functioning adequately, or it may occur in cases where surgical removal of the adrenal glands is indicated.

symptoms   The onset is usually very slow, and the course of the disease can vary from relatively slow to relentlessly progressive. There are complaints of muscle weakness and a fatigue which tends to be progressive until bed rest is required. There is loss of appetite, weight loss, nausea and vomiting—this last may be accompanied by vague, crampy, but sometimes severe abdominal pains.

An obvious sign is the change which occurs in the skin pigment. Brown or tan darkenings or clouds of freckles appear over many parts of the body, particularly over pressure points and areas that normally have clear flesh tones.

Examination often reveals low blood pressure, low blood sugar, and other chemical changes. Mental changes can be quite striking. The patient may become lethargic and irritable, showing increased signs of apprehension. His sex urge is reduced and there is a decrease in the growth of body hair. In time he presents the picture of a patient with severe malnutrition.

complications   When this disease is unrecognized and untreated, secondary infections tend to become overwhelming. Complications can include progressive disability, weakness, and death.

When the cause is established as active tuberculosis, the outlook is very poor.

prevention (or lessening of impact)   Now that cortical steroids have been discovered and put to use, patients with Addison's disease show remarkable improvement. The hormonal and chemical balance of the body can be regulated by diet and drugs prescribed by the doctor. Patients are taught to recognize the symptoms of too little or too much medication, and ways to cope with infection and periods of unusual stress.

With proper treatment patients are considerably improved, generally return to normal functions, and have a bright outlook.

Addison's Disease (Underactivity of the Adrenal Cortex)

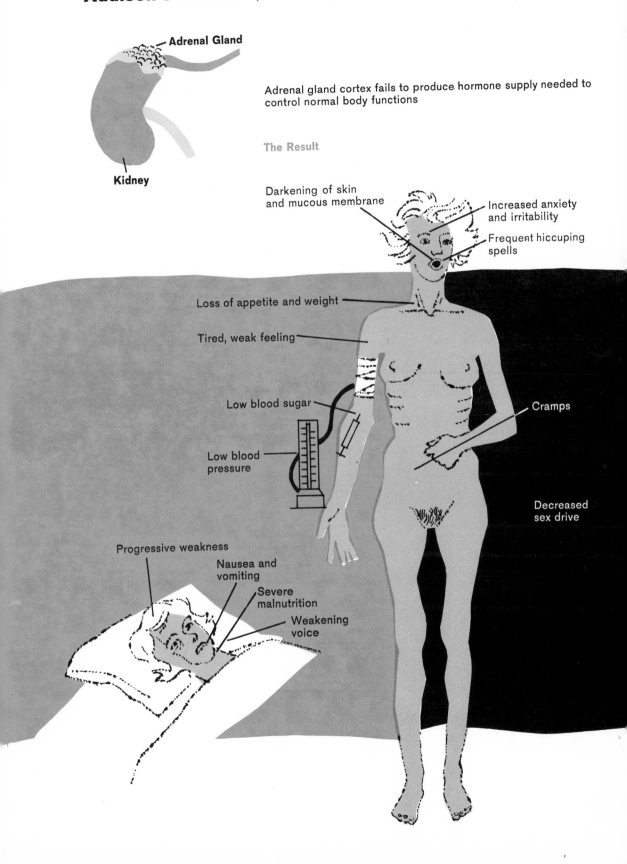

Adrenal Gland

Kidney

Adrenal gland cortex fails to produce hormone supply needed to control normal body functions

The Result

Darkening of skin and mucous membrane

Increased anxiety and irritability

Frequent hiccuping spells

Loss of appetite and weight

Tired, weak feeling

Low blood sugar

Cramps

Low blood pressure

Decreased sex drive

Progressive weakness

Nausea and vomiting

Severe malnutrition

Weakening voice

the disease and its cause An alcoholic is one so dependent on drinking alcoholic beverages—such as whiskey, gin, vodka, rum, wine, beer, and brandy—that they affect his health and interfere with his social and economic relationships. Alcoholism is a widespread disease, affecting over 5 million Americans alone. The effects of this disease on society—in terms of accidents, crimes, breakup of family life, and loss of productivity—are tremendous.

Many people brighten up after small doses of alcohol and act more freely than usual, because the restraining influence they usually exercise has been diminished. This is because alcohol depresses the functions of the brain and central nervous system and therefore reduces the person's self-control. However, excessive amounts of alcohol also act as a poison and can seriously damage the body. But the alcoholic has a compulsive need for alcohol. He cannot control his drinking, and becomes physically dependent on alcohol.

symptoms Drunken behavior is, of course, a preeminent symptom of alcoholism. Some alcoholics need many drinks before they develop signs of intoxication; others have become so sensitized to alcohol that only one or two drinks will precipitate them into drunken behavior. The loss of restraint while drunk will manifest itself in varying degrees of exhilaration, talkativeness, slurred speech, and loss of coordination. Irrational and destructive acts are also typical of this state.

complications Some alcoholics develop delirium tremens—a state in which they suffer from uncontrollable tremors and are tortured by terrifying hallucinations. During such seizures, they can seriously injure themselves in an effort to escape from these hallucinations.

Another peril of alcoholism is extreme drowsiness and lethargy which, with very large amounts of alcohol, can lead to coma and death.

efforts to break the habit Treatment of the confirmed alcoholic is long and difficult. Antabuse—which makes the body react adversely to alcoholic drinks—and tranquilizing drugs have sometimes proved helpful in breaking the alcoholic cycle.

After the first stages of recovery, psychological support can be effective —particularly from groups like Alcoholics Anonymous. A proper diet and the avoidance of even small amounts of alcohol are essential. This means that the active cooperation of the alcoholic is needed to effect his cure.

Alcoholism

Compulsive, excessive drinking,
which can cause damage to . . .

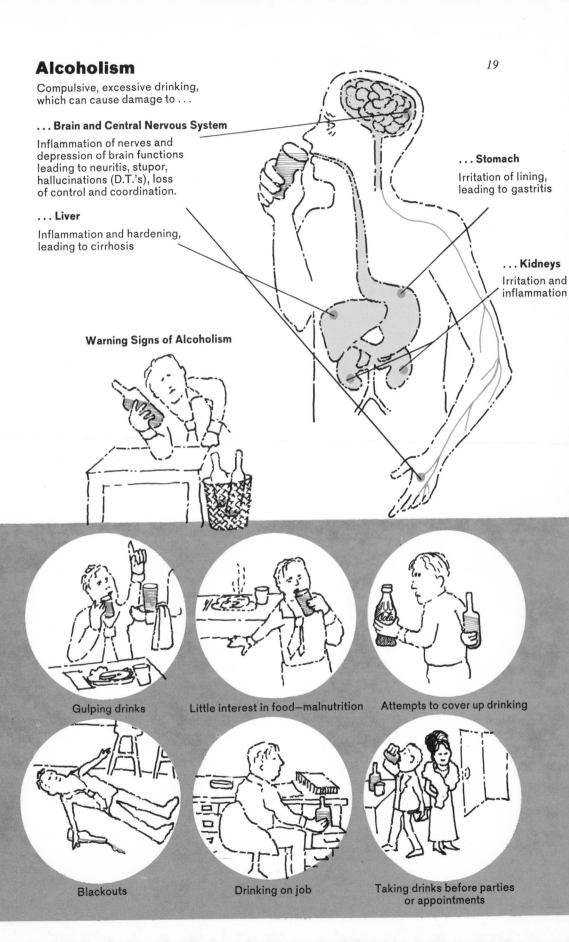

. . . Brain and Central Nervous System

Inflammation of nerves and
depression of brain functions
leading to neuritis, stupor,
hallucinations (D.T.'s), loss
of control and coordination.

. . . Liver

Inflammation and hardening,
leading to cirrhosis

. . . Stomach

Irritation of lining,
leading to gastritis

. . . Kidneys

Irritation and
inflammation

Warning Signs of Alcoholism

Gulping drinks

Little interest in food—malnutrition

Attempts to cover up drinking

Blackouts

Drinking on job

Taking drinks before parties
or appointments

the disease and its causes Amebiasis or amebic dysentery is caused by amebae—microscopic one-celled animals. This disease affects about 10% of the population of the United States and is found throughout the world, particularly in warmer climates. Primarily, the bowels are involved, but the disease may affect other organ systems, particularly the liver and the lungs.

Infected flies, water, and food are among the transmitting agents. Infected food handlers are particularly responsible. The disease is common in areas where human waste is used for fertilizer.

Once the ameba has been eaten, or otherwise taken internally, it lodges in the lower end of the small intestine. Here it develops, multiplies, and ultimately becomes capable of penetrating the bowel wall and spreading to other parts of the body. Some of these amebae may be excreted with the stool. In the cyst form the disease is contagious.

The incubation period varies from a few days, which is the usual time, to from nine to eighty days.

symptoms There is great variation in the severity of the symptoms. Many individuals who are carriers never know it and never have any symptoms. In the acute form, the onset is sudden. There is severe abdominal pain, nausea, vomiting, and liquid stools with blood and mucus excreted up to 15-20 times a day. Marked rectal pain accompanies the bowel movements. If there is any fever it is mild, but the patient feels weaker and weaker.

In most cases, the attack leaves the patient with chronic amebic dysentery with characteristic bouts of diarrhea from time to time, gas, loss of appetite and weight, weakness, usually some anemia and periods of low-grade fever. Without treatment the condition may last for years and the patient can become a chronic invalid.

complications Liver involvement occurs in about 5% of all cases of amebiasis, with abscess of the liver the most serious and common complication. When the abscess ruptures there is peritonitis and the outlook becomes much more serious.

Another complication is involvement of the right lung and pleural cavity, usually by direct extension from amebic liver disease. The patient develops lung abscess and empyema (which is an accumulation of pus in the pleural sac).

The pericardium, which is the sac containing the heart, can be affected. Painful, destructive skin lesions can also occur.

prevention (or lessening of impact) The doctor can detect amebic infection by stool examination, or proctoscopic study. Specific drugs are available to eradicate amebae from the large bowel and treat any liver involvement.

In areas where amebic infection exists, care must be given to the protection of the water supply and to proper sewage disposal. People in these areas should also avoid eating fresh, uncleaned vegetables, and should protect food from flies.

Amebiasis and Amebic Dysentery

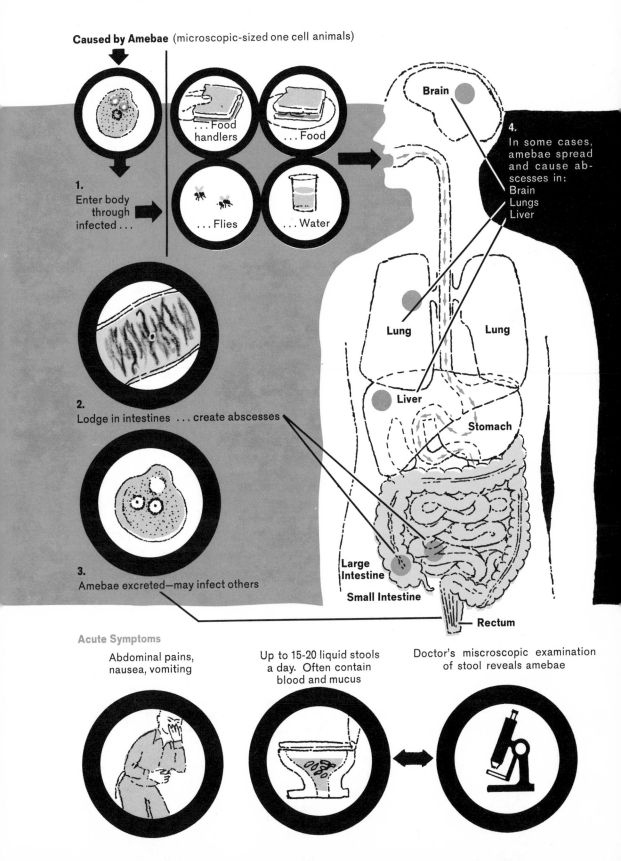

Caused by Amebae (microscopic-sized one cell animals)

1.
Enter body through infected . . .

. . .Food handlers

. . .Food

. . .Flies

. . .Water

Brain

4.
In some cases, amebae spread and cause abscesses in:
Brain
Lungs
Liver

Lung

Lung

Liver

Stomach

2.
Lodge in intestines . . . create abscesses

3.
Amebae excreted—may infect others

Large Intestine

Small Intestine

Rectum

Acute Symptoms

Abdominal pains, nausea, vomiting

Up to 15-20 liquid stools a day. Often contain blood and mucus

Doctor's miscroscopic examination of stool reveals amebae

Aneurysms

the disease and its causes   An aneurysm is a sac formed by the enlargement of the wall of a blood vessel. This is caused by the destruction of elastic tissue in the artery or vein involved during the course of diseases such as arteriosclerosis, hypertension, and syphilis. The most important aneurysms are those which affect the important aortic artery, the main trunk of the entire arterial system.

Aneurysms vary in degree from slight widening of the blood vessel to an enlargement great enough to involve the ribs, esophagus, and lungs. They may be single or multiple, and of varying shapes. Frequently they are filled with large thrombi, or blood clots.

Older people subject to the diseases noted above are affected, as a rule, with a slightly higher frequency of aneurysms occurring in men than in women.

symptoms   Symptoms depend upon the size and location of the aneurysm, although many aneurysms are present without any symptoms at all. However, when there is compression, or displacement, or interference with circulation to adjacent body structures, the aneurysm causes chronic disabilities. Those on the front part of the aorta may cause erosion of the ribs and even some bulging of the front chest wall. Chronic cough, frequent pneumonias, blood spitting, and a picture that resembles lung cancer may reveal the presence of an aneurysm in the arch of the aorta that is compressing the bronchial tubes. Further symptoms may be hoarseness, difficulty in swallowing, swelling of the neck, and perhaps swelling of an upper extremity.

Still other aneurysms can cause pain in the spine and nerves, high blood pressure, or kidney failure—as shown in the Medi-Graph.

complications   The most serious complication occurs when the sac bursts. The result is hemorrhage and death. Depending upon the size and site of the aneurysm, other complications can develop. These include pulmonary infection, congestive heart failure, kidney failure, and circulatory problems of the extremities.

prevention (or lessening of impact)   Aneurysms resulting from syphilis can be prevented by therapy with anti-syphilitic drugs during the early stages of this illness. Once a syphilitic aneurysm has formed, the doctor still prescribes treatment with these anti-syphilitic drugs—but how effective they will be depends upon how far along the disease has progressed. The drugs may relieve some of the symptoms and slow down further enlargement, but they will not cure the deformity already there.

There is no known way of preventing aneurysms that result from arteriosclerosis. The only treatment at present is surgery in which the diseased part of the blood vessel is replaced. Associated symptoms and complications are treated as they become evident.

Aneurysms

Bulging of blood vessel wall because of weak spot or loss of elasticity that develops. Bursting of sac can cause death

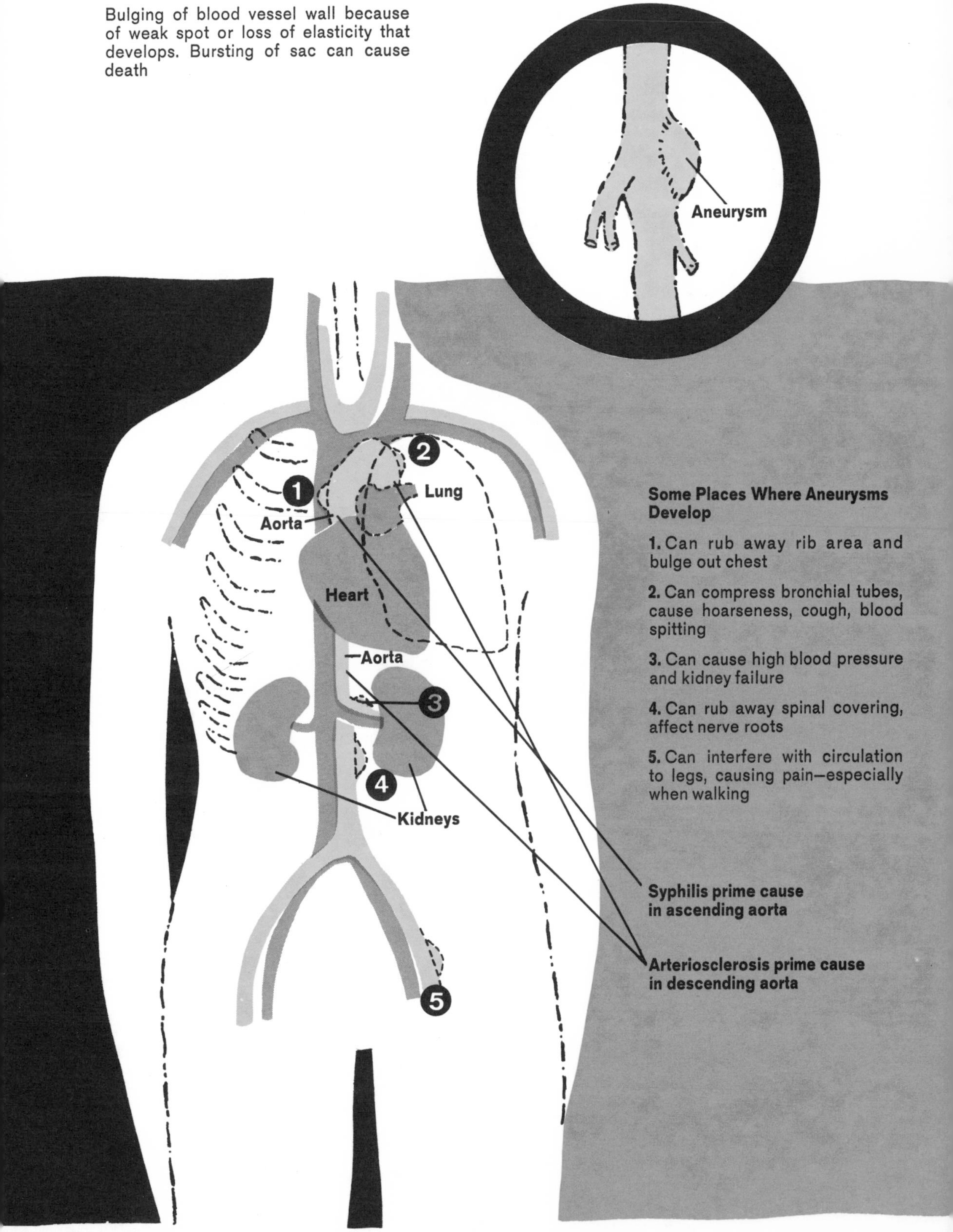

Aneurysm

Some Places Where Aneurysms Develop

1. Can rub away rib area and bulge out chest

2. Can compress bronchial tubes, cause hoarseness, cough, blood spitting

3. Can cause high blood pressure and kidney failure

4. Can rub away spinal covering, affect nerve roots

5. Can interfere with circulation to legs, causing pain—especially when walking

Lung

Aorta

Heart

Aorta

Kidneys

Syphilis prime cause in ascending aorta

Arteriosclerosis prime cause in descending aorta

Anthracosis (Coal Miner's Pneumoconiosis) and Asbestosis

the diseases and their causes   Anthracosis and asbestosis are occupational diseases caused by breathing certain dusts for long periods. As the names indicate, coal dust is the cause of anthracosis and asbestos dust the cause of asbestosis. We are discussing these diseases together because they exhibit similar symptoms—though the changes that occur within the body because of them differ in important aspects.

In anthracosis, the dust particles take hold throughout the lungs causing small scattered areas of infiltration and irritation, particularly in the lymph areas. Black masses of carbon build up in the lungs over the years.

In asbestosis, the inhalation of asbestos fibers produces fibrous changes in the lungs—causing hardening and shrinking of the lung tissue. This represents an attempt by the tissue of the lung to wall off this foreign substance. The degree of this fibrosis is much more severe and scattered than in anthracosis. In asbestosis, the lymph glands are frequently involved, too. The lining (pleura) of the lungs often becomes inflamed—so that pleurisy is common and chronic.

Both diseases are diagnosed through the victim's history of exposure to these noxious dusts and through typical lung patterns visible on X rays.

symptoms   The symptoms—which appear after a worker has had prolonged exposure to these dusts—are similar for both diseases. These include cough, shortness of breath, and progressively more severe breathing difficulties. Victims of asbestosis also begin to spit out a brownish substance containing the fibers and spiky needles associated with asbestos.

complications   If these diseases are allowed to go unchecked, pulmonary heart disease and heart failure are frequent complications. Even removing the worker from the offending environment will not actually cure the diseases but will only prevent them from becoming more acute.

prevention (or lessening of impact)   Prevention depends on the proper venting of the troublemaking dust—so that it is removed from the work area without being inhaled by the workers. Protective masks are of some help, but their use limits the efficiency of coal and asbestos workers.

Anthracosis (Coal Miner's Pneumoconiosis) and Asbestosis

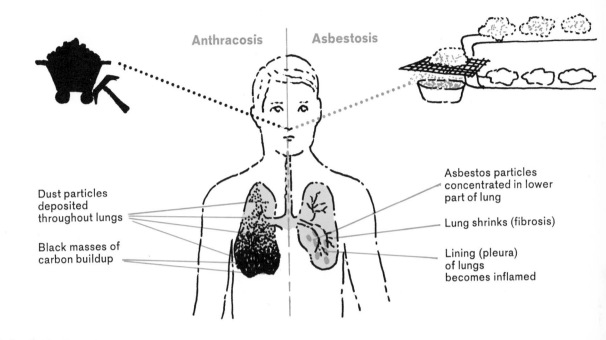

Anthracosis

Asbestosis

Dust particles deposited throughout lungs

Black masses of carbon buildup

Asbestos particles concentrated in lower part of lung

Lung shrinks (fibrosis)

Lining (pleura) of lungs becomes inflamed

Symptoms for both diseases

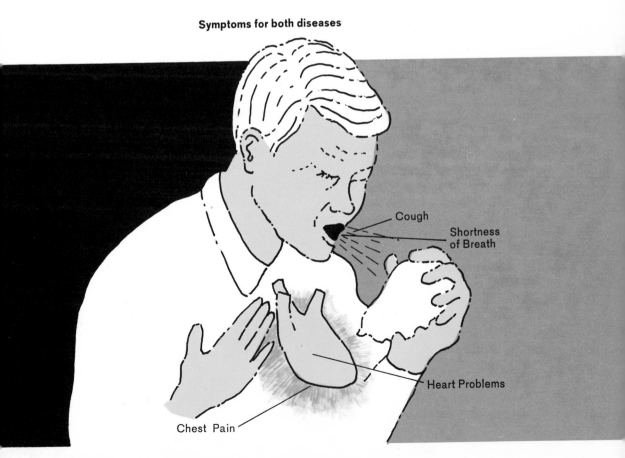

Cough

Shortness of Breath

Heart Problems

Chest Pain

the disease and its causes   This disease most often comes to public attention when an anthrax epidemic breaks out among animals: cattle, sheep and horses. However, this infectious disease attacks humans as well. It is a bacterial infection which is transmitted to man by contact with infected animals. Anthrax crops up most frequently among people working in the meat industry as butchers or others who handle the carcasses of infected animals—or work as handlers of contaminated wool, hair, or hides.
The germs enter most frequently through the skin via a wound, scratch or insect bite. It is also possible to be infected by anthrax bacteria by inhaling or by ingesting them with contaminated food or liquids.

symptoms   A case of anthrax is frequently heralded by an attack of painful itching. Several hours later, the first visible sign of anthrax develops in the form of a characteristic pimple or boil on the part of the skin exposed to the bacteria. This pimple is painless, itching, and has a purple center. It swells up and discharges a thick blood pus. The nearby lymph glands swell up, and the veins become inflamed.
The first boil is followed by many others. Headache, fever and a feeling of weakness are other symptoms that develop.
After discharging their pus, the boils ulcerate to form black scars.
Diagnosis of the disease is usually made by finding anthrax bacteria in the lesion or boil produced by the bacteria.

complications   Severe cases may rapidly develop a high temperature and pneumonia, and may prove fatal. Anthrax of the lungs is particularly dangerous in this regard. Other complications can include secondary infection around the boils and meningitis.

prevention (or lessening of impact)   Elimination of anthrax among animals is the best way of removing this danger to humans. In situations where there is a chance of contact with contaminated animal products, precautions must be taken to guard against this contact. Processing plants handling wool, hair, brushes and similar material need strict controls of both local and imported material. Sterilization of these materials before handling has proved helpful in preventing the spreading of anthrax. Protective clothing—such as overalls, rubber aprons and gloves which protect the skin—may be worn by a worker handling this material. Any person sorting wool or hair should wear breathing devices which will prevent him from inhaling anthrax bacteria.
Vaccines have been developed which have been reasonably effective in preventing the disease among humans in an area where an epidemic of anthrax has broken out. The vaccine should also be used by workers who are constantly exposed to possibly contaminated materials. And a wide range of sulfa drugs and antibiotics have proved effective in treatment—particularly in preventing secondary infections. Prompt diagnosis is the key, and should assure early recovery.

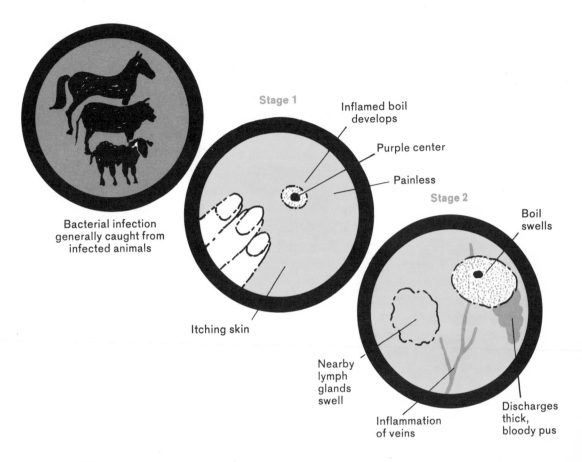

Bacterial infection
generally caught from
infected animals

Stage 1

Inflamed boil
develops

Purple center

Painless

Itching skin

Stage 2

Boil
swells

Nearby
lymph
glands
swell

Inflammation
of veins

Discharges
thick,
bloody pus

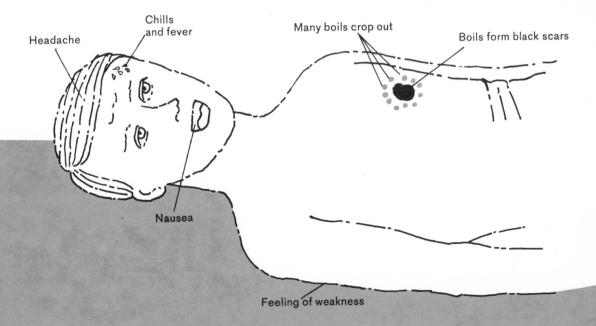

Stage 3

Headache

Chills
and fever

Many boils crop out

Boils form black scars

Nausea

Feeling of weakness

the disease and its causes Appendicitis is an inflammatory disease of the appendix. It can occur at any age but appears most often in young adults of both sexes.

The exact cause is unknown, but one of the explanations offered is the bacterial cause, that is, bacterial infection elsewhere in the body may be carried by the blood or by food to the appendix. A more acceptable theory is based on a mechanical cause, in which the appendix is blocked, usually by stool or, rarely, by swallowed foreign bodies.

Occasionally worms may lodge in the appendix and cause infection.

In all cases the symptoms are the same: the appendix is infected and swollen, and acts like an abscess on any part of the body.

symptoms The accompanying Medi-Graph diagrams one specific appendicitis attack. However, it must be emphasized that there is *no* typical case of acute appendicitis. The appendix may be in an unusual location and the area of pain may be completely different from that described. Occasionally the pain is located on the left side of the abdomen. For very old people appendicitis may be almost painless. Since it is difficult to make a diagnosis, no increasing abdominal pain should be disregarded.

complications The common complication is rupture of the appendix. When this happens the infection can spread to the membrane lining of the abdomen. The resulting peritonitis can severely infect the whole abdominal area. Before the rupture there is a great increase in pain and a spread of the area of pain.

Another complication is that the appendix may perforate and an abscess form in the area of the infection. This may burst into other organs or even open through the skin surface in the form of a fistula.

Abscess of the liver and abscess below the right diaphragm also are possible complications.

prevention (or lessening of impact) There is no way to prevent appendicitis. Once the attack begins, prompt medical care and surgery are essential in order to avoid serious complications and speed recovery. The patient should avoid taking any laxatives, because they can cause the infected appendix to rupture. Ice packs may ease the pain, and even slow the process, but surgery is the only cure. So-called chronic appendicitis, in which there are repeated attacks, is very unusual, and most physicians do not believe such a condition exists.

Appendicitis and Peritonitis

1. Appendicitis . . .

A. In typical cases, starts with off-and-on pain near navel.

B. Pain radiates down to right lower abdomen over appendix. Becomes constant and progressively more severe. Spot is tender to touch.

C. Nausea and occasionally vomiting follows. Sequence may take anywhere from several hours to 1-2 days.

D. Blood test reveals inflammation.

E. Attack may pass by itself. But if it gets worse . . .

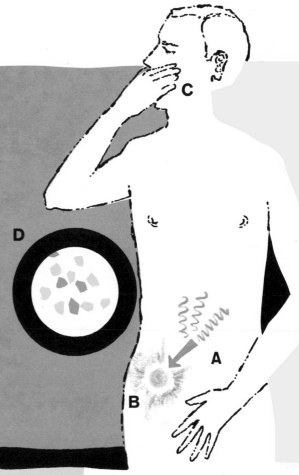

2. . . . and Peritonitis

. . . infection from badly inflamed or bursting appendix may spread to peritoneum (membrane lining of abdomen). Resulting peritonitis may severely infect whole abdominal area.

Small Intestine

Large Intestine

Appendix

Peritoneum

the disease and its causes   Arteriosclerosis is the name given to the loss of elasticity and the hardening of the arteries of the body. It occurs at all ages but is more truly a degenerative disease, affecting people in the older age group as their bodies begin to wear out.

Some men and women have an inherited tendency toward this illness, but it is more likely to be severe in patients with diabetes, sluggish thyroid, and those with high blood cholesterol. Most frequently it affects the arteries supplying blood to the brain, the extremities, and the heart. The aorta (the major artery supplying the body) is also frequently involved.

Cholesterol, saturated fats, and particularly excessive intake of refined carbohydrates such as sugar are believed to play an important role in the development of this disease. Certain diets raise blood cholesterol, cause fat to be deposited on the inner wall of the arteries, and hasten the clotting of blood. Thus, the formation of blood clots may be related to both the arteriosclerosis and the blood changes caused by diets rich in cholesterol. It would seem that diet is important both as a cause and a preventive in the most important form of arteriosclerosis—that involving the primary arteries.

symptoms   When the disease is generalized there may be few or no symptoms. Symptoms of the extremities are illustrated in the Medi-Graph. When the brain is involved, there may be decrease in mental activity, loss of memory, dizziness, and confusion. Coronary arteriosclerosis, perhaps the most important form, results when the arteries feeding the heart become so narrowed that sufficient blood cannot get through.

complications   Stroke, heart failure, gangrene of the legs, and the development of blood clots in the larger blood vessels of the body are possible complications.

prevention (or lessening of impact)   Much can be done today to delay or control arteriosclerosis. Patients with a family history of high blood cholesterol or blood vessel disorders should be conscious of the importance of diet. They are urged to avoid the overuse of foods rich in refined carbohydrates, such as pies, cakes, and soft drinks, and concentrate on lean meat, fish, milk, and vegetable products. Smoking should be avoided. Exercise, as prescribed by the physician, should be a routine part of living. The doctor will also prescribe the proper thyroid extract for patients with hypothyroidism and high blood cholesterol. Any underlying disorder that might contribute to the development of arteriosclerosis should be treated promptly. In some cases, where the legs are involved, the diseased artery may be replaced surgically.

Vascular (blood vessel) diseases in diabetics are controlled where possible by treatment of the diabetes itself. For arteriosclerosis occurring without clear-cut contributing disorders, some drugs of limited effectiveness are available to moderate the disease.

Two Main Types of Arteriosclerosis

1. Hardening or Calcification

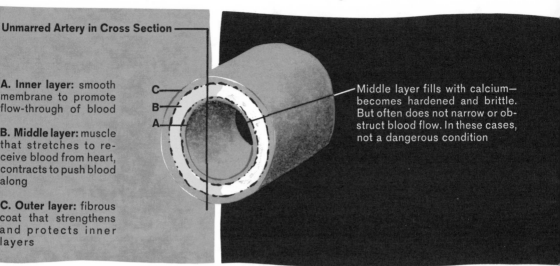

Unmarred Artery in Cross Section

A. Inner layer: smooth membrane to promote flow-through of blood

B. Middle layer: muscle that stretches to receive blood from heart, contracts to push blood along

C. Outer layer: fibrous coat that strengthens and protects inner layers

Middle layer fills with calcium—becomes hardened and brittle. But often does not narrow or obstruct blood flow. In these cases, not a dangerous condition

2. Atherosclerosis

A. Deposits—mainly of cholesterol—build up on inner layer, thickening and roughening it
B. Thickening reduces the channel, cuts down easy flow of blood
C. Roughened surface promotes formation of blood clots—which further obstruct flow of blood
D. Thickening and roughening tend to go on progressively over the years

When atherosclerosis attacks the body's major systems, other diseases may appear

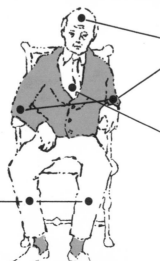

Central Nervous System: Stroke, paralysis of arms and legs

Central Heart-Blood Vessel System: High blood pressure, heart attack (coronary artery disease)

Outlying Blood Vessels: Gangrene of the legs (arteriosclerosis obliterans)

the disease and its causes   In this illness the arteries to the legs become so narrowed that an insufficient blood supply passes through and the legs are deprived of essential nutrients. The causes are not completely understood, but the disease is considered a part of the aging process. Men are affected more often than women, and the disease occurs more frequently in patients who have diabetes.

symptoms   The outstanding symptom is pain which occurs, as a rule, in the calves of the legs. When the patient exercises his legs, there is pain. When he rests, the pain disappears. This pattern of pain and rest is known as claudication. Usually the color of the leg involved is abnormal and it is cooler to the touch than the unaffected one. If the involved leg is elevated or exposed to cold, it turns pale. If it is warmed, it regains its color. If it is allowed to hang down after being elevated, it will first turn blue, and then red.
Often the patient complains of sharp shooting pains up and down the leg, particularly· at night. The skin becomes very thin and shiny. A minor injury may cause it to ulcerate.

complications   With the progression of the disease there are skin infections; brittle, slow-growing nails; and associated neuritic pain. In the final stages of a severe arteriosclerosis of the leg, gangrene may develop. Occasionally, osteomyelitis (an inflammation of the bone) results secondary to the infection. Amputation may be necessary.

prevention (or lessening of impact)   There is no known preventive for peripheral arteriosclerosis. Patients should avoid smoking and take care not to become overweight. They should avoid injury and exposure to cold. An underlying disease such as diabetes should be adequately controlled. Foot care to avoid infection is most important. Athlete's foot and ingrown nails need particular attention. Once there is evidence of infection, energetic treatment should be employed. The physician will discuss with the patient who has peripheral arteriosclerosis various treatment techniques including nerve block, exercises, and surgery.

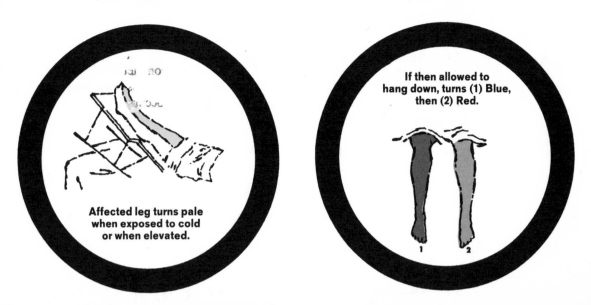

Affected leg turns pale when exposed to cold or when elevated.

If then allowed to hang down, turns (1) Blue, then (2) Red.

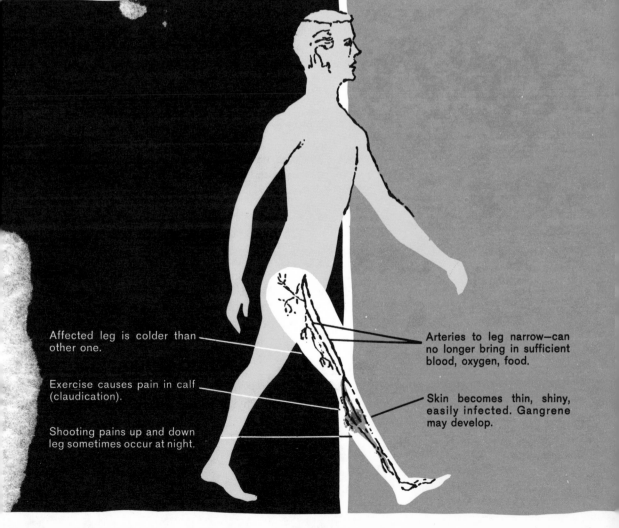

Affected leg is colder than other one.

Exercise causes pain in calf (claudication).

Shooting pains up and down leg sometimes occur at night.

Arteries to leg narrow—can no longer bring in sufficient blood, oxygen, food.

Skin becomes thin, shiny, easily infected. Gangrene may develop.

the disease and its causes   Arthritis is an inflammation of the joints. Rheumatoid arthritis is an acute and chronic form which can involve many joints. It has an extremely variable course and results in characteristic deformities. The specific cause is not known, but it occurs most often in cold, damp climates in the temperate zone. There are those who believe that the streptococcus bacteria are responsible, and others who hold to the "focus of infection" theory and insist on having bad teeth and tonsils removed. Still others speak of fatigue, shock, and allergy as possible causes. Twice as many women as men get rheumatoid arthritis, usually in the age group 30 to 40. But it can even occur in children just a few months old.

It has not been established whether this disease runs in families or whether it often occurs among several members in a family because of a common environment.

symptoms   It is characteristic of this disease that the symptoms vary greatly. Some patients have fever, severe inflammation, and develop deformities rapidly. Others have little fever and only mild discomfort. The accompanying Medi-Graph illustrates the more common symptoms, in both the early and later stages. In addition, patients may show signs of wasting away. In the mornings they are likely to experience stiffness of the joints. Occasionally there are changes in the eyes and lymph glands. About 15% of all patients develop firm nodules under the skin, something like buckshot.

About a quarter of all people who get rheumatoid arthritis recover from the first attack without serious symptoms. Half suffer only minor discomfort, while the remaining quarter go on to chronic, progressive, disabling arthritis.

The physician establishes that the patient has this disease by making certain blood tests, taking X rays, and by observing the course of the illness.

complications   When the joints become disabled or immobilized, the complication is serious. The patient's muscles can waste away, and he or she can become crippled and bedridden.

prevention (or lessening of impact)   There is no known cure or preventive for rheumatoid arthritis. Deformities should be prevented where possible, and corrected if possible. Specific drugs are available to minimize pain and control acute attacks. They do little to affect the course of the illness, but they can do much to help make the rheumatoid patient a useful individual.

A patient with the disease should get adequate rest and exercise. A balanced diet, elimination of sources of infection, and maintenance of general good health are important. Physiotherapy and rehabilitation should be explored.

Rheumatoid Arthritis

Early Stage

Weakness,
weight loss,
poor appetite,
temperature

Mild joint and
muscle pain

Excessive
sweating
of hands
and feet

Inflammation of joints — most commonly the hands.
Also can involve wrists, knees, ankles, feet

Later Stage

Fever

Deformity of joints

Skin darkens above
affected joint

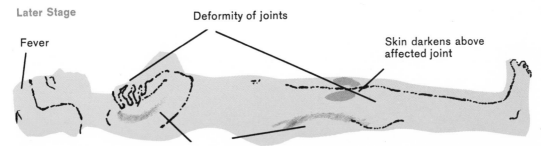

Muscles near inflamed joints develop spastic rigidity.　　Fusion of joints, leading to progressive disability.

the disease and its causes   Bell's palsy is an inflammatory disease of the facial
nerve which controls the muscles of facial expression. The cause is
unknown, but it is thought that there may be some relation to upper
respiratory infections or exposure to cold. Other causes of facial palsy
are tumors which invade the skull bone and interfere with the nerve;
a skin and nerve disease called herpes zoster (shingles); and certain
vascular injuries. However, it is not too difficult to distinguish these
conditions from true Bell's palsy, and the course of these illnesses is
different from Bell's palsy.

The effects of Bell's palsy vary, depending upon the exact point at
which the facial nerve is involved. Most often it is at the point behind
the ear where the nerve makes its exit from the skull. When there is
involvement within the skull, facial paralysis is greater, with changes
in taste and hearing, and tearing of the eyes.

symptoms   As shown in the Medi-Graph, the attack is preceded by pain below
and behind the ear. Sometimes there is some gland swelling in the
angle of the jaw. As a rule, paralysis is sudden and complete, but at
other times it can take from 24 to 36 hours to develop. The side of
the face that is affected sags visibly because all the muscles on that side
are affected. The patient may have no sense of taste on two-thirds of
his tongue on the paralyzed side. His eyes may tear. He may drool.
He cannot whistle or blow out his cheek. Loud noises or clicking
sounds disturb him. Occasionally there is deafness, ringing in the ears,
or sleepiness. When he tries to close his eyes he cannot control the
paralyzed side. He has some feeling of sensation throughout, but the
affected side feels numb or heavy.

In most cases recovery begins to take place during the 2nd and 3rd
weeks. Complete recovery may take as long as three months, or even
longer. In some cases, recovery may not be complete and facial
deformities can remain.

complications   When full recovery does not take place, the most serious complication is the facial deformity. Also, a patient can develop painful ulceration of the cornea of the eye if he is unable to close it while he sleeps.
It is important that the correct diagnosis be made to avoid the possibility of neglecting a tumor within the skull.

prevention (or lessening of impact)   There is no known cure for Bell's palsy,
but the great majority of cases recover by themselves. Treatment with
massage, heat, and electrical stimulation seems to be helpful in preventing degeneration of the muscles, muscle contraction, and permanent
muscle weakness. The eyes should be protected during sleep, and a
splint used to prevent drooping of the lower face. There are medicines
available which appear to shorten the length of the illness.

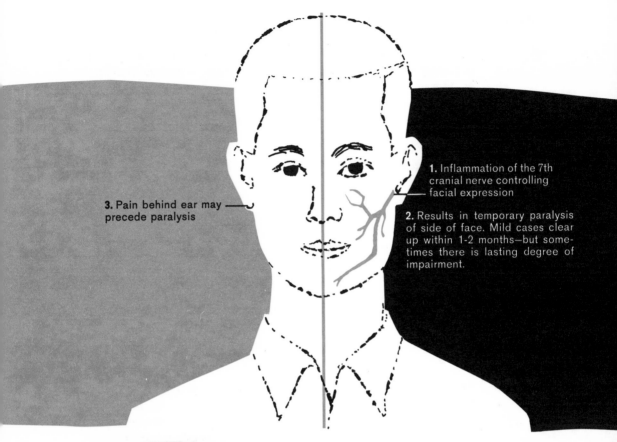

1. Inflammation of the 7th cranial nerve controlling facial expression

2. Results in temporary paralysis of side of face. Mild cases clear up within 1-2 months—but sometimes there is lasting degree of impairment.

3. Pain behind ear may precede paralysis

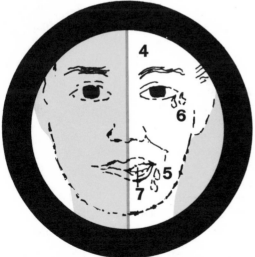

4. Paralysis usually sudden and complete

5. Drooling

6. Tearing

7. Taste dulled. Difficulty chewing and swallowing

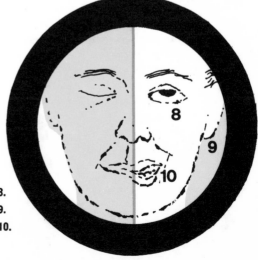

Inability to close eye **8.**

May be sensitive to sound **9.**

Cannot whistle or blow out cheek **10.**

the disease and its causes   Beriberi is a disease commonly seen in the Far East
and less frequently seen, in a milder form, in the United States. It
occurs when a person does not get enough vitamin B_1 (thiamine). The
deficiency can result from a diet low in foods containing vitamin B_1,
or from the body's inability to make use of some of the foods it takes in.
Vitamin B_1 is present in high amounts in fresh vegetables, fruits, beans,
whole wheat flour, barley, peas, liver, and wheat germ extracts. The
amount of vitamin B_1 an individual needs depends on his metabolism
and body weight. Large, active people may require more than small,
sedentary people.
Patients with beriberi may have been living on a diet with too much
milled rice, wheat, or corn, and not enough proteins, minerals, and
vitamins. Other patients develop beriberi as the result of organic
diseases that affect the appetite or prevent the assimilation and utiliza-
tion of vitamin B_1. Among these diseases are gastrointestinal illnesses,
any chronic debilitating disease, or a condition that causes severe, persistent vomiting.
Certain people need more than the amount of vitamin B_1 available in
the normal diet. These include children during the period of rapid
growth, women during pregnancy, individuals with illnesses accompanied by prolonged fever, hyperthyroid patients, alcoholics, and
diabetics.

symptoms   The varied symptoms are illustrated in the accompanying Medi-Graph.
However, beriberi can escape detection for a long time because patients
can have few noticeable symptoms for months or years despite a partial
vitamin B_1 deficiency. In infants there is frequently loss of the voice,
hoarseness, and vomiting. A severe attack of the disease may be
triggered by unusual physical exertion or an acute case of some other
disease.

complications   Complications such as severe multiple neuritis and congestive heart
failure are the result of the progressive involvement of the organ systems affected by beriberi. There is also greater susceptibility to
secondary infections. Sudden death can occur on rare occasions.

prevention (or lessening of impact)   This disease can be prevented easily by
eating a well-balanced diet which includes satisfactory amounts of
vitamin B_1. Commercial products are also available.
In addition to prescribing a balanced diet for a patient with beriberi,
the doctor gives special orders for the patient who has developed a
cardiac disorder as a result of the disease. Bed rest is vital at this
point to avoid heart failure.

Beriberi

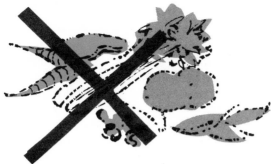

Disease occurring because of low intake or inability of body to use Vitamin B$_1$ (Thiamine) which is found in high amounts in fresh vegetables, fruits, beans, peas, liver, whole wheat flour, barley, wheat germ extract

In fully developed cases, Beriberi may affect...

... Nervous System

... Heart

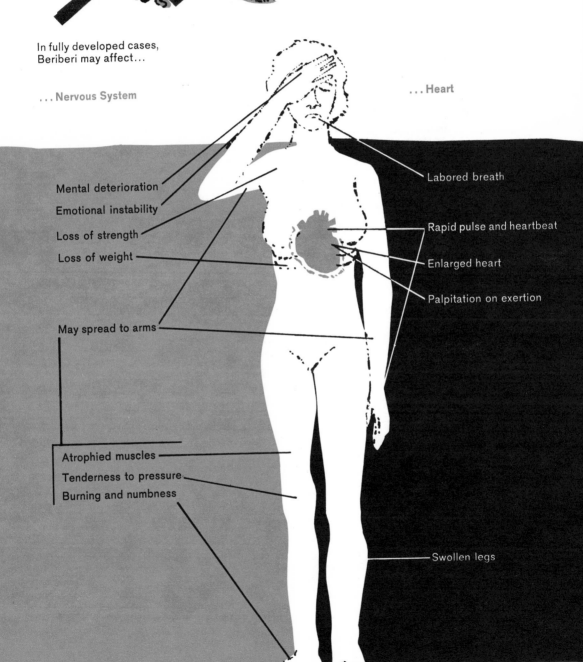

Mental deterioration

Emotional instability

Loss of strength

Loss of weight

May spread to arms

Atrophied muscles

Tenderness to pressure

Burning and numbness

Labored breath

Rapid pulse and heartbeat

Enlarged heart

Palpitation on exertion

Swollen legs

the disease and its cause   This is the most dangerous of all food poisonings. It is caused by eating canned or preserved foods contaminated by the bacterium *Clostridium botulinum*. This germ is found in soils throughout the world and so is a potential contaminant in every food product grown. The germs produce a variety of toxins which themselves are the poisonous element. The proper pressure steaming and boiling of canned and preserved foods destroys the bacteria and their toxins.

Home canned and preserved products, improperly treated, are still responsible for a number of botulism deaths each year. Occasional spectacular cases of botulism have also been caused by commercial food packers who have not taken adequate precautions. On rare occasions, a wound contaminated with botulism bacteria may serve as the infection point.

symptoms   These usually begin within 18–36 hours of eating the contaminated food—but this period can vary from as little as 4 hours to as long as 8 days. The earlier the symptoms appear, the more serious the disease.

The poisonous toxins attack the nervous system, causing weakness and paralysis. The first symptom is fatigue, followed by visual disturbances, difficulty in swallowing and speaking, weakness of neck and respiratory muscles, and finally extreme weakness of all muscles. Vomiting and diarrhea occur in about one out of three cases. Since the temperature remains normal, absence of fever is a strong indication that botulism may be present.

complications   If the disease is not diagnosed early, paralysis of the breathing apparatus can occur very quickly, with heart arrest and death.

prevention (or lessening of impact)   Proper heating and boiling of all canned and preserved foods—both at home and in the factory—is the best method of preventing botulism. These foods should be heated for 6 minutes at 120°C (248°F) to kill the spores of the bacteria or for 30 minutes at 80°C (176°F) to destroy the toxins.

Once the disease has been contracted and diagnosed, breathing may have to be maintained by use of a respirator if respiratory paralysis seems impending. Prompt treatment with antitoxins is needed. Even with these measures, the death rate may be as high as 65%. Recovery for those who survive is slow, but there are no permanent aftereffects.

Botulism

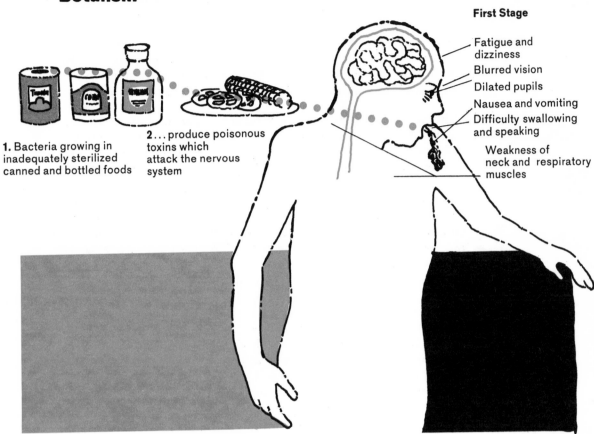

1. Bacteria growing in inadequately sterilized canned and bottled foods

2 ...produce poisonous toxins which attack the nervous system

First Stage

Fatigue and dizziness

Blurred vision

Dilated pupils

Nausea and vomiting

Difficulty swallowing and speaking

Weakness of neck and respiratory muscles

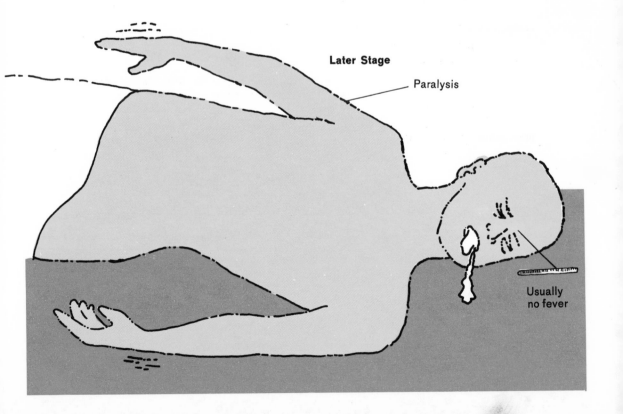

Later Stage

Paralysis

Usually no fever

the disease and its causes   Tumors of the brain are relatively common, accounting for some 5% of all malignant diseases. Any age group can be affected, although brain tumors are found most frequently in the forties, and slightly more often in males than in females. The cause is unknown.

symptoms   The type of tumor, its rate of growth, and its particular location in the brain all bear upon the appearance of symptoms and the order in which they appear. There is no simple sequence that reveals the presence of a brain tumor. Often it comes to light only after a thorough neurological examination.

There are mental changes, such as loss of concentration, irritability, forgetfulness, and lack of interest. The patient has what appears to be ordinary, simple headaches which are slightly painful, dull, and temporary, or he may find them severe and almost unbearable. They should be viewed with suspicion when they are recurrent and persistent.

Forceful vomiting may occur without any preceding nausea and without any relation to the food eaten by the patient. Dizziness unrelated to the position of the patient can be a symptom of brain tumor.

Convulsive seizures resembling epilepsy are often the first indication of tumor. Blurring or interference with vision, flashing spots before the eyes, double vision, the development of blind spots, and loss of peripheral vision all call for investigation. Temporary or permanent changes in sensation, weakness of an extremity, facial weaknesses, changes in the sense of smell, ringing in the ears, and the sudden onset of deafness are further possible indications of brain tumor.

As the disease progresses, the patient becomes more apathetic and drowsy, and eventually may fall into a coma.

complications   The complications are the same as for malignant disease in any part of the body. The tumor may develop with great speed, and quickly become unresponsive to any form of therapy.

A calamitous complication is hemorrhage into the brain tumor, caused by the erosion of a blood vessel by the tumor. The effects are similar to a stroke.

prevention (or lessening of impact)   There is no known way of preventing the development of this malignant disease. The only hope lies in early recognition. Surgery can be effective when the tumors are located in favorable sites and are either benign or have low grades of malignancy. It is absolutely imperative that any single symptom or cluster of symptoms be reported and investigated promptly.

Brain Tumors

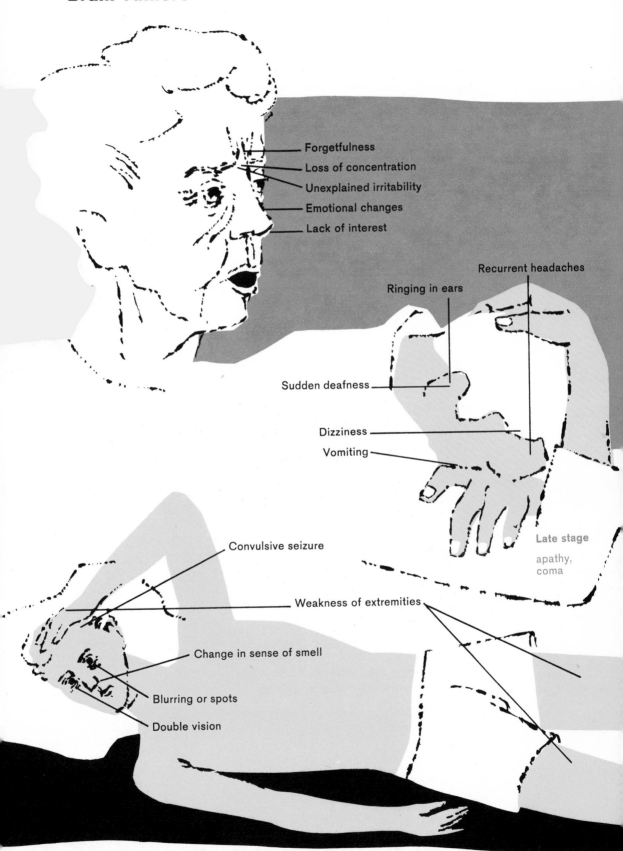

Forgetfulness

Loss of concentration

Unexplained irritability

Emotional changes

Lack of interest

Recurrent headaches

Ringing in ears

Sudden deafness

Dizziness

Vomiting

Late stage

apathy, coma

Convulsive seizure

Weakness of extremities

Change in sense of smell

Blurring or spots

Double vision

the disease and its causes   This tumor, usually benign, occurs in the bronchial tree
—the main branches which come out of the trachea and form the underlying structure of the lungs. Bronchial adenoma occurs in both sexes,
and most frequently strikes in younger middle age (around 45).
Because of its slow growth and the chronic nature of its symptoms, it is
often confused with other lung disorders. It makes up about 2% of all
lung tumors.

symptoms   The most common are coughing and spitting up of blood. Repeated
bouts of pneumonia are also characteristic, and the victim is likely to
suffer from fever, wheezing, shortness of breath and pleurisy-type lung
pains.
In about 5% of the cases there are no apparent symptoms—but the
disease comes to light on a chest X ray. This may also reveal the secondary effects of the tumor—such as lung collapse or pneumonitis.
Positive diagnosis of the disease is made by biopsy of the lesion during
bronchoscopy (taking a slice of tissue out during an instrument examination of the lungs).

complications   Severe bleeding may be a problem—and can be precipitated by
a biopsy procedure. In the rare case where a bronchial adenoma is
malignant, it can spread to other parts of the body.

prevention (or lessening of impact)   Since the cause of these tumors is unknown,
there is also no known way to prevent them. However, prompt diagnosis
and surgical removal result in a cure for the benign types of bronchial
adenomas. This procedure will also be effective in the rare malignant
types. Chemotherapy also helps in certain forms.

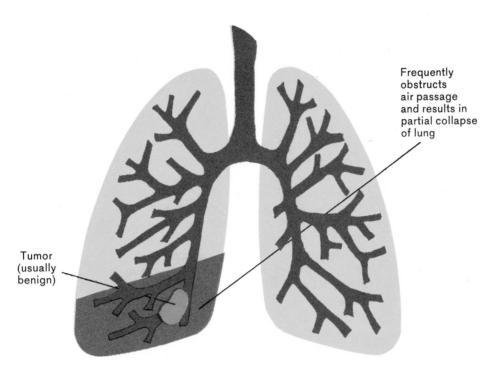

Frequently
obstructs
air passage
and results in
partial collapse
of lung

Tumor
(usually
benign)

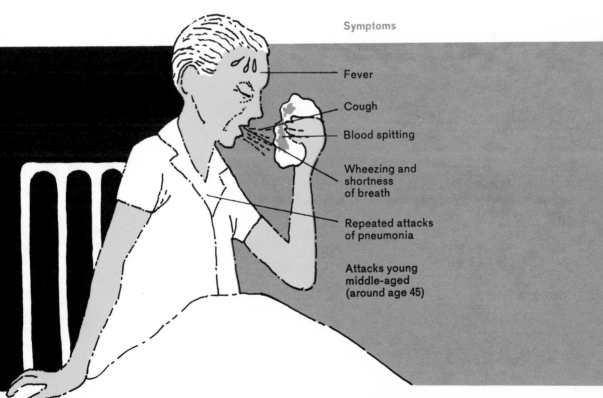

Symptoms

Fever

Cough

Blood spitting

Wheezing and
shortness
of breath

Repeated attacks
of pneumonia

Attacks young
middle-aged
(around age 45)

the disease and its causes Asthma of any kind is really a symptom, not a disease. Bronchial asthma is an illness caused by the reaction of the bronchi to some irritating substance which the patient has inhaled. The attacks occur irregularly, and are marked by wheezing, cough, and shortness of breath. They usually follow exposure to air-borne pollen, animal hairs, house dust, fungi, or vegetable dusts. Many people are also allergic to their own infections.

Bronchial asthma is quite common, affects both sexes equally, and tends to run in families. When it is caused by a specific pollen, it occurs during the season of growth of that particular plant.

symptoms Attacks of bronchial asthma can be of varying degrees of severity, lasting from minutes to days. If there is no accompanying infection of the sinuses or lungs, the patient can be quite comfortable between attacks. If there is an accompanying infection, he will have symptoms associated with the particular area of infection.

An attack of bronchial asthma is likely to start at night with a sudden shortness of breath and coughing. The exhaling of air becomes difficult and the patient gasps for breath. Sometimes by sitting up he can use his abdominal and neck muscles to breathe in air more easily. His wheeze is loud and plain to hear. His cough starts out dry but later produces large amounts of stringy mucus. In severe attacks he may become cyanotic, a condition in which the body turns blue because it is suffering from lack of sufficient fresh oxygen. Coma may result.

complications Chronic lung disease—such as emphysema, chronic bronchitis, and bronchiectasis—are frequently long-term results of asthma.

prevention (or lessening of impact) The most successful means used by the doctor in dealing with bronchial asthma is to remove the cause or causes of the allergy. This includes correction of infections and removal of any associated nasal growths or polyps or mechanical obstructions. Filtration systems to remove air-borne pollens are sometimes helpful. Allergy covers for bedding are readily available. Some patients profit by desensitization by injection. In this procedure the patient is given increasing doses of the offending material until, it is hoped, his body builds up a tolerance for it and no longer rejects it by way of an asthmatic attack.

When the primary cause of an infection is identified, bacterial vaccines can be used with some success. Patients allergic to their own infections are sometimes successfully desensitized.

Medications for the prevention and treatment of this illness are available and will be prescribed by the physician.

Bronchial Asthma

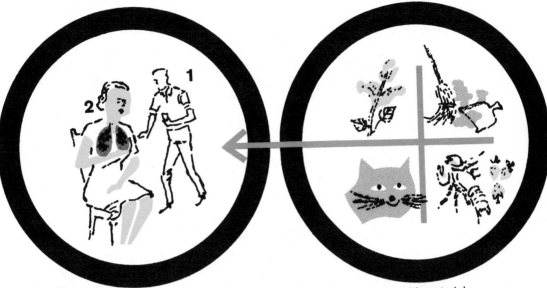

Spasms of wheezing

Gasping for breath

Dry coughing (later bringing up mucus)

Attacks May Be Started by:

1. Emotional upset

2. Respiratory infection

3. Contact with materials causing allergic reaction

During Asthmatic Attack:

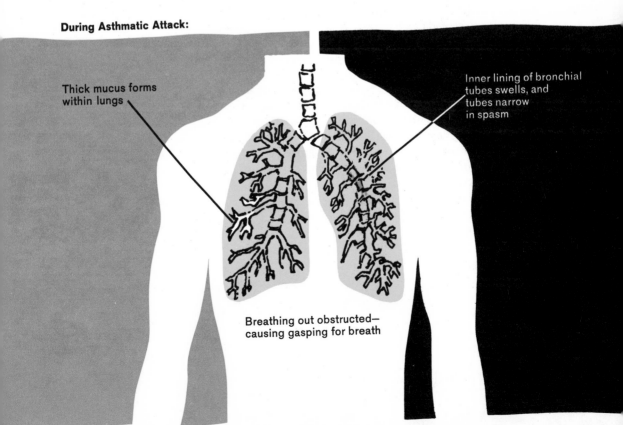

Thick mucus forms within lungs

Inner lining of bronchial tubes swells, and tubes narrow in spasm

Breathing out obstructed— causing gasping for breath

the disease and its causes Bronchiectasis is often the end result of chronic
bronchitis. In this disease, the lungs are prevented from properly clearing out secretions which become lodged in them. This is because their
bronchial tubes and bronchi (the air channels in the lungs) become enlarged and lose their flexibility. Some people are born with this condition. Others acquire it as the result of chronic infections, or as the
result of obstruction of a bronchus by a foreign body or tumor.
Bronchiectasis patients usually have a previous history of repeated
attacks of pneumonia, frequent colds, or bronchitis, and a gradual decline in general health.

symptoms The early symptoms are usually mild and resemble bronchitis. There
is a dry or slightly productive cough. Occasionally small amounts of
blood are brought up during a coughing spell. As the disease progresses,
the cough gets more persistent, is worse in the morning, and frequently
is brought on by lying down. The patient begins to produce a great
deal of yellow sputum. Occasionally this is foul smelling. Blood
begins to appear more frequently in the sputum and may become substantial in amount. There is low-grade fever, and the patient often
complains of pleuritic-type chest pains. As with any chronic infection,
there is weight loss and weakness, as well as shortness of breath on
exertion. The fingers frequently become "clubbed," as illustrated.

complications A complication known as emphysema can develop, in which there
is fibrosis (loss of elasticity) of lung tissue. This condition interferes
with the entire breathing mechanism. Associated chemical changes take
place and can be severe enough to produce coma.
Lung abscess in association with, or as a result of, bronchiectasis is the
other common complication.

prevention (or lessening of impact) Early recognition of bronchiectasis is important in order to limit the extension of the disease through proper
medical and surgical care. Infections in the respiratory tract must be
energetically treated. Early removal of the underlying causes of infection can result in cure or retardation of this illness. The use of antibiotics is of great help in controlling and lessening the frequency of
infections.
Bronchial obstructions must be removed. Postural drainage of the infected matter and the maintenance of good general health are most
important.

Bronchiectasis

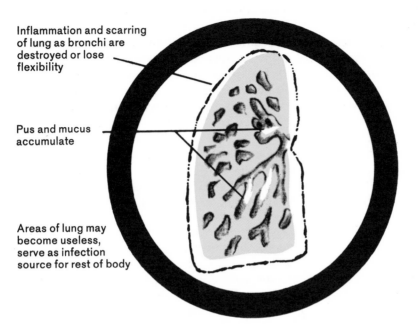

Inflammation and scarring of lung as bronchi are destroyed or lose flexibility

Pus and mucus accumulate

Areas of lung may become useless, serve as infection source for rest of body

Causes

- Chronic infection—severe and repeated sinusitis, bronchitis, pneumonia, tuberculosis

- Birth defects

- Blockage of bronchial tube by substance lodged within it

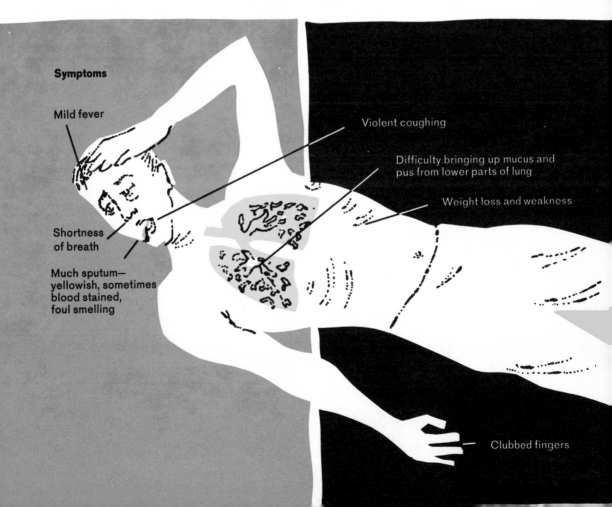

Symptoms

Mild fever

Shortness of breath

Much sputum—yellowish, sometimes blood stained, foul smelling

Violent coughing

Difficulty bringing up mucus and pus from lower parts of lung

Weight loss and weakness

Clubbed fingers

the disease and its causes   ACUTE BRONCHITIS   Acute bronchitis occurs when the windpipe and bronchial tubes become inflamed or infected. Both viruses and bacteria can be responsible, generally attacking after a patient has had a simple head cold, sinusitis, or pharyngitis (sore throat). Measles, whooping cough, and influenza also open the way to bronchitis. The acute form is usually mild and rarely lasts over a week, although the cough may persist for 4 to 6 weeks. Acute bronchitis occurs most often in the spring and fall when the weather is changeable, and is common in small children.

CHRONIC BRONCHITIS   Chronic bronchitis can result when irritation from excessive smoking or breathing in of irritating dust or fumes cause the bronchial tubes to become inflamed. Tuberculosis can similarly inflame the bronchial tubes and bring about a type of chronic bronchitis.

symptoms   ACUTE BRONCHITIS   In the acute form there is mild fever and some soreness under the breastbone, which is aggravated by a tight, dry cough. It is frequently associated with symptoms of head cold.

As the disease progresses, the tightness becomes less marked. The cough becomes looser, and produces a thick yellow or green mucus.

CHRONIC BRONCHITIS   Chronic bronchitis presents symptoms that are similar, but the illness does not progress as satisfactorily. The bronchi become thick and inelastic. Instead of being coughed up, the mucus and pus accumulate in the lower part of the lungs. As a result, there is a chronic cough, shortness of breath, sometimes spasm, and frequent reinfection.

complications   Generally there are no serious complications to acute bronchitis unless the condition is neglected and pneumonia develops.

In chronic bronchitis, lung abscess, emphysema, and bronchiectasis may result.

prevention (or lessening of impact)   CHRONIC BRONCHITIS   In chronic bronchitis the bronchial tubes become inflamed or infected following an illness involving the mouth, nasal passages, windpipe, and trachea. Therefore, it is important to eliminate the primary source of infection. If contact with hostile substances (such as those noted in the beginning of this article) is the cause of the irritation to the bronchial lining membranes, the patient must take steps to avoid such contacts. Elimination of cigarette smoking is particularly important when chronic bronchitis has developed.

ACUTE BRONCHITIS   Acute bronchitis is a mild illness that usually runs its course within 4 to 7 days. Once the disease has begun, its duration and severity can be minimized by care devoted to its symptoms, rest, fresh air, and nutritious foods.

Bronchitis

Inflammation of windpipe (trachea) **A**
and its branches into
the lungs—bronchi **B**
and bronchial tubes **C**.

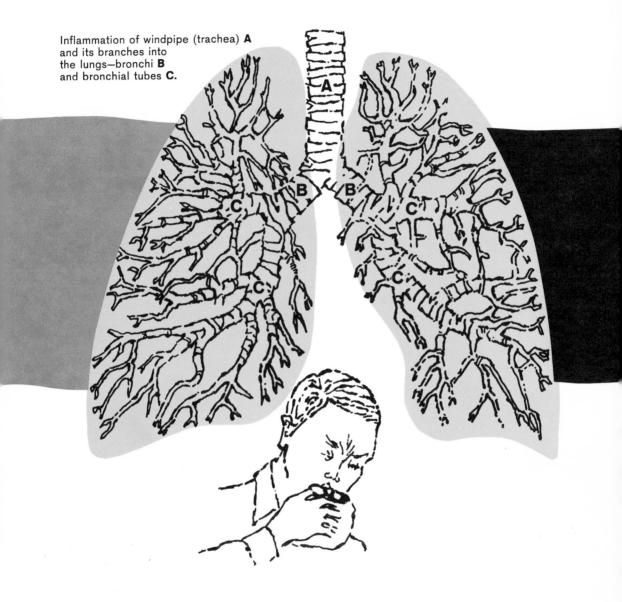

Acute Bronchitis
1. Mild fever

2. Soreness under breastbone, aggravated by coughing.

3. Dry cough at first

4. Cough later begins to bring up green and yellow mucus

5. Cough may persist 4-6 weeks.

Chronic Bronchitis
1. Produced by other chronic problem: sinusitis, smoking, TB, etc.

2. Bronchi become thick, inelastic, accumulate mucus and pus in lower part of lungs instead of bringing discharges up and out.

3. Result is chronic cough, shortness of breath, sometimes spasm, frequent infection.

the disease and its causes   This is a chronic disease of the arteries and veins. Although it affects the extremities most often, it can involve any blood vessels of the body. A gradual thrombosis—narrowing of the blood vessel—eventually interferes with the blood supply to the affected part, and gangrene results. The disease is thought to be hereditary. Patients are almost always men, and most have a history of heavy smoking. Another unexplained fact about Buerger's disease is that 50% of the victims are of Jewish parentage.

symptoms   The first symptom is usually a crampy pain in the calves or arches brought on by walking or running. As the disease progresses, it takes less and less activity to produce this pain—and after a while it is almost constant. Phlebitis—inflammation in which the veins become swollen, red, and painful to touch—is usually associated with Buerger's. The nails become brittle and grow slowly, and there is ulceration of the toes. Color changes take place. In the beginning the extremity is usually cold to touch and pale in color. Later on, depending upon where the disease is established, the affected part may be deep red or blue—depending on its position. When it is elevated, it may turn white; when it is hanging down, it becomes dark.

As time passes there is a tendency for the skin to infect easily. There are ulcerations. Eventually gangrene may develop, accompanied by severe, persistent pain.

complications   The main complication is the amputation of the affected part, surgically or spontaneously. Another serious complication is severe infection with eventual gangrene. There have been some reports of coronary or cerebral artery involvements resulting in stroke or coronary attacks.

prevention (or lessening of impact)   Patients must be put on a strict program which will improve the circulation picture. This program has to be strictly observed. Smoking is forbidden. Specific exercises are prescribed. The affected extremity must be kept warm, and special care taken to avoid injury or chilling of the feet. Infections must be treated immediately.

Medications, nerve blocks, and surgery are all available and are used by the physician as the situation warrants.

Buerger's Disease (Thrombo-angiitis Obliterans)

Test for Arterial Diseases:

Elevated leg becomes white . . .

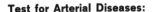

. . . turns blue or dark red when switched
to hanging down position

Inflammation of blood vessels leads to clots which
slow or stop blood supply

Most often affects legs. But
can involve blood vessels
in arms and elsewhere

Heavy smoking seems to
promote disease

Spreads from one leg to
other. Legs become pale
color and noticeably cool.
Veins become swollen, red,
painful (phlebitis)

Early Symptom: pain in
calves or arches while running or walking

Later Stages: Easy infection, open sores, gangrene

Nails become brittle—grow
slowly

the disease and its causes   Wherever there is a joint, there is a sac filled with fluid which acts as a cushion and lubricant, and prevents friction. This is called a bursa, and there are at least 140 different ones in the body. When bursitis develops, particles of calcium are deposited in the sac. The result is inflammation and pain. Bursitis can occur in any joint but is found most often in the shoulder, hip, heel, elbow, and knee. The cause is unknown, but it is believed to be related to some injury to the joint affected. However, it has been found where there was no history of injury. The disease is common in both men and women in their adult years. Although athletic people do get bursitis when they injure a bursa, many people who are unathletic and live very sedentary lives also get it.

symptoms   There are two forms of bursitis—acute and chronic. The patient with the acute form complains of a sudden, severe pain and is reluctant to move the affected joint. In the shoulder bursa, which is the one most usually involved, the pain can be excruciating, radiating up to the neck or down to the fingertips. Pressure on the site of the bursa causes great pain. In order to relieve his pain, a patient often finds it helpful to hold his arm bent as if it were in a sling. Motion of the arm or shoulder joint makes him very uncomfortable.

X ray examination shows calcium deposits in half of these cases. When the attack is over, the patient has little or no discomfort until the next attack, which may not occur for months or years.

Chronic bursitis is an on-and-off affair, which is brought on by such factors as changes in the weather or excessive use of the joint. It may be the result of acute bursitis or it may take this form right from the start.

complications   There are no serious complications. The patient may have to limit his activities and this, in turn, may have some effect upon the work he does for a living.

prevention (or lessening of impact)   There is no way of preventing bursitis. Once it has developed, it is helpful to immobilize the affected part as much as possible. If this is not done, pain is likely to increase and cause even greater disability.

Drugs are available that give effective relief. Direct injection of cortisone into the troubled area also gives relief. There is no cure. But as a rule patients are quite comfortable between attacks and are able to do most things they did previously. When there are signs of a fresh attack, prompt treatment can minimize discomfort.

Bursitis

Acute attack — probably brought on by injury to nearby muscle or tendon

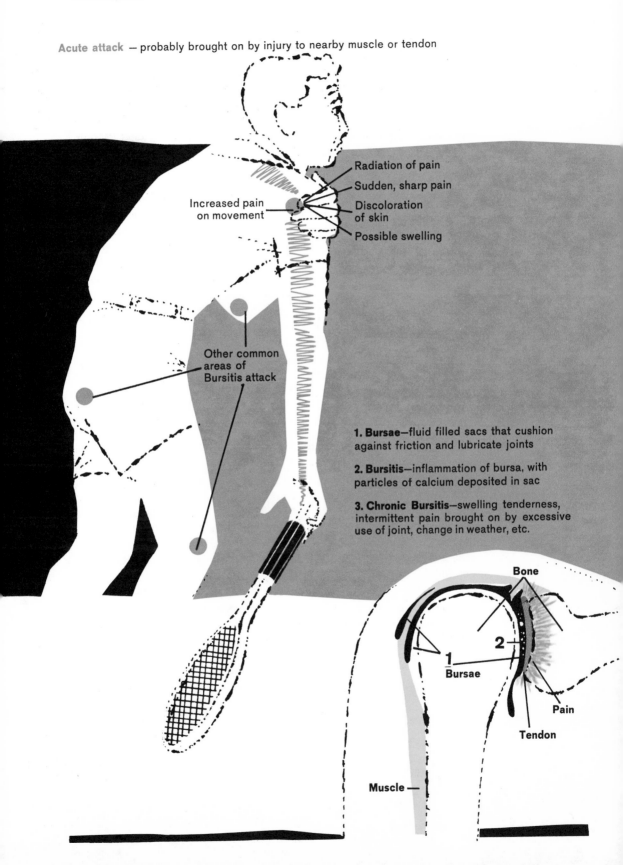

Radiation of pain

Sudden, sharp pain

Discoloration of skin

Possible swelling

Increased pain on movement

Other common areas of Bursitis attack

1. Bursae—fluid filled sacs that cushion against friction and lubricate joints

2. Bursitis—inflammation of bursa, with particles of calcium deposited in sac

3. Chronic Bursitis—swelling tenderness, intermittent pain brought on by excessive use of joint, change in weather, etc.

Bone

2

1

Bursae

Pain

Tendon

Muscle—

the disease and its causes   Breast cancer is the most common form of cancer found among women, accounting for 25% of all the cancers in women. It occurs at all ages but is most common between the ages of 45 and 49. The cause is unknown. However, there always have been some questions about the relationship of a female hormone called estrogen to cancer, when estrogen is used in treating pre-menopausal women. Although this relationship is not firmly established, most doctors now think it best to avoid the use of estrogen in younger patients who have a family history of breast cancer.

symptoms   There are few early symptoms. The first is usually a painless lump in the breast found accidentally or on routine examination. The size may vary but generally it is small and quite hard, and it may be attached to the skin. The nipples may be sore or there may be some discharge from them. (The discharge may be bloody.) Occasionally the veins in the skin over the tumor become quite prominent. The skin becomes tight and resembles an orange in texture.

As the growth gets larger, there may be swelling of the upper arm on the side involved, chest pain, and pain in the armpit with noticeable swelling in that area. Finally, there is weakness, weight loss, and general symptoms of illness.

complications   Complications are the same as for any malignancy—when' the cancer spreads to other organs, there is generalized deterioration and eventual death.

prevention (or lessening of impact)   Routine breast examination by a trained observer is the only effective means of preventing the deadly progression of this illness. Any breast lump or swelling should be investigated, since there is no way of distinguishing a benign tumor from a malignant one in the early stages. In women over 30, the investigation should probably be done surgically. There is no known means other than biopsy (examination of a piece of tissue removed from the breast) to establish a certain diagnosis. Special X ray studies have been found helpful as a diagnostic aid. If neglected, the malignant lump can spread to the point where little can be done. It is far better to remove a benign mass (one that will *not* have a cancerous growth) than to take the chance of allowing a malignant one to develop beyond the early stage.

Once the diagnosis of cancer is established by means of a biopsy, all suspicious areas and beyond are promptly removed surgically.

Early diagnosis and therapy offer the only hope of eliminating this disease.

Breast Cancer

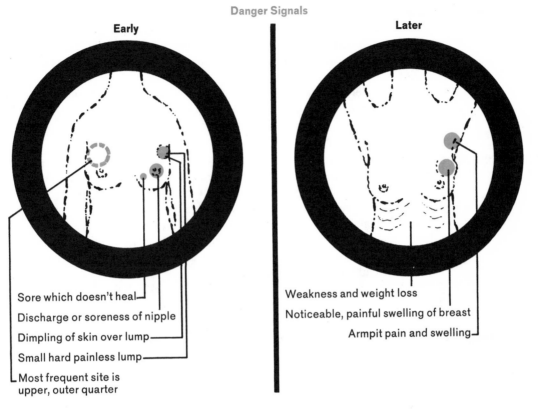

Danger Signals

Early

Sore which doesn't heal
Discharge or soreness of nipple
Dimpling of skin over lump
Small hard painless lump
Most frequent site is upper, outer quarter

Later

Weakness and weight loss
Noticeable, painful swelling of breast
Armpit pain and swelling

Two Signs of Breast Cancer

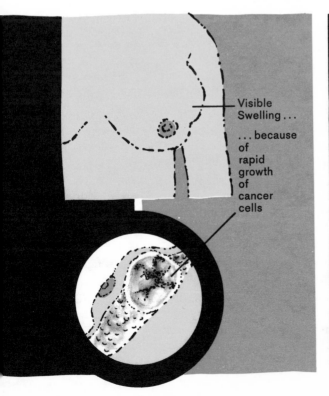

Visible Swelling...

...because of rapid growth of cancer cells

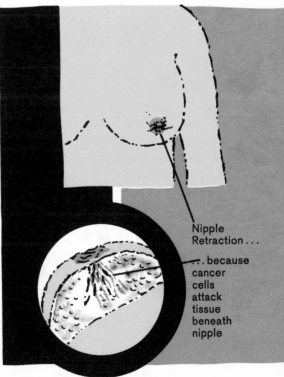

Nipple Retraction...

...because cancer cells attack tissue beneath nipple

the disease and its causes   Approximately 15,000 women die of cancer of the cervix each year, making it one of our most important gynecological problems. The cervix, a small tubelike structure situated at the bottom of the uterus, is a passage which protects the rest of the uterus—especially during pregnancy.

Like all cancers, the cause of cancer of the cervix is at present unknown. Women who go for regular checkups stand a good chance that their doctor will detect this disease early when the prospects of dealing with it successfully are good.

symptoms   In the majority of cases, the first symptom is bleeding—usually between menstrual periods. This bleeding may be precipitated by exertion, sexual intercourse, or straining at defecation. It becomes more frequent and heavy as the disease progresses. Another symptom is a watery discharge from the vagina, often tinged with blood.

Later symptoms include increased bleeding, rectal and bladder discomfort, and heavy aching pain—generally because the disease has spread to the rectal and bladder areas.

The doctor is usually able to make a diagnosis of cancer of the cervix quickly by the simple *Pap test,* as well as by his examination and a biopsy (microscopic examination of a piece of cervical tissue).

complications   Invasion of the bladder and rectum by the tumor, with the formation of *fistulas,* is possible if the disease is not caught early. It can also spread to distant organs which become secondarily infected.

prevention   (or lessening of impact)   This very much depends on early diagnosis. When found early, cancer of the cervix can generally be successfully treated by surgery, X ray treatment, chemotherapy, or a combination of all three.

CANCER OF THE UTERUS

the disease and its causes   Though a substantial problem, this type of cancer occurs only about one-tenth as often as cancer of the cervix. About two-thirds of the cases occur in women past the menopause. The average age of victims is about 56.

symptoms   The most common symptom is abnormal bleeding. In menopausal women this may take the form of recommencement of bleeding after regular periods have stopped. In women still menstruating, the periods may become very heavy or prolonged, or there may be bleeding between periods.

Another symptom is watery vaginal discharge, frequently mixed with blood. Pain, weight loss and anemia are frequent later symptoms. Your doctor usually makes the diagnosis by removing tissue from the uterus for examination—a form of biopsy known as *curettage.*

complications   Complications are similar to those of cancer in general—the spread of the disease to other organs of the body.

prevention (or lessening of impact)   Early diagnosis is vital in limiting the illness. And again surgery, X ray therapy and chemotherapy make up a generally successful battery of weapons when brought into play early.

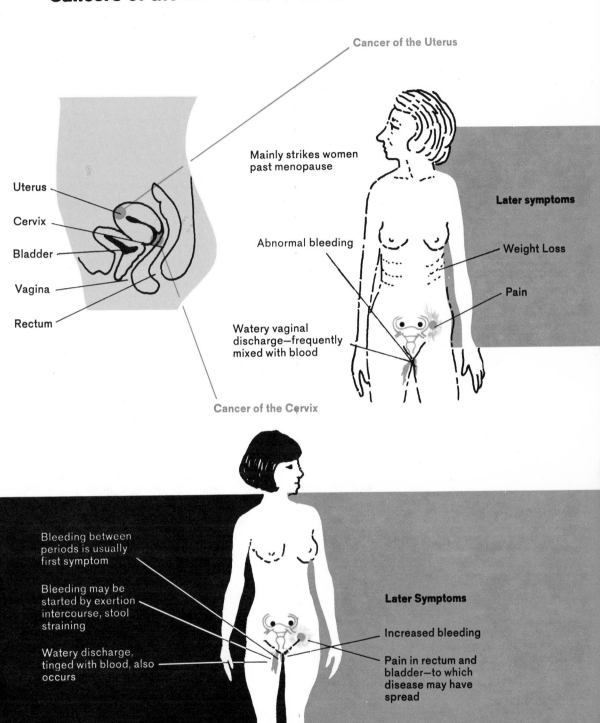

Cancer of the Uterus

Mainly strikes women past menopause

Uterus

Cervix

Bladder

Vagina

Rectum

Abnormal bleeding

Later symptoms

Weight Loss

Pain

Watery vaginal discharge—frequently mixed with blood

Cancer of the Cervix

Bleeding between periods is usually first symptom

Bleeding may be started by exertion intercourse, stool straining

Watery discharge, tinged with blood, also occurs

Later Symptoms

Increased bleeding

Pain in rectum and bladder—to which disease may have spread

the disease and its causes Cancer of the colon and rectum are responsible for 15% of all deaths from cancer. They are more common in men than in women, and occur in the age group 50 to 70. There is no known cause, and it is an open question as to whether there is any inherited tendency.

Rectal polyps, which are stalk-like growths, are regarded most often as pre-malignant conditions—foreshadowing the possible future development of cancer.

There is no evidence that diverticulitis, parasites, or hemorrhoids predispose to cancer in this area.

As shown in the Medi-Graph, about 75% of all large-bowel cancers occur on the left side: 50% in the rectum; 25% in the sigmoid colon.

symptoms In the early stages of this illness there may be no characteristic symptoms, and the patient scarcely heeds his mild abdominal distress, gassiness, and constipation. When the cancer occurs in the left half of the colon—which is part of the large intestine—the symptoms are usually those of bowel obstruction: a change in bowel habit, or alternating diarrhea and constipation along with increased gassiness and abdominal discomfort.

There may be bright red blood mixed with mucus in the stool, some rectal pain, and the sensation of an incomplete bowel movement. The stool may change in size until it becomes pencil-shaped.

As the cancer develops there is progressive constipation until there is complete obstruction.

When the cancer occurs on the right side of the bowel the symptoms are less specific. Constipation and diarrhea are less common. The pain is sometimes mistaken for appendicitis. And usually the accompanying anemia (lowering of the red blood cell count) causes the patient to complain of weakness and fatigue.

complications The complications of cancer of the colon are usually responsible for the symptoms that appear. Obstruction is one such complication. There can be ulceration or breakdown of the cancer, with spreading infection, and even perforation and peritonitis. Bleeding may be a serious problem.

prevention (or lessening of impact) There is no known way to prevent this disease. The only hope is early recognition and treatment, with proper surgical and medical care. A patient with symptoms suggesting this illness should arrange promptly for a rectal examination, including sigmoidoscopic and X ray studies.

Cancer of the Colon and Rectum

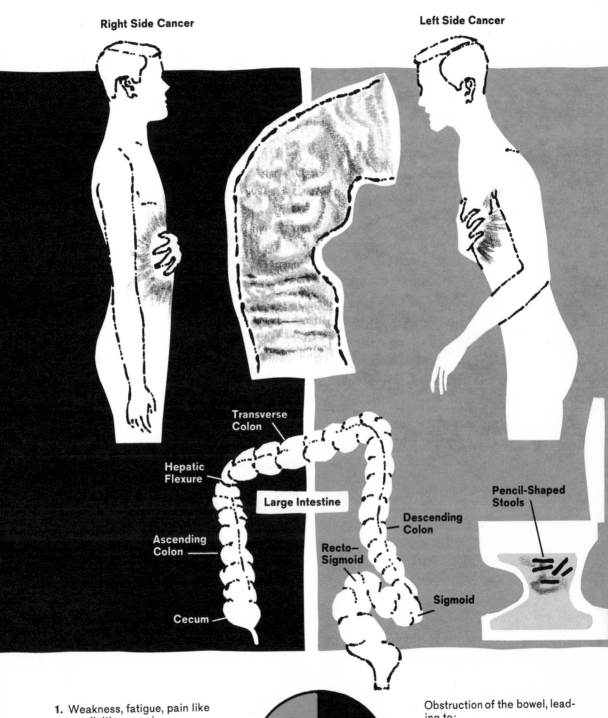

Right Side Cancer

Left Side Cancer

Transverse Colon

Hepatic Flexure

Large Intestine

Ascending Colon

Cecum

Descending Colon

Recto–Sigmoid

Sigmoid

Pencil-Shaped Stools

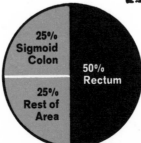

1. Weakness, fatigue, pain like appendicitis, anemia.

25% Sigmoid Colon

50% Rectum

25% Rest of Area

Obstruction of the bowel, leading to:

1. Alternating diarrhea and constipation, plus gassiness and abdominal pain

2. Blood mixed with mucus appears in stool. Stool changes to pencil shape

the disease and its causes   The great majority of lung cancers originate within the walls of the bronchi, the tree-like structures of tubes which carry air to the lungs. That is why lung cancers are more correctly known as bronchogenic cancers.

The direct cause of this form of cancer, like all other cancers, is unknown. However, there is much evidence to show that cigarette smoking is a responsible factor, as well as inhalation of certain irritating dusts (including cobalt and chromates) and fumes.

Lung cancer cases have increased, and now account for about 15% of all cancers. The disease occurs in middle life or later, with greater frequency in men.

symptoms   Symptoms vary with the size and location of the tumor. As shown in the Medi-Graph, the patient develops a cough early in the illness. It is usually dry but there may be blood in the mucus. There is chest pain similar to that of pleurisy. The patient is often short of breath and wheezes as he breathes. His finger joints swell painfully. There can be swelling of the face and upper extremities, and swallowing difficulties, depending upon where the tumor is located.

complications   Complications include collapse of the lung, recurrent pneumonias, bronchiectasis, and lung abscess. However, the real danger is the fatal spread of this tumor to other parts of the body.

prevention (or lessening of impact)   The main hope is to identify the tumor before the symptoms appear. For that reason, all men over 40, and particularly those who smoke, should have routine chest X rays. A patient who has a persistent cough, or spits blood, should notify his doctor promptly. People who have repeated bouts of pneumonia, or a case of pneumonia that does not respond to treatment, should be checked to rule out the possibility of underlying malignant disease. It may also be suspected in any case of unresponding lung disease for which no cause is apparent.

Early recognition and surgery to eradicate the disease are vital. Delay that permits the cancer to spread beyond the confines of the lung is fatal.

Lung Cancer

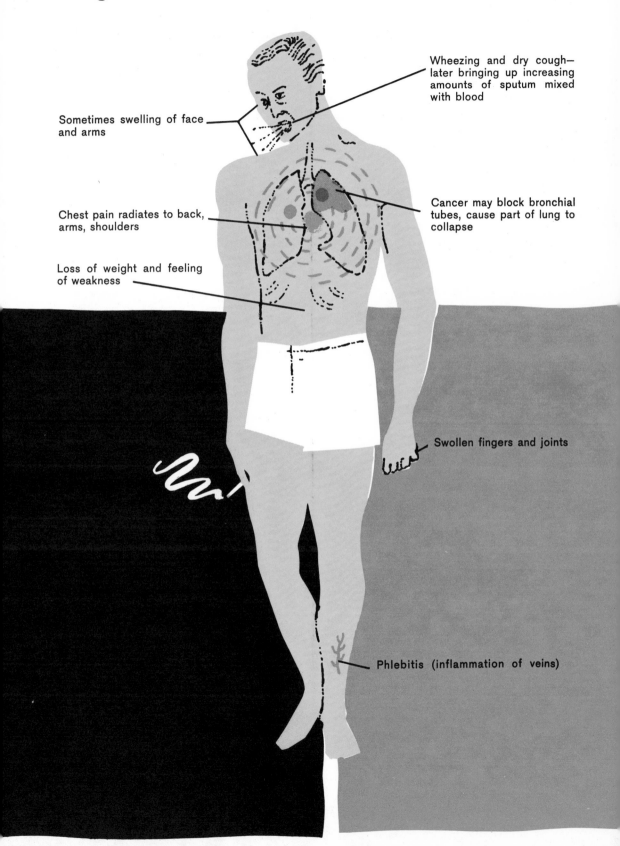

Wheezing and dry cough— later bringing up increasing amounts of sputum mixed with blood

Sometimes swelling of face and arms

Cancer may block bronchial tubes, cause part of lung to collapse

Chest pain radiates to back, arms, shoulders

Loss of weight and feeling of weakness

Swollen fingers and joints

Phlebitis (inflammation of veins)

the disease and its causes Cancer of the pancreas occurs most often in patients over 45, and affects men twice as often as women. It is believed that diabetic patients are more susceptible. The cause is unknown.

symptoms The symptoms are vague and for the most part deceptive. There is weight loss, some abdominal pain, and jaundice. The patient notes digestive disorders such as loss of appetite, nausea, a feeling of fullness after eating even small amounts of food, diarrhea, and more frequently, constipation.

The location of the tumor within the pancreas determines the nature of the symptoms. When it is at the head of the pancreas and obstructs the bile ducts, jaundice results. When, less frequently, it is in the body or tail of the pancreas, there is severe back pain. And, as shown in the Medi-Graph, it can spread to the small intestine or to the spleen, lymph nodes, and liver.

Late findings such as swelling of the abdomen with fluid, enlargement of the liver, and unexplained, frequent vein inflammation (thrombophlebitis) usually indicate the patient is beyond cure.

Diagnosis of cancer of the pancreas is difficult to make early because it rarely can be made from a GI series and symptoms alone. Frequently, exploratory surgery leads to its discovery.

complications The most serious complications result from the spread of the cancer through the bloodstream to other organs.

The cancer growth, as has been mentioned, can obstruct the drainage of bile.

Phlebitis and other problems related to the clotting of blood are further complications.

The outlook for patients with cancer of the pancreas is, as a rule, quite poor.

prevention (or lessening of impact) There is no way to prevent this illness. Prompt recognition and proper surgical-medical care are the only hopes for cure.

Cancer of the Pancreas

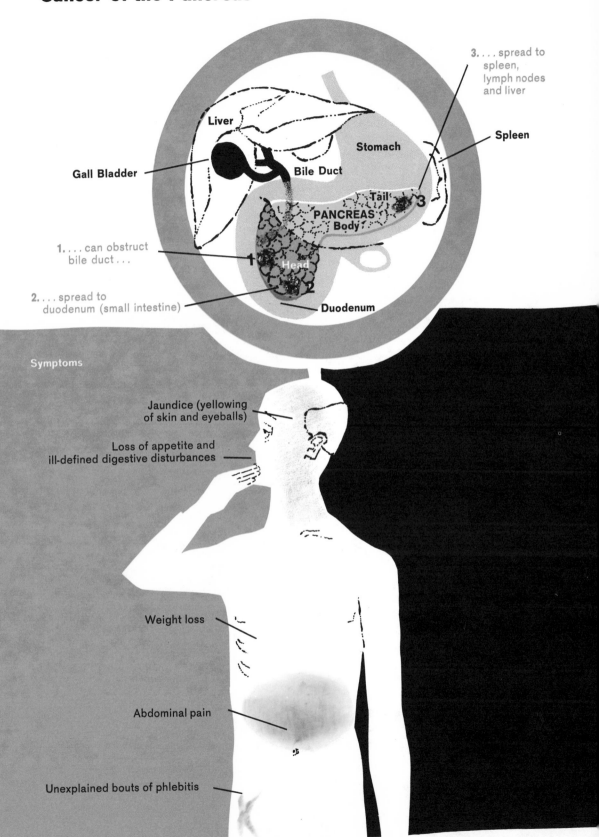

3.... spread to spleen, lymph nodes and liver

Liver

Stomach

Spleen

Gall Bladder

Bile Duct

PANCREAS
Body

Tail

3

1.... can obstruct bile duct...

1

Head

2

2.... spread to duodenum (small intestine)

Duodenum

Symptoms

Jaundice (yellowing of skin and eyeballs)

Loss of appetite and ill-defined digestive disturbances

Weight loss

Abdominal pain

Unexplained bouts of phlebitis

the disease and its causes Skin cancer is probably the most common form of cancer a doctor sees. As a rule, it responds to treatment and is the form of cancer most often cured. The exact cause is unknown. Occurring slightly more often in males than in females, it strikes hardest in the older age group.

There may be some relationship to skin cancer among people with light complexions or those heavily exposed to the sun. Exposure to X ray radiation and chronic exposure to certain chemicals are also considered to be factors in skin cancer.

The most common area for skin cancer is the face, extending over the cheeks from the nose to the ears.

symptoms There are two types of skin cancer: one, basal cell carcinoma, appears in its early form as small, hard nodules of waxy appearance. They grow very slowly and are often present for years before their presence is questioned. Although the nodules are small, they can be identified readily by a trained person.

A more serious form of this type of skin cancer, known as rodent cancer, is characterized by ulceration of the immediate area. It is rapidly destructive, penetrating the skin and involving the local area.

As with most skin tumors, basal cell cancer frequently arises from areas of thickened skin.

Another type of skin cancer is called epidermoid cancer. This form attacks principally the cheeks, ears, and back of the hands. It begins as a warty growth which bleeds easily when the surface is removed. Usually it ulcerates and is often hidden by a secondary infection. Sometimes there is local pain as it penetrates the skin. Depending upon where the malignancy is, the neighboring lymph glands may be involved.

complications There are few complications in skin cancer, provided treatment is rapid and adequate. Of course, as with any malignant disease, there is a possibility that it can spread widely. Ulceration with secondary infection is a possible complication. However, this is not nearly as important as the skin cancer itself.

prevention (or lessening of impact) There is no known way of preventing the development of skin cancer. Once the nodules are observed, investigation should follow promptly. The diagnosis can be established easily by biopsy or complete removal of the section. The doctor will urge the removal of any suspicious area. When it is indicated, X ray can be used most effectively.

Pre-cancerous moles, or areas of skin which have become thickened and are known to be pre-malignant, should be removed before the change occurs.

Skin cancer does not have to be a matter of concern and worry for the patient, provided it is not neglected.

Skin Cancer

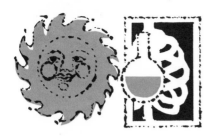

Contributing Factors
X-ray radiation, contact with
industrial chemicals, chronic
irritation; too much sunlight

Two Types of Skin Cancer

Most Frequent Sites

1. Basal Cell — Small, hard, waxy nodules
Grow slowly

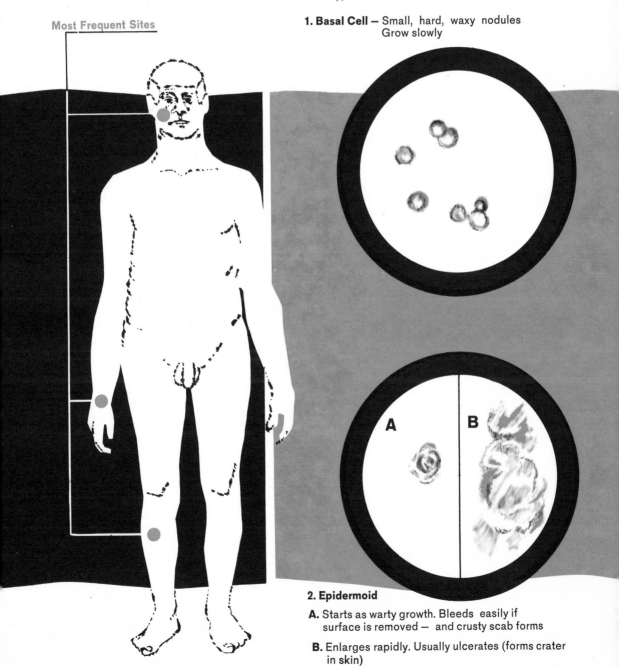

2. Epidermoid

A. Starts as warty growth. Bleeds easily if
surface is removed — and crusty scab forms

B. Enlarges rapidly. Usually ulcerates (forms crater
in skin)

the disease and its causes   Cancer of the stomach, one of the commonest forms of all cancers, accounts for about 30% of all cancer deaths. It occurs at either the upper end of the stomach where the esophagus empties into it, or at the lower end at the exit to the small intestine. The disease develops at any age but appears most often in middle or later middle life. Males are affected three times as often as females.

symptoms   Unfortunately, stomach cancer can be present for as long as two to three years before there are obvious symptoms. Finally the patient complains of discomfort over his abdomen, loses weight and strength, and has no appetite for certain foods, particularly meat. Simultaneously, he shows signs of dyspepsia: discomfort after eating; a feeling of fullness or gas; nausea; and vomiting. Occasionally his history suggests a peptic ulcer.

A patient may have these symptoms for months or years, but at some point the weakness and weight loss become pronounced, and an examination reveals the stomach cancer.

Signs of obstruction may indicate the location of the cancer. By the time it can be felt through the outer abdominal wall, it is usually too late for any cure or effective treatment.

complications   Among the complications of stomach cancer are massive hemorrhage from erosion of a stomach blood vessel, intestinal obstruction, spread of the disease to involve distant organs, and eventually death.

prevention (or lessening of impact)   As yet there is no known preventive for cancer of any type. Hope lies in early discovery and prompt treatment. A patient who has had the symptoms described for any length of time should see a doctor at once. If a diagnosis of stomach cancer is established, arrangements will be made for surgery. Chances of recovery are good only if action is taken early enough.

Cancer of the Stomach

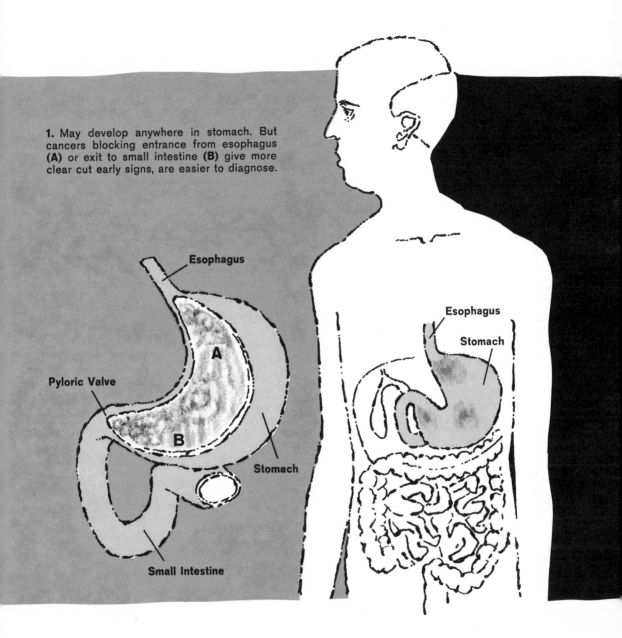

1. May develop anywhere in stomach. But cancers blocking entrance from esophagus **(A)** or exit to small intestine **(B)** give more clear cut early signs, are easier to diagnose.

Esophagus

A

B

Pyloric Valve

Stomach

Small Intestine

Esophagus

Stomach

2. General symptoms: loss of weight, strength, appetite (particularly for meat), fullness and gas after eating, discomfort over abdomen. In later stages fully developed cancer can be felt through abdominal wall.

Carbuncles, Furuncles (Boils) and Folliculitis

(Bacterial infections of the skin)

the disease and its causes FOLLICULITIS This is a skin infection usually caused by streptococcus or staphylococcus bacteria. It occurs most often on the scalp in the form of scattered pustules or pimples and crusts around the hair follicles. Nearby lymph glands may become enlarged and tender. Another form of folliculitis is commonly known as barber's itch because it occurs on the bearded areas of a man's face. In this case, the infection is spread by shaving.

Sometimes folliculitis follows such primary skin disorders as scabies, contact rashes, and lice. Occasionally it is related to certain medicines taken internally, such as iodides and bromides.

FURUNCLES Furuncles are small, superficial abscesses which usually occur singly or in crops at the site of the hair follicles. They are deeper than simple follicular infections. Commonly, they are found around the hairy parts of the body, particularly the neck, scalp, face, buttocks, and thighs. Unfortunately, they tend to recur frequently.

Furunculosis is often related to generalized diseases of the system, such as diabetes, blood disorders, or any other condition which causes weakness and lowered resistance. It may also be a secondary infection following any other skin disorder.

CARBUNCLES This is a larger, deeper abscess than a furuncle and is commonly found on the back of the neck. It usually appears singly but has several heads. Carbuncles are common in patients suffering from diabetes or any other illness that weakens the body.

symptoms FOLLICULITIS The main symptom of folliculitis is itching.

FURUNCLES A furuncle begins as a small area of pain and swelling. This enlarges, becomes hard, and develops into a pimple or pustule. After several days it may soften and open by itself, draining pus-like material. If it does not open or subside, it may have to be lanced.

CARBUNCLES The area around a carbuncle is large, red, and very painful. Chills, fever, and weakness accompany its appearance. After several days it begins to discharge blood and pus from several openings.

complications FOLLICULITIS The only complication is the spread of the infection from hair follicle to hair follicle.

FURUNCLES On rare occasions abscesses develop in other parts of the body. There can be blood poisoning.

CARBUNCLES Abscesses in other parts of the body can develop. In critical areas they can be very dangerous, due to the spread deep into local tissues. Occasionally there is blood poisoning.

prevention (or lessening of impact) Because of the infectious nature of these forms of skin disease, it is imperative to observe good hygiene habits and keep the skin scrupulously clean. Avoid contact with infected people or materials they handle. Avoid barber shops that employ common shaving and hair cutting equipment without sterilization for each customer. General and local antibiotics will be prescribed by the doctor when treating these infections. Many people also find that the use of special anti-bacterial soaps will prevent outbreaks of infections.

Carbuncles, Furuncles (Boils) and Folliculitis

(Bacterial infections of the skin)

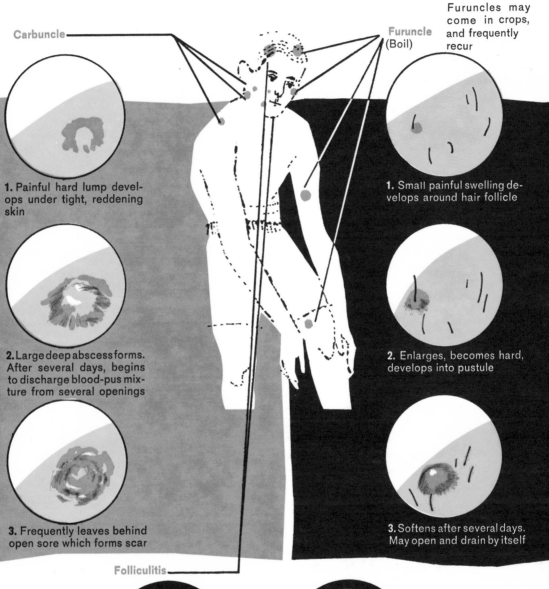

Carbuncle

Furuncle (Boil)

Furuncles may come in crops, and frequently recur

1. Painful hard lump develops under tight, reddening skin

2. Large deep abscess forms. After several days, begins to discharge blood-pus mixture from several openings

3. Frequently leaves behind open sore which forms scar

1. Small painful swelling develops around hair follicle

2. Enlarges, becomes hard, develops into pustule

3. Softens after several days. May open and drain by itself

Folliculitis

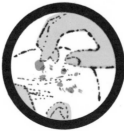

Magnified

1. Small, itchy pustules and crusts form around hair follicles

2. Scratching frequently spreads disease

the disease and its causes A patient with a cataract has an eye condition in which the lens of the eye becomes clouded over. When the lens becomes completely opaque, no longer allowing light to pass through to the retina, sight is completely lost.

This clouding of the lens is seen most frequently after middle age, as the tissues of the eye lenses degenerate. But some people are born with cataracts and others may inherit the disease or a tendency toward it. Cataracts are also caused by nutritional diseases such as diabetes and rickets, an injury to the eye lens or lens capsule, and by diseases of the eye. Certain drugs, and exposure to radium or X ray, can also cause toxic cataracts.

The disease may start in one eye, but eventually it will affect both. This is not because it is "catching" or infectious. What it signifies is that the same physical breakdown takes place in the second eye. From start to finish the development of cataracts can take about two years. Usually it is seen without any other sign of eye disease.

symptoms Regardless of the cause, the symptoms of most cataracts are the same. With time, the patient sees less and less, and his sensitivity to light decreases. He may develop double vision and nearsightedness. Often he will complain of spots before his eyes or have unexplained daytime headaches. On close examination the pupil of the affected eye, normally black, takes on a milky gray or whitish color.

complications Slow but continuously increasing loss of vision is the most serious complication which develops as the cataract grows. An eye disease in which the cataract is a secondary condition can cause blindness if the primary infection or injury is not properly treated.

prevention (or lessening of impact) Most cataracts accompany old age and there is little that can be done to prevent their development. When they are secondary to injury or infection their development can be prevented with prompt care.

Surgery—in which the cataract-covered lens of the eye is removed—is considered the only effective treatment for cataracts once they have developed. After the operation, the patient wears special cataract glasses or contact lenses which effectively replace the clouded eye lens removed in the operation. However, it usually takes several months after the operation before the patient gets used to this and adequate vision returns.

Cataracts

Normal Eye

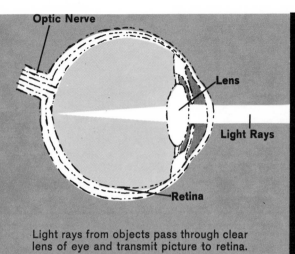

Optic Nerve

Lens

Light Rays

Retina

Light rays from objects pass through clear lens of eye and transmit picture to retina.

Eye with Cataract

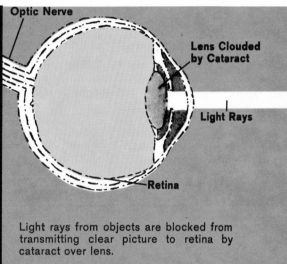

Optic Nerve

Lens Clouded by Cataract

Light Rays

Retina

Light rays from objects are blocked from transmitting clear picture to retina by cataract over lens.

Symptoms of Cataracts

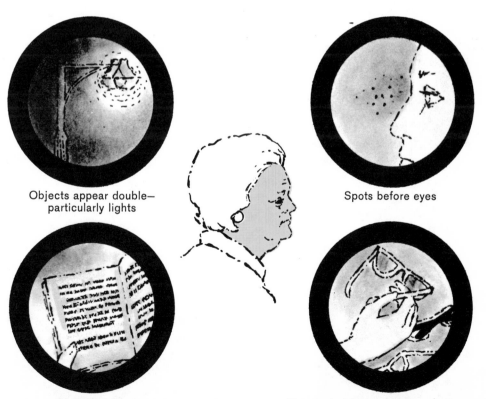

Objects appear double—particularly lights

Spots before eyes

Blurred vision

Frequent change of glasses because of progressive loss of vision

the disease and its cause   This digestive disease primarily affects children under 5 years of age, the age of onset typically being 6 to 18 months. Symptoms may sometimes reappear from ages 20 to 50.

Persons who have this disease are unable to utilize a large part of the normal diet—fats, starches, and sometimes sugars. Sensitivity to gluten, a protein found in wheat, rye, barley, and oats, is the factor which causes the digestive problems of these celiac victims.

The disease has been noted to run in families, pointing to the possibility of a genetic defect as the cause.

symptoms   Though the symptoms are variable, severe diarrhea is almost always present—sometimes 5–6 movements a day. Stomach cramps, weight loss, swollen stomach, and the other symptoms shown in the accompanying illustration are a possibility. Because celiac children are sick and not getting adequate nourishment, they sleep poorly, cry a great deal, and can be difficult to manage.

complications   If the illness is not diagnosed, the child's normal development is delayed and growth is retarded. The failure of normal digestion can lead to the loss of vitamins and iron—leading in turn to such dietary deficiency diseases as rickets, scurvy and anemia. Fractures occur more easily because of calcium deficiency. Skin hemorrhages are common because of vitamin K deficiency. The rundown child is also susceptible to secondary infections.

prevention (or lessening of impact)   Since celiac disease is probably genetic in character, there is no way to prevent its occurrence at present.

However, early treatment can stop the disease from becoming a serious problem. A doctor can tailor a diet to the case—one primarily high in protein foods which can be eaten with no ill effects. These include skim milk, egg whites, lean meat, fish, liver, and protein-rich vegetables. Rice, corn, and soy can be substituted for wheat and other grains. Bread, cake, ice cream, whole milk, and other foods high in starches, sugars, and fats must be avoided. The addition of vitamins to the diet, and iron if there is anemia, also help to promote normal growth.

Celiac Disease (Nontropical Sprue)

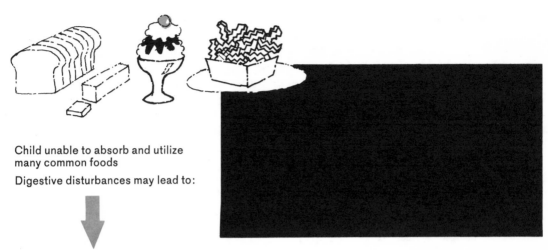

Child unable to absorb and utilize many common foods

Digestive disturbances may lead to:

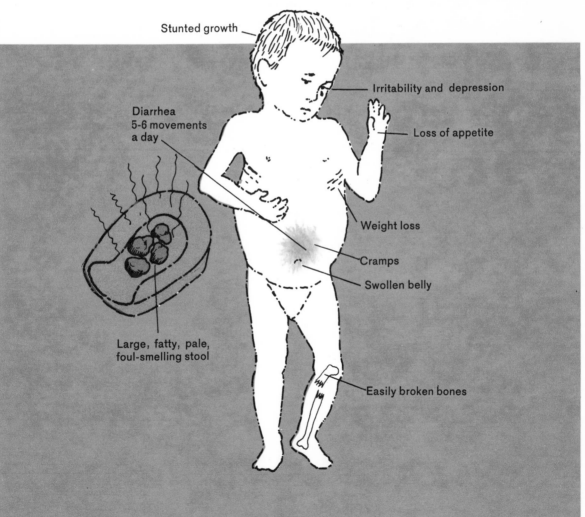

Stunted growth

Irritability and depression

Loss of appetite

Diarrhea
5-6 movements
a day

Weight loss

Cramps

Swollen belly

Large, fatty, pale,
foul-smelling stool

Easily broken bones

the disease and its causes Cerebral palsy is the term given to a wide variety of non-contagious and usually non-progressive defects in the nervous system present from the time of birth or from early childhood. The defects may be inherited or acquired; they may be related to injury at birth; they may be the result of an illness which affected the baby while it was still in the womb; or they may be the result of an illness contracted in very early infancy. Frequently the cause is uncertain.

There are several general categories into which patients fall, and classification is usually based on the type of defect present. The disease is broadly divided into three groups: (1) rigid (spastic) paralysis; (2) tremors, localized rigidity of a muscle group, and an unsteady gait; (3) generalized paralysis without rigidity, involving large areas, or localized as in facial palsy or arm palsy.

symptoms Because cerebral palsy includes such a wide variety of neurological defects, the symptoms are extremely varied and relate to the damage. Patients with the spastic type of cerebral palsy usually have all four extremities involved to some degree. Another form of cerebral palsy causes complete or partial paralysis of one side of the body. Sometimes there is just a weakening of one side of the body. Still another type is characterized by weakness on both sides of the body as well as on the face. In such cases mental development is almost always retarded.

A second group includes children who are so mildly affected that their abnormal movements may be misinterpreted as restlessness. Others are plagued by involuntary twisting, grimacing, drooling, and a whole array of bizarre movements. Mental development may or may not be interfered with, but most often it is not. In this group, the less severely affected patient can make some adjustment to his illness. Heavily handicapped ones must, of course, be cared for.

A third group is made up of patients who show signs of paralysis without muscle spasm. Such infants usually are feeble from the day of birth. There is motion of all muscle groups but weakness of motion is apparent from the beginning. Mental development is interfered with. Few of the severely affected children in this group live to puberty.

Milder versions of this form of cerebral palsy are known by different names, depending on the extent of damage.

There are many other manifestations of cerebral palsy. Further information concerning these can be obtained from your local cerebral palsy chapter.

complications These depend entirely on the extent of damage and the areas affected. Infants severely involved are prone to secondary infections and die early.

prevention (or lessening of impact) There is no known way to prevent cerebral palsy. Physical therapy and speech therapy should be begun as soon as practicable. Patients with mild cases can be treated and helped to care for themselves.

Cerebral Palsy

1. Brain damage — usually occurring before, during, or shortly after birth—results in inability to control and coordinate muscles

2. Mother or medical attendants familiar with normal child development may recognize disability in infant. Treatment and training can help

3. Wide range of conditions labeled Cerebral Palsy. Not contagious and usually non-deteriorating. Many cases are mild, without impairment visible to untrained eye

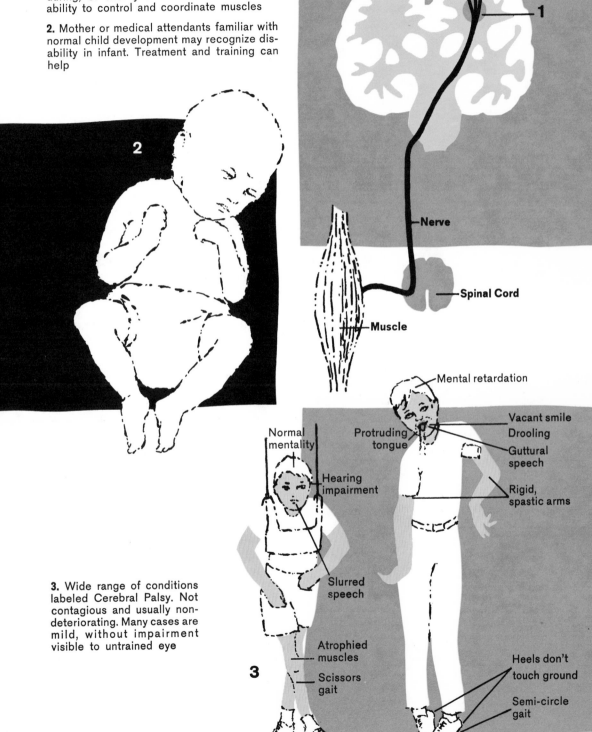

the disease and its causes   This is an acute illness, caused by a protozoa *(Trypanosomacruzi)*, affecting mostly children. Various animals harbor the disease, including cats, dogs, bats, foxes, opossum and squirrels. Chagas' disease is transmitted from them to humans through the bite of the *Reduviid bug* (kissing bug). The bite is painless and frequently inflicted about the lips (hence the name kissing bug) or the eyes.

The bug excretes the infectious protozoa while it is biting, and the victim rubs it into the wound. The incubation period is about 2 weeks.

This disease is widely found in South and Central America, and even has been seen in Texas and the southwestern U.S.

symptoms   About 2 days after the bite, a red nodule (pimple) appears at the site. The lymph glands in the area may also swell up.

In about 2 weeks the victim develops a high fever which often lasts for weeks. Other symptoms are a swelling of the face—particularly about the eyes—and a diffuse skin rash. The sufferer's liver and spleen enlarge and become tender.

The disease either causes the victim's death in 2–4 weeks, or it goes into a chronic stage. In this stage, the parasites in the body spread to involve the muscles, heart or nervous system. The doctor diagnoses the disease by means of a blood test or biopsy (examination of slices of tissue) of the lymph glands or liver.

complications   These include heart failure, convulsive (shake-like) symptoms, and delirium and other psychic disturbances.

prevention (or lessening of impact)   The outlook for victims of this illness is dim— since there is no effective treatment known at this time. Prevention is the best weapon—and is accomplished by the elimination of the transmitting bug. The use of insecticides, netting to protect children from the bite while sleeping, and generally good sanitary principles applied to the home and the community are the most effective measures possible.

Chagas' Disease

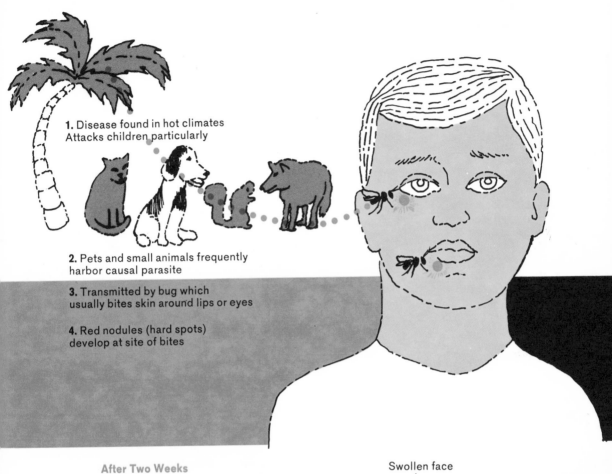

1. Disease found in hot climates
Attacks children particularly

2. Pets and small animals frequently
harbor causal parasite

3. Transmitted by bug which
usually bites skin around lips or eyes

4. Red nodules (hard spots)
develop at site of bites

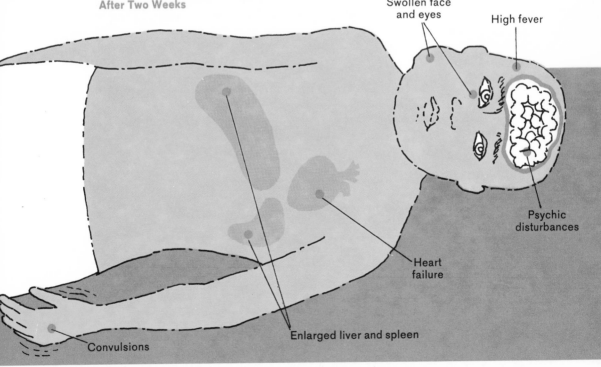

After Two Weeks

Swollen face
and eyes

High fever

Psychic
disturbances

Heart
failure

Convulsions

Enlarged liver and spleen

the disease and its causes   Chickenpox is a generalized disease caused by a virus, involving the skin and mucous membranes of the entire body. It is spread by direct contact with someone infected with the disease, by contact with objects handled by an infected person, or by a carrier. One attack carries lifelong immunity to this disease. It occurs most generally in the fall and winter, with an incubation period of 2 weeks, although it may be as long as 3 weeks. The contagious stage lasts about 10 days and is over when the pox lesions dry up and begin to fall off. They should be allowed to fall off by themselves, because if the scabs are removed the patient will be left with ugly scars. Tub baths should be avoided until the skin lesions are in the final dry stage.

symptoms   Chickenpox begins suddenly with the appearance of the rash, as illustrated. It starts on the trunk, spreads to the face, and then to the extremities, in that order. There is temperature in the 102° range and it lasts throughout the period of breakout. The rash is quite itchy but usually becomes dry and crusted, and falls off in about 1 week. It leaves scars only if the pox become infected or are badly scratched or forcibly removed. All parts of the body may be involved, including the mouth, nose, and rectum.

complications   These are not common, but they do occur. Infections of the skin, such as furuncles, boils, or impetigo, are often seen. More rare are nephritis and encephalitis, but they do occur.

prevention (or lessening of impact)   There is no vaccine for chickenpox and no way to insure a mild case, as with some other childhood diseases. If the itching is severe, a lotion or drug is available to give relief. To avoid the danger of infection, the patient's fingernails should be cut short and scrubbed thoroughly with soap, water, and alcohol. Virus diseases tend to lower resistance and so it is helpful to provide an especially nourishing diet to build up the body and encourage healing. If there are other young children in the house, the patient with chickenpox should be isolated as long as there is fever and new blisters continue to appear. Supportive care of this kind under the family doctor's direction is all that is usually required in this illness.

Chickenpox

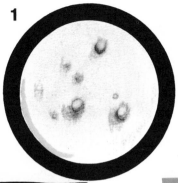

1. First Day
Red spots suddenly appear on body. Some spots develop into blisters. Patient runs fever.

2. Second Day
Spots and blisters spread to face, arms and legs. Rash may be quite itchy.

3. Fourth Day
Rash starts to lose color and dry up. Scales drop off within week—leave scars only if infected or badly scratched.

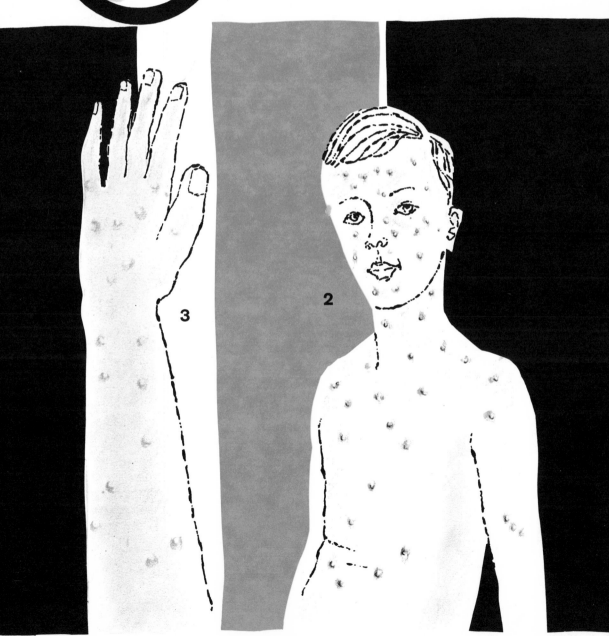

the disease and its causes   This bacterial infection of man usually crops out in
epidemic waves. The disease is characterized by severe diarrhea and
dehydration. It is thought that a toxin produced by the bacteria acts on
the small intestine in such a way as to prevent sodium from being absorbed. The unabsorbed sodium acts as a laxative that causes the severe
diarrhea and dehydration.

The germ *(Vibrio comma)* which causes the disease gains entrance to
the body through polluted drinking water or food. Some of these cholera
germs later leave the body through material that is vomited or defecated.
Cholera most frequently crops up in hot, humid climates, like India,
Pakistan, and Southeast Asia—aided by poor sanitation which promotes
contamination. Epidemics also occur periodically in Egypt and other
parts of Africa.

symptoms   Symptoms break out suddenly, 5–6 days after infection with the cholera
germ. The patient is hit by a sudden, severe, watery diarrhea, frequently
accompanied by vomiting and muscle cramps. The diarrhea can be so
severe that the victim is rapidly dehydrated. Several quarts of fluid may
be lost in a few hours. The dehydration may be so severe that the victim
will go into shock.

The disease is relatively easy to diagnose during epidemics because of
the characteristic symptoms, substantiated by a microscopic analysis of
the victim's feces or vomit—which shows the presence of the bacteria.

complications   If severe cases are not treated, there can be death from shock,
anemia or blood chemical disturbances.

prevention (or lessening of impact)   Good sanitation in a community prevents the
outbreak or spread of a cholera epidemic. Where the disease does break
out, its spread can be prevented by isolating the patient and destroying
all of his waste materials.

People in an area where cholera breaks out should take care only to eat
cooked food, and to drink water that has been boiled or—preferably—
chlorinated. This food and water should not be permitted to stand for
any length of time since it may thus become contaminated.

A serum has been developed which can give partial protection to those
who live in or must travel through cholera-ridden areas. Victims of
cholera also respond to antibiotics. Cases treated in this way generally
make a good recovery.

Cholera

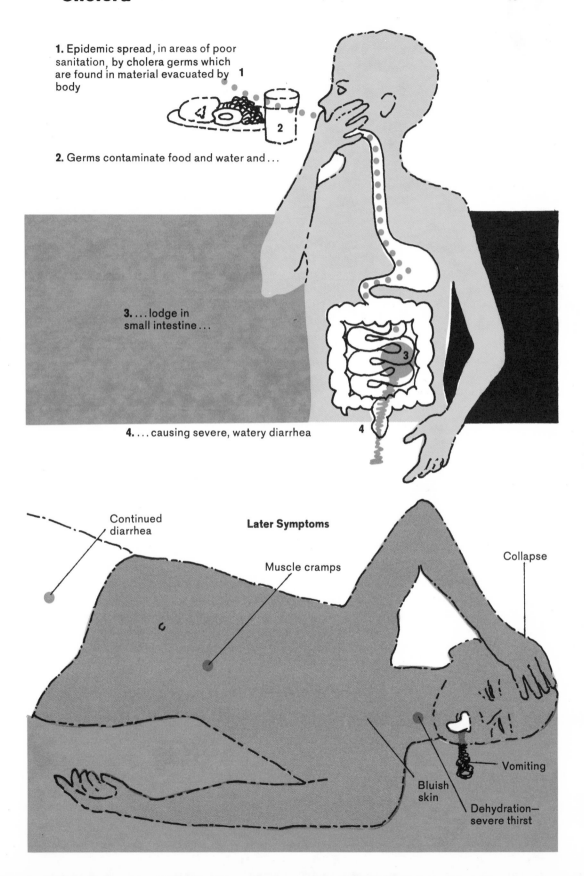

1. Epidemic spread, in areas of poor sanitation, by cholera germs which are found in material evacuated by body

2. Germs contaminate food and water and...

3. ...lodge in small intestine...

4. ...causing severe, watery diarrhea

Later Symptoms

Continued diarrhea

Muscle cramps

Collapse

Vomiting

Bluish skin

Dehydration— severe thirst

the disease and its causes   Cirrhosis of the liver is a chronic disease of the liver which results in its hardening because of scar formation. Its causes and the exact mechanism of its development are uncertain. The disease is believed to be the result of chronic alcoholism and poor diet. Occasionally it is a complication of other diseases where malnutrition is a factor, as for example, diabetes, chronic dysentery, and some thyroid disorders.

A form of cirrhosis is also caused by the hepatitis virus.

symptoms   The disease usually develops very slowly and the initial complaints are generalized, as illustrated in the Medi-Graph. The specific symptoms of the advanced stage may not appear for months or even years. As the disease advances, signs of liver failure develop. Jaundice, swelling of the feet and abdomen, and bleeding tendencies are seen. The skin is sallow and the veins over the face are larger, presenting the typical "alcoholic" face. There is also loss of hair in the armpits and pubic areas. The breasts in the male may enlarge and impotence may develop. As the disease progresses further, the patient becomes more anemic, his abdomen swells further and, in the final stages, he is likely to fall into a coma. The liver, which is enlarged when the disease begins, shrinks as it progresses.

complications   Varicose veins can develop in the esophagus (the passageway between the mouth and stomach). This can result in bleeding from the intestinal tract. There can be severe secondary infections. Cancer of the liver can develop. Other complications are pancreatitis and peptic ulcer, but these are more likely to be related to the alcoholism and poor diet than to the liver cirrhosis. Liver coma is the most serious complication. It occurs late and may end fatally.

prevention (or lessening of impact)   As with so many other diseases, early recognition and vigorous treatment can give good results. The approach includes control of drinking, adequate diet, and vitamin therapy. Secondary infections which appear must be dealt with and eliminated. Where there is abdominal fluid to be drained or bleeding to be stopped or any other specific symptom to treat, the signs and symptoms will determine the kind of treatment to be given. If the patient is in a coma, the attending physician will issue specific instructions for his care.

Again it is important to emphasize the grave consequences of indifference and delay in treating this disease.

Cirrhosis of the Liver

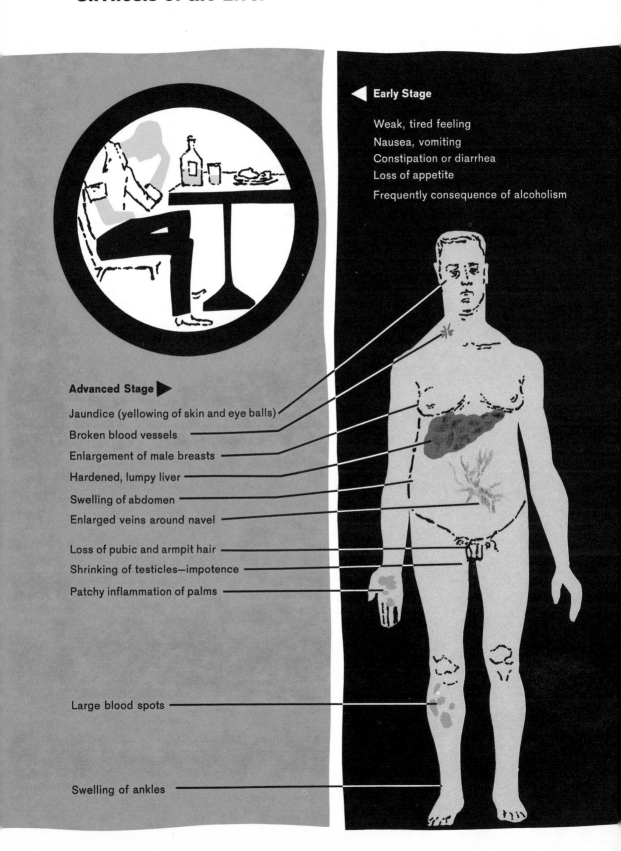

Early Stage

Weak, tired feeling
Nausea, vomiting
Constipation or diarrhea
Loss of appetite
Frequently consequence of alcoholism

Advanced Stage ▶

Jaundice (yellowing of skin and eye balls)
Broken blood vessels
Enlargement of male breasts
Hardened, lumpy liver
Swelling of abdomen
Enlarged veins around navel

Loss of pubic and armpit hair
Shrinking of testicles—impotence
Patchy inflammation of palms

Large blood spots

Swelling of ankles

Cold Sores (Herpes Simplex . . . Fever Blisters)

the disease and its causes   Cold sores are groups of small, watery blisters which are frequently related to a common cold or diseases causing high fever. Another name for this condition is herpes simplex. This acute infection of the skin is caused by a virus. Most often the sores appear on the lips and nose, but they may occur on other areas of the body such as the eyelids, penis, and vagina.

symptoms   Small painful swellings appear. These soon develop into red areas with small, watery blisters which eventually break and become crusty. Gradual healing follows, the whole cycle lasting from ten days to two weeks. Some people tend to get cold sores repeatedly.

Occasionally the local lymph glands are involved. These become swollen and slightly tender.

complications   The most common complication is secondary infection and impetigo, which is an infection of the skin.

prevention (or lessening of impact)   It is difficult to know when cold sores will develop, and nothing can be done to stop them from developing. Some patients who get cold sores repeatedly have been treated with smallpox vaccination with occasional success. Care should be taken to avoid secondary infections.

Cold Sores (Herpes Simplex ... Fever Blisters)

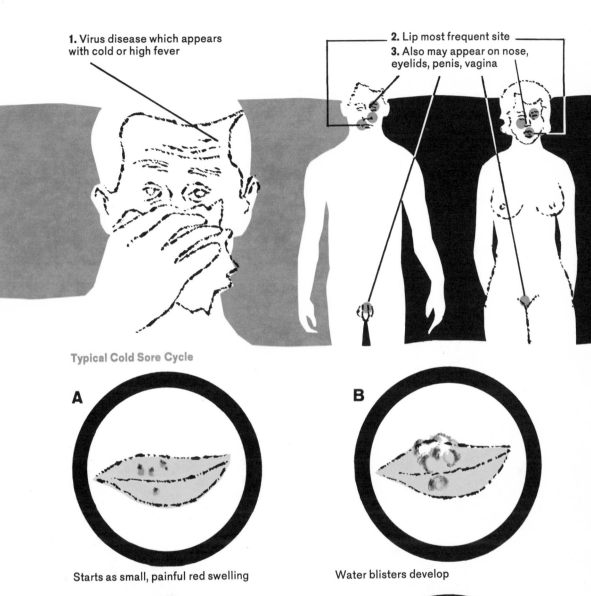

1. Virus disease which appears with cold or high fever

2. Lip most frequent site

3. Also may appear on nose, eyelids, penis, vagina

Typical Cold Sore Cycle

A

Starts as small, painful red swelling

B

Water blisters develop

C

Blisters break, scab forms in hollow left by breaking of blister

D

Usually heals and disappears within 10 days—2 weeks. May become recurrent problem

the disease and its causes   Ulcerative colitis is a disease generally located in the
rectal and the sigmoid portion of the large intestine. However, all of the
colon may be involved, and occasionally this disease even extends into
the end of the small intestine. There is ulceration, inflammation, and
thickening of the bowel wall, and also a generalized inflammation involving joints and skin.

This disease is relatively common and is found equally in men and
women. It can occur in childhood, but the usual age group is from
20 to 40. The cause is not known, but there are many theories. Various
bacteria are thought to be responsible. Allergies, viral infections, and
nutritional deficiencies have all been mentioned as possible causes.
Emotional problems and anxieties have also been held responsible, particularly since they are definitely associated with flare-ups of this disease.

symptoms   The illness may begin slowly or suddenly, and it may proceed halt-
ingly or explosively. Few patients are permanently cured, and it tends to
be chronic, flaring up frequently and then quieting down. Most patients
are affected on and off throughout their lives.

Symptoms depend upon the extent and severity of the inflammation and
its location. If it begins in the rectum, the only symptom may be the
passage of bright red blood and mucus in the stool, along with some
constipation or diarrhea. There may be a normal number of stools a
day or up to 15 or 20. With a bowel movement there may be pus,
accompanied by pain and cramps. There can be fever, loss of appetite,
and marked loss of weight. There may or may not be discomfort in the
abdomen.

As the disease progresses and becomes chronic, the patient becomes
wasted and weak. His stools may now occur 3 to 5 times a day in a
semi-solid form, with bright red blood. In severe cases, there is high
fever, weakness, and other evidence of serious illness.

complications   Serious complications are perforation (puncture) of the bowel wall,
with peritonitis (infection), and massive bleeding. The patient is chronically ill and disabled.

Another complication in as much as 10% of the cases is the development of cancer in the area involved. Rectal fissures or abscesses can
appear. And there are complications having to do with acute arthritis,
skin changes, anemia, and phlebitis.

prevention (or lessening of impact)   There is no known way of preventing this
illness. Periodic examinations are essential to avoid some of the serious
complications. Many symptoms can be controlled with the help of
medicine and a suitable diet. Since repeated attacks are clearly linked
to anxiety and frustration, psychotherapy is often mentioned and frequently used to help patients deal with their problems and thereby avoid
recurrence of the disease.

Ulcerative Colitis

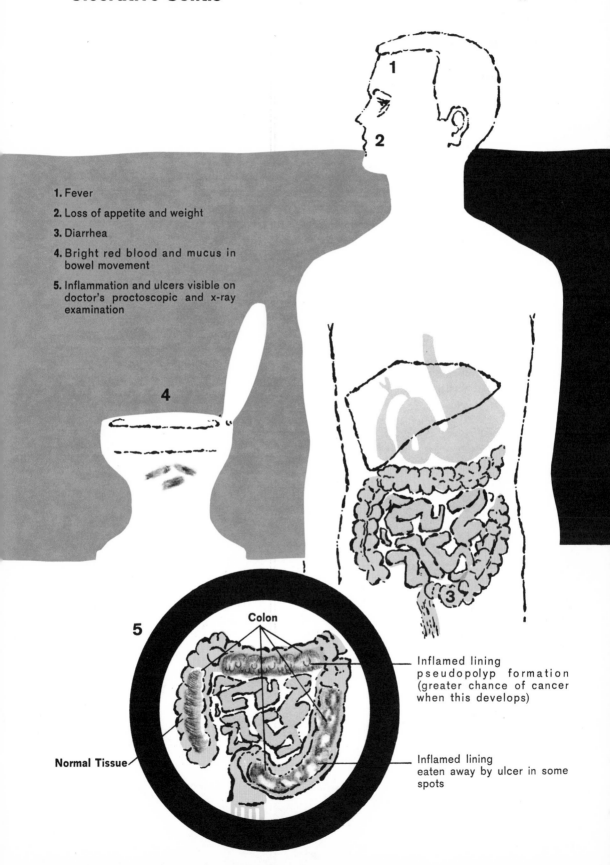

1. Fever

2. Loss of appetite and weight

3. Diarrhea

4. Bright red blood and mucus in bowel movement

5. Inflammation and ulcers visible on doctor's proctoscopic and x-ray examination

Colon

Normal Tissue

Inflamed lining pseudopolyp formation (greater chance of cancer when this develops)

Inflamed lining eaten away by ulcer in some spots

Conjunctivitis (Including Pink Eye)

the disease and its causes   This is an acute infection of the conjunctiva, which is the delicate lining of the eyeball and eyelids. A wide variety of bacteria and viruses cause this highly infectious and contagious disease. It is readily spread in families and schoolrooms by contact with towels, handkerchiefs, or fingers of patients who have it. Other forms of conjunctivitis are caused by foreign bodies in the eye, allergy, exposure to smoke or intense light, and certain contagious diseases.

symptoms   The eyes produce a secretion which is watery at first but soon becomes a thick, yellowish pus. Overnight this secretion dries and the patient's lids are pasted together when he wakes in the morning.
The eyelids usually itch and burn as if there were something in the eye. Sometimes there is sensitivity to light and blurred vision, depending upon how much infectious secretion is present. These symptoms tend to worsen toward evening. Usually one eye is involved at first, but conjunctivitis can and does spread to the other. The eyes get red and the lids swell.

complications   Conjunctivitis is usually a mild illness unless the cornea is attacked. In this event, there is corneal ulceration which can be serious and have a permanent effect on vision.
Treatment is important if the disease is not to become chronic and resistant to therapy. When it is caused by certain bacteria, as for example, bacteria responsible for gonorrhea, it can be quite serious and may even end in blindness.

prevention (or lessening of impact)   Since conjunctivitis is so very contagious, personal hygiene must be stressed. Every member of the family should use a separate towel. Hands should be washed frequently and thoroughly. It is well to avoid contact with the infectious eye discharge. Fortunately, this disease responds quickly to a simple routine of specific ointments and eye drops.

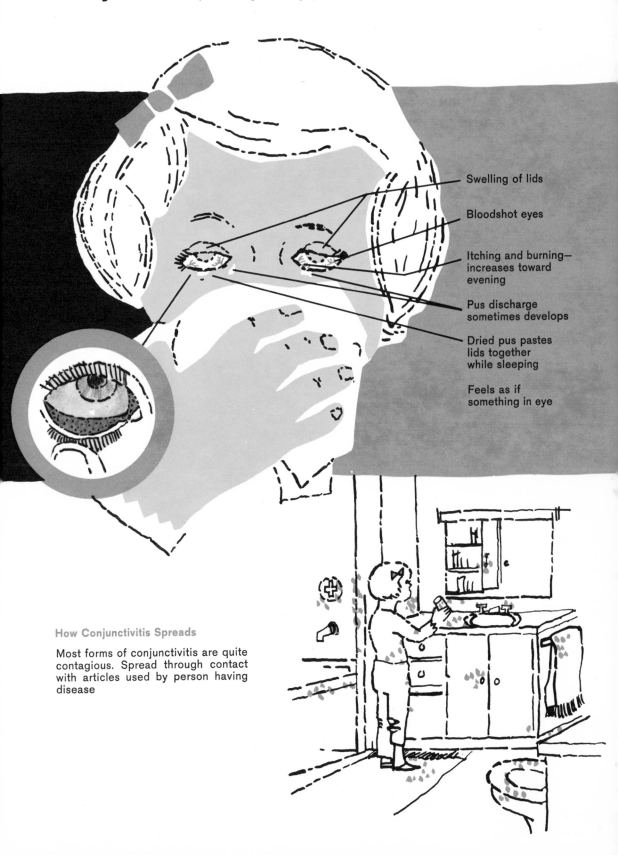

Swelling of lids

Bloodshot eyes

Itching and burning—
increases toward
evening

Pus discharge
sometimes develops

Dried pus pastes
lids together
while sleeping

Feels as if
something in eye

How Conjunctivitis Spreads

Most forms of conjunctivitis are quite contagious. Spread through contact with articles used by person having disease

Contact Dermatitis and Drug Reactions

(Allergic Diseases of the Skin)

the disease and its causes There are many possible causes of contact dermatitis and drug reactions—two allergic diseases of the skin. These causes include many chemicals used industrially, such as certain dyes, formalin, etc.; cosmetic preparations, such as lipstick, nail polish, and hair dyes; household items, such as paints, plastics, nickel, and even wood; many common plants, including poison ivy, oak, and sumac; externally applied medications, such as the penicillin and sulfa groups; certain drugs taken by mouth; soaps and detergents; clothing; starches and cleaning fluids.

symptoms The severity of the symptoms depends upon each individual's sensitivity to the offending material. Generally, the reactions are of two types: *contact* reactions occur at the points at which the individual comes into contact with the material causing the reaction. The rash that results can, however, be spread to other parts of the body by the patient himself. *Drug* reactions tend to appear all over the body.

In contact reactions, a rash appears, accompanied by redness, swelling, blistering, and crusting of the skin areas involved. There is usually itching and burning. Secondary infections can be caused by scratching or rubbing. When this happens, the rash becomes pussy.

While drug eruptions may simulate any skin disorder, in general they are characterized by the even distribution of the rash on both sides of the trunk. Frequently, the skin of the hands and feet is involved.

Drugs taken by mouth can cause not only the dermatitis described above, but also a severe type called exfoliative dermatitis. This can begin suddenly, with or without fever, starting off with a slightly raised rash and followed by peeling. Loss of nails and hair is not unusual. The disease varies in severity depending on sensitivity. It can follow other skin disorders or be related to a generalized illness.

complications There are usually no serious complications to contact dermatitis. Secondary infections are not unusual, but fortunately respond to treatment. Where large parts of the body are involved, there can be such symptoms of generalized illness as fever, weakness, and perhaps prolonged disability. Exfoliative dermatitis, when severe, can cause death.

prevention (or lessening of impact) The offending agent must be found—a task that can be difficult in light of the many causes. Patch tests of skin reactions may be attempted by the doctor. The materials handled by the patient should be itemized and considered. The only form of desensitization that is at all satisfactory is for the plant contact group, including poison ivy, oak, and sumac. Both a vaccine and an oral preparation are available which tend to lessen the severity of the illness or prevent it entirely.

Once the cause of the reaction is found there are many forms of treatment available to lessen the serious effects. These include the use of anti-histamine drugs which, in many cases, give good results. Protective gloves and other clothing can prevent contact with allergy-causing industrial and household materials.

Contact Dermatitis and Drug Reactions

(Allergic Diseases of the Skin)

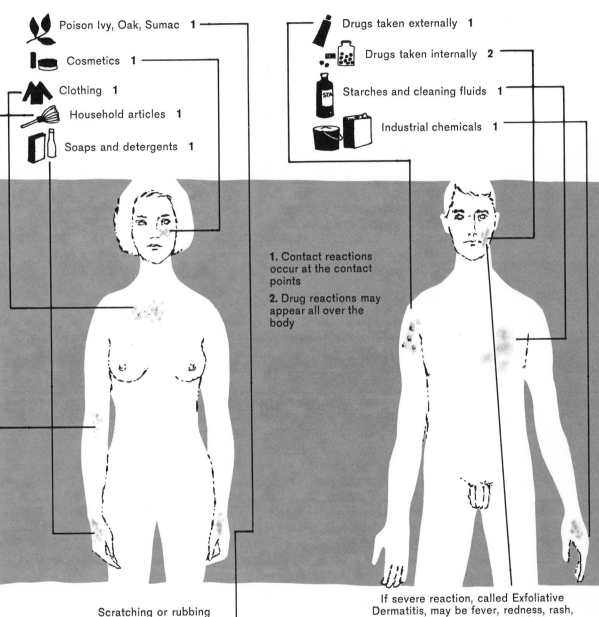

Poison Ivy, Oak, Sumac 1

Cosmetics 1

Clothing 1

Household articles 1

Soaps and detergents 1

Drugs taken externally 1

Drugs taken internally 2

Starches and cleaning fluids 1

Industrial chemicals 1

1. Contact reactions occur at the contact points

2. Drug reactions may appear all over the body

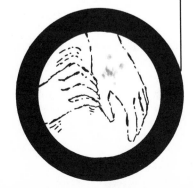

Scratching or rubbing causes secondary infection

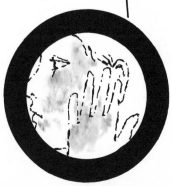

If severe reaction, called Exfoliative Dermatitis, may be fever, redness, rash, peeling, loss of nails and hair

the disease and its causes In coronary artery disease, there is narrowing or clogging of the coronary arteries which bring blood to the heart. As a result, the heart area supplied by the coronary artery is cut off both from its blood supply and from the oxygen and nourishment carried by the blood. The deprived area becomes severely damaged or destroyed (infarcted).

The narrowing or clogging of an artery is usually due to arteriosclerosis (hardening of the arteries): the inner walls of the artery are roughened or thickened, and fat deposits accumulate. Only a little, inadequate supply of blood can trickle through this hardened and roughened area— or the blood supply may be stopped completely. This is called coronary thrombosis.

The arteriosclerosis bringing on coronary artery disease may, in turn, have been brought about by a number of long-term factors, either singly or in combination: inheritance of a tendency toward hardening of the arteries and heart trouble; use of tobacco and other stimulants; inability to relax from the tension and stress of modern life; obesity, diabetes, high blood pressure. But a specific coronary artery attack may be precipitated by overeating, emotional upset, or unusual physical effort.

Coronary artery disease is a very common problem and occurs most often in the over-40 age group.

symptoms The symptoms—and severity—of coronary artery disease depend upon the size of the artery cut off . . . how big an area of the heart is injured or destroyed . . . the vigor and reserve power of the undamaged areas of the heart . . . the demands made upon the heart at the time, and many other factors. In 10% of the cases, there may be no pain.

As a result, the symptoms may vary. Some patients may have only a mild type of discomfort in the middle of the chest, similar to mild indigestion. In others, the pain may be very severe, starting from the chest area and radiating up into the neck and face, to the back, and down into the left arm. In the more severe forms, the patient may also develop shortness of breath, blue lips, and even enter a state of shock.

complications If the attack is severe or the patient not treated promptly, the complications are heart failure, change in rhythm and rate of the heart beat, shock, or death.

prevention (or lessening of impact) A life of moderation is the best way to prevent the occurrence of coronary artery disease. This means keeping one's weight down; avoiding overeating; taking regular exercise—but not to the point where one becomes overtired; avoiding tobacco and other stimulants; and making a conscious attempt to relax from the daily demands of work and the pressures of modern life. A patient who is already suffering from coronary artery disease will probably find his doctor prescribing an approach like this as he recovers from the illness.

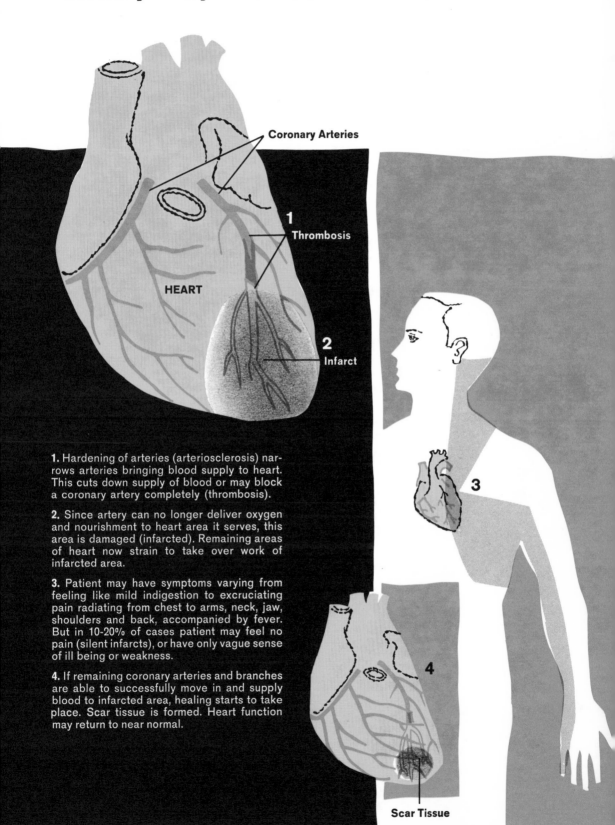

Coronary Arteries

1 **Thrombosis**

HEART

2 **Infarct**

3

1. Hardening of arteries (arteriosclerosis) narrows arteries bringing blood supply to heart. This cuts down supply of blood or may block a coronary artery completely (thrombosis).

2. Since artery can no longer deliver oxygen and nourishment to heart area it serves, this area is damaged (infarcted). Remaining areas of heart now strain to take over work of infarcted area.

3. Patient may have symptoms varying from feeling like mild indigestion to excruciating pain radiating from chest to arms, neck, jaw, shoulders and back, accompanied by fever. But in 10-20% of cases patient may feel no pain (silent infarcts), or have only vague sense of ill being or weakness.

4. If remaining coronary arteries and branches are able to successfully move in and supply blood to infarcted area, healing starts to take place. Scar tissue is formed. Heart function may return to near normal.

4

Scar Tissue

Cretinism and Myxedema

(Hypothyroid—Underactive Thyroid Gland—Diseases)

the disease and its causes   These diseases arise because not enough thyroid hormone is made available to the tissues of the body. The prime reasons for this are stated in the accompanying Medi-Graph. Other possible causes are glandular defects, particularly those of the pituitary, the use of radioactive drugs, and exposure to X ray.

The age groups involved are usually between 30 and 60, and the diseases occur more frequently in females than in males. When symptoms appear shortly after birth, the disease is called cretinism. In children and adults this disease is known as myxedema. The course of the illness differs, depending upon the age at which it starts.

symptoms   The symptoms of cretinism and juvenile myxedema are quite similar. The effects of the disease on mentality and bone growth are determined by the age at which a child becomes involved. The effects of the hormone deficiency are more apparent in the cretin because it begins so much earlier. These patients are usually short and fat, as shown in the Medi-Graph.

Characteristic symptoms of the adult patient with myxedema are shown in the accompanying Medi-Graph. Some additional symptoms are anemia and premature graying. The outer third of the eyebrow may be missing. There are often vague muscle pains and weakness, and persistent upper respiratory infection.

complications   In the untreated adult hypothyroid patient, heart disease may develop. There are occupational and emotional problems for the patient and family. Without adequate and early therapy, the loss of mental ability and bone growth in the infant and child may go beyond reversal.

prevention (or lessening of impact)   Early diagnosis of this particular disorder is of extreme importance because bone growth and mental development can be stimulated by the proper use of thyroid hormone. Although the patient may be on medication all his life, the treatment is most effective, and he can at least be a functioning human being.

Cretinism and Myxedema

(Hypothyroid—Underactive Thyroid Gland—Diseases)

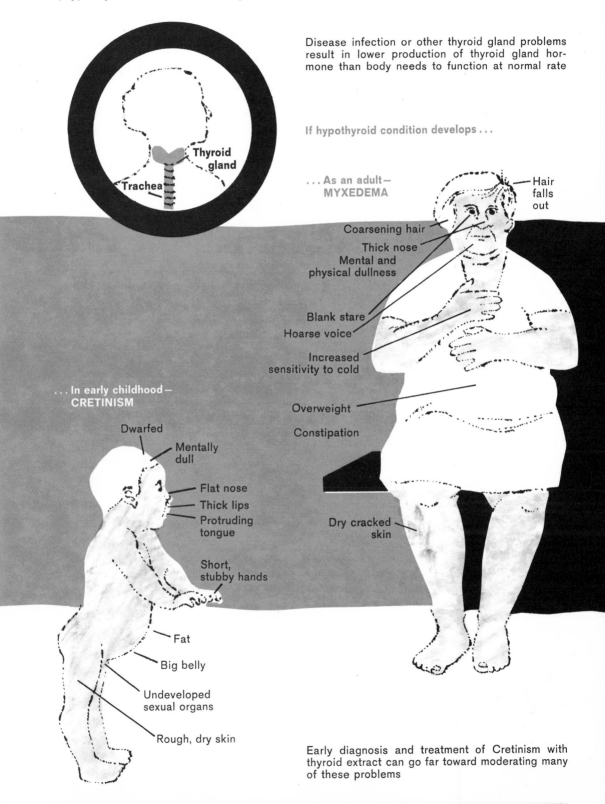

Thyroid gland

Trachea

Disease infection or other thyroid gland problems result in lower production of thyroid gland hormone than body needs to function at normal rate

If hypothyroid condition develops . . .

. . . As an adult—
MYXEDEMA

Hair falls out

Coarsening hair

Thick nose
Mental and physical dullness

Blank stare

Hoarse voice

Increased sensitivity to cold

Overweight

Constipation

. . . In early childhood—
CRETINISM

Dwarfed

Mentally dull

Flat nose

Thick lips

Protruding tongue

Short, stubby hands

Dry cracked skin

Fat

Big belly

Undeveloped sexual organs

Rough, dry skin

Early diagnosis and treatment of Cretinism with thyroid extract can go far toward moderating many of these problems

the disease and its causes   Cushing's syndrome is caused by the overproduction of the hormones of the adrenal cortex. The adrenal cortex, which is the outer sheath of a gland at the upper end of the kidney, is responsible for the formation and secretion of more than 30 steroid hormones, among which cortisone is the best known.

Cushing's syndrome is relatively rare, and is seen more often in females than in males. While it occurs most often in the third and fourth decades of life, it can occur at any age. In 60% of the cases noted, the disease is caused by an excessive growth of the adrenal cortex. A third of the cases of this disease result from benign or malignant tumors of the cortex. In 10% of all cases, there is no demonstrable cause.

This illness may be related to a tumor within the pituitary gland itself which, in turn, affects the secretions of the adrenal gland.

When, on occasion, the adrenal cortex is found to be the source of a cancer associated with Cushing's disease, it usually proves to be highly malignant and spreads quickly to adjacent structures as well as the liver and lungs.

symptoms   The earliest symptom is usually an increase in the weight of the patient, followed by the growth of hair over the face and other parts of the body. A high percentage of women patients stop menstruating. Some develop markedly masculine characteristics, as shown in the Medi-Graph (lower left).

The weight increase is marked by a complete redistribution of body fat, as shown in the Medi-Graph. The patient's face and neck redden. The skin becomes thin and fragile, and bruises easily. Red or purplish streaks may appear over the abdomen, breasts, and buttocks.

Other common complaints include backache and recurrent, severe headaches. There can be such mental disturbances as depression, confusion, and extreme irritability.

The diagnosis of this disease is established by means of examination, laboratory studies of 24 hour urine specimens, and blood chemistries and specific blood counts.

About a third of Cushing's syndrome patients develop diabetes and calcium deficiency in their bones. Fractures occur easily and frequently. Tumor in the adrenal gland is sometimes revealed by X ray studies.

complications   Patients with Cushing's syndrome do not always die, but the mortality is high. Causes of death include secondary infections, strokes, heart failure, and kidney failure. When there is a cancer present, death results from the spread of that cancer. Patients with this disease require care by a very competent surgical-medical team.

prevention (or lessening of impact)   If a diagnosis is made relatively early, before the onset of heart and kidney involvement, a patient can be helped. When the adrenal gland becomes enlarged, a cure may be effected with surgery. In a third or half of the cases where the pituitary gland is involved, X ray therapy can halt or slow the progress of the disease.

Cushing's Syndrome (Overactivity of the Adrenal Glands)

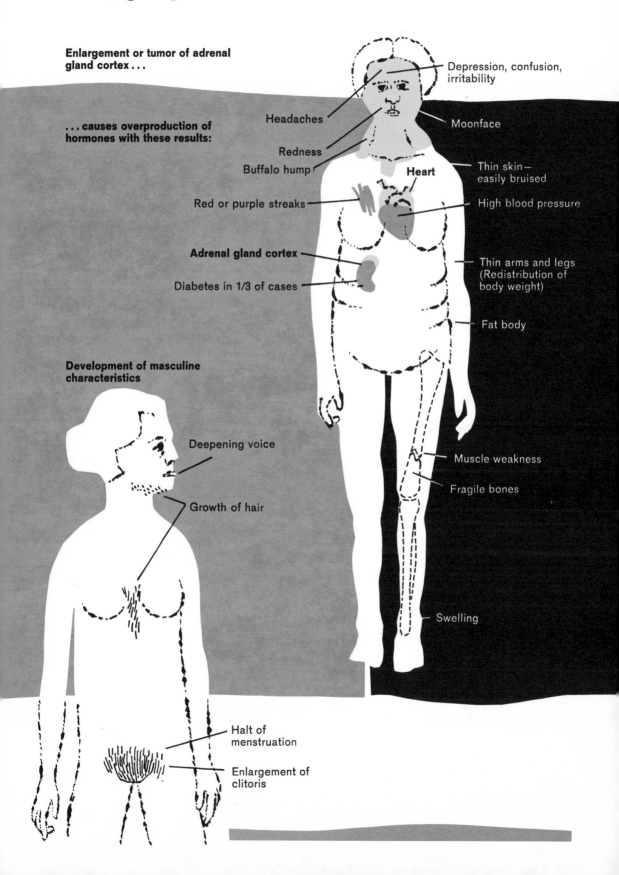

Enlargement or tumor of adrenal gland cortex...

... causes overproduction of hormones with these results:

Headaches

Redness

Buffalo hump

Red or purple streaks

Adrenal gland cortex

Diabetes in 1/3 of cases

Depression, confusion, irritability

Moonface

Heart

Thin skin — easily bruised

High blood pressure

Thin arms and legs (Redistribution of body weight)

Fat body

Muscle weakness

Fragile bones

Swelling

Development of masculine characteristics

Deepening voice

Growth of hair

Halt of menstruation

Enlargement of clitoris

the condition and its causes   The nasal septum is a partition that normally divides the nose into two equal parts. The lower part, toward the tip of the nose, is composed of relatively pliable cartilage, while the upper part is composed of bone. This septum is subject to many problems—with deviation (distortion to one side) being among the most common.

This deviation may be present at birth—often inherited. Or it may be caused by injury—particularly to a young child whose tissues are soft and can be more easily pushed out of line. Nasal tumors or polyps may also push the septum out of shape. Men are more often affected than women, perhaps because the rougher games they play as children make them more susceptible to injury.

symptoms   Minor deviations rarely produce symptoms. But when the deviation is marked, there may be external deformity of the nose.

One of the internal problems is chronic nasal congestion, which may cause repeated nose and throat infections. Due to the obstruction, neuralgic head pains, headaches, and cough due to postnasal drip may also be present.

As sometimes happens with a stuffed nose, the voice can become nasalized. Defective hearing may result because the Eustachian tube on the blocked side tends to be more susceptible to repeated infections.

complications   No serious complications usually occur. But chronic nasal stuffiness may interfere with breathing, and repeated minor respiratory infections can be annoying.

prevention (or lessening of impact)   If the problems arising from the deviated septum become too serious, surgical correction is simple and effective.

Deviated Septum

Cutaway view of nose

Normal Nose	**Types of Deviated Septum**

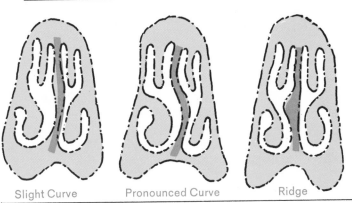

Septum—Partition of bone and cartilage dividing nose into two equal passages

Slight Curve   Pronounced Curve   Ridge

Caused by Birth Defect, Injury or Polyp or Tumor

Side View

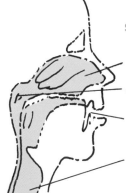

Septum

Auditory (Eustachian) Tube

Mouth

Larynx

Possible Results of Deviated Septum

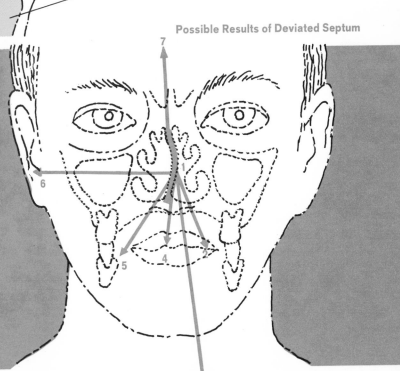

1 Chronic nasal congestion because of blocked passageway

2 Cough due to post-nasal drip

3 Upper respiratory illness stimulated by cough and drip

4 Nasalized voice because of nasal block

5 Toothaches stimulated by infection

6 Hearing impaired because of blockage of auditory tube

7 Headaches and neuralgic head pains stimulated by infection

the disease and its causes In a normal body, food sugar and starches are converted into a sugar form that is readily used as fuel by the muscles. In a diabetic, the pancreas does not produce enough insulin to turn food sugar and starches into this usable form. Instead of serving as fuel, they create a surplus of blood sugar that spills over into the urine. The proteins and fats consumed are not burned up as they should be, and the chemical balance of the body is affected.

Diabetes is common. It can occur at any age but affects the older group most—women slightly more often than men. It affects all races in varying degrees. The disease seems to run in families. And being overweight also seems to play a significant role.

The exact reason why the pancreas fails to function properly and produce the necessary amount of insulin is not known. But in addition to the influence of obesity and heredity, there appears to be a correlation with certain conditions increasing the body's need for insulin. Among these are infections and other hormonal disturbances.

symptoms The onset may be slow or rapid. Children usually develop it suddenly and more severely. In adults the course is slower. There is a need to urinate frequently, and the patient complains of excessive thirst and hunger. There may be a slight loss of weight and strength. A clue may be repeated skin infections such as furuncles and carbuncles. A common complaint is itching of the external genitalia.

As the disease progresses there is marked weight loss. A frequent and characteristic symptom is a sweetish breath odor.

On examination, the urine reveals the presence of sugar, and the blood sugar is abnormally high.

complications As shown in the Medi-Graph, complications are multiple and severe. Insulin shock can be a complication of concern to a patient who takes this drug.

The patient and his family should learn from their doctor to distinguish between *diabetic coma,* which results from uncontrolled diabetes brought about by a variety of factors such as insufficient insulin, infection, or perhaps prolonged vomiting or diarrhea; and *insulin shock,* which can follow by several hours the injection of insulin. Although in both cases the patient falls into a deep coma, the treatment is different and the life of the patient depends upon administering the correct treatment promptly.

prevention (or lessening of impact) While a person can do very little to avoid getting diabetes, there are certain rules anyone can and should follow if he has a strong family history of this disease. He should have regular physical examinations with blood and urine checks. He should guard against overweight. He should have any infection promptly treated. And a patient who develops diabetes should minimize possible complications by strictly following the program of diet and medication prescribed by his doctor.

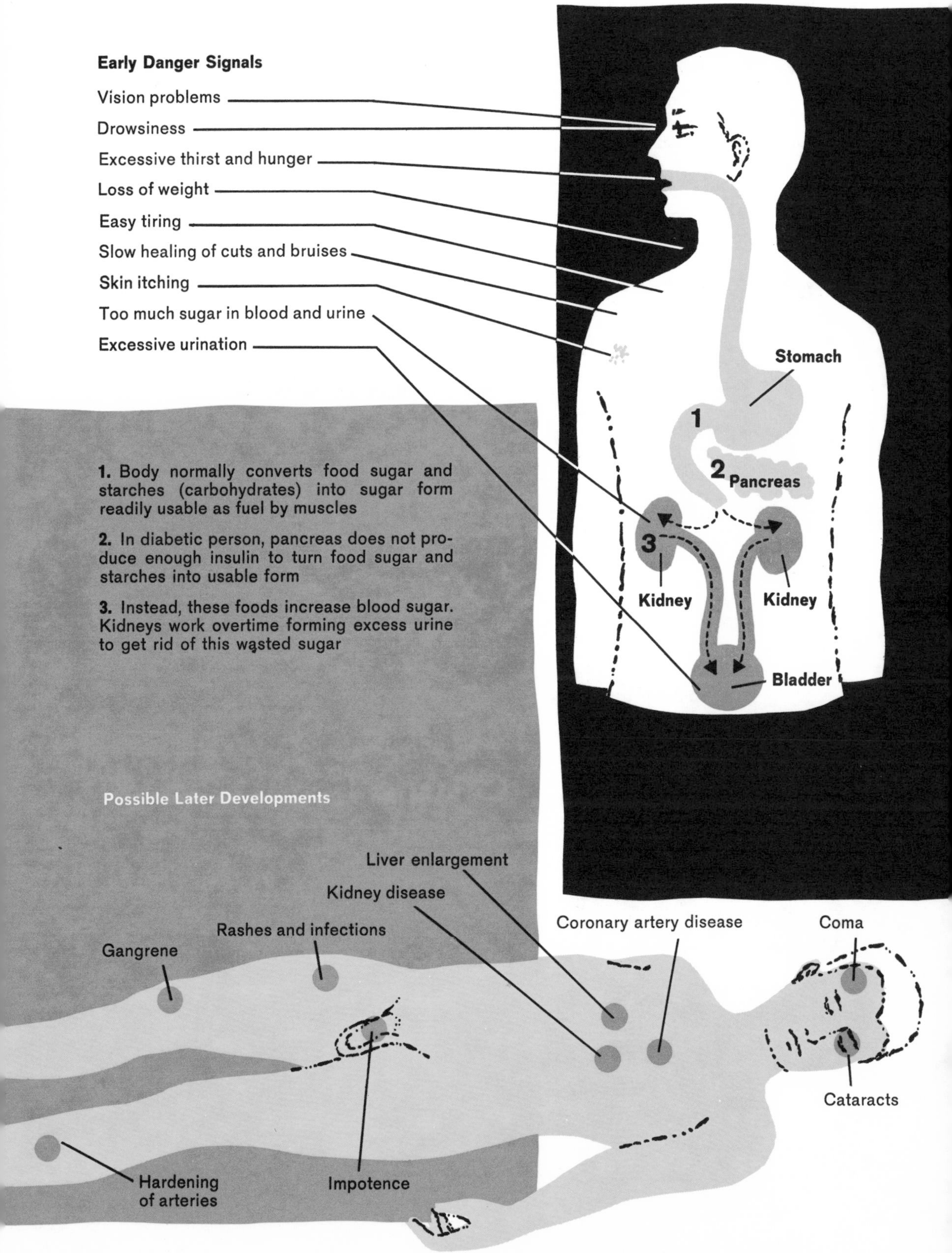

Diabetes

Early Danger Signals

Vision problems

Drowsiness

Excessive thirst and hunger

Loss of weight

Easy tiring

Slow healing of cuts and bruises

Skin itching

Too much sugar in blood and urine

Excessive urination

1. Body normally converts food sugar and starches (carbohydrates) into sugar form readily usable as fuel by muscles

2. In diabetic person, pancreas does not produce enough insulin to turn food sugar and starches into usable form

3. Instead, these foods increase blood sugar. Kidneys work overtime forming excess urine to get rid of this wasted sugar

Stomach

1

2 **Pancreas**

3

Kidney   **Kidney**

Bladder

Possible Later Developments

Liver enlargement

Kidney disease

Rashes and infections

Coronary artery disease

Coma

Gangrene

Hardening of arteries

Impotence

Cataracts

the disease and its causes   Diphtheria is an acute (which is to say quick-developing), severe contagious illness caused by a specific type of bacteria. It involves mainly the respiratory system. The disease is spread by direct contact with an infected patient, with a carrier who may be perfectly healthy himself, or through contact with infected objects or from unpasteurized milk. It occurs mainly during the winter months, and usually affects children who have been ill with an infection of the nose or throat. Babies up to 6 months have some immunity. The disease has an incubation period of 2 to 5 days. The contagious period of the disease may last as long as from 2 to 4 weeks.

symptoms   The disease begins with temperatures in the 101° range, headache, and sore throat. The symptoms vary depending upon the severity of the case and the areas involved. The throat is usually covered with a grayish membrane which may extend to the roof of the mouth and even up into the nose. The mouth odor is foul, the voice becomes hoarse, and swallowing difficult. The glands of the neck become enlarged and painful. Nosebleeds may occur. Breathing may be difficult and noisy. The usual course is 7 to 14 days, and milder cases may improve even more quickly.

complications   In the 2nd to 4th weeks of this illness, severe complications can develop that involve the heart, lung, kidneys, and nervous systems. These include inflammation of the heart muscle, bronchopneumonia, nephritis, and paralysis affecting the muscles of speech, eye movements, arms and legs.

prevention (or lessening of impact)   A diphtheria vaccine is available which should be given to every child by the time he is ready for school. Booster injections are given until the age of 12 to maintain immunity. The Schick Test is used to reveal whether or not an individual is immune to the disease. Anyone who is not immune, or who has been exposed to the disease, should be immunized promptly with diphtheria toxoid or given booster shots of the vaccine. Antibiotic drugs are used in the treatment of the disease and in some of its complications.
Since the diphtheria germ attacks the body by producing a poison known as diphtheria toxin, an early diagnosis is very important. The longer the delay in administering the antitoxin or the toxoid, the more poison is absorbed by the body. Breathing can become difficult, and the patient may suffocate.
Diphtheria antitoxin is available for those not previously immunized with toxoid. In these patients it should be used early, and may be lifesaving.

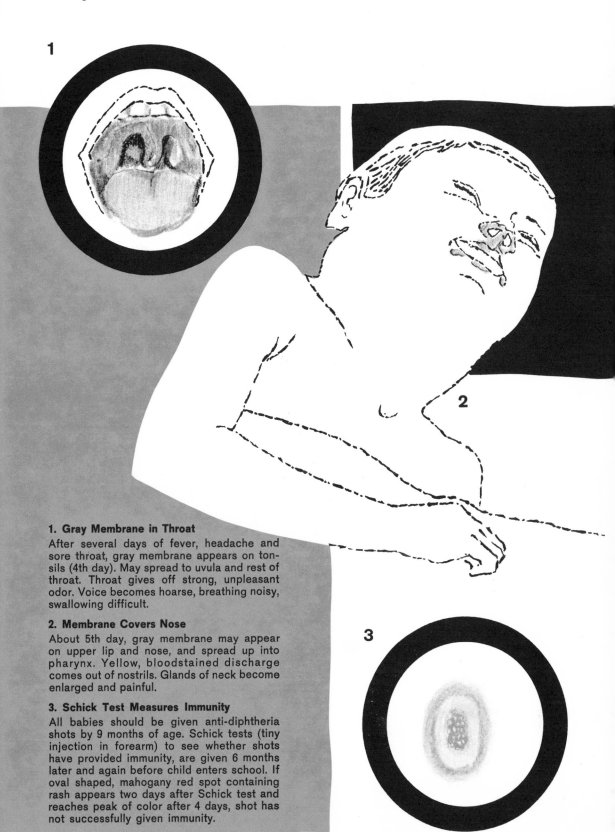

1. Gray Membrane in Throat

After several days of fever, headache and sore throat, gray membrane appears on tonsils (4th day). May spread to uvula and rest of throat. Throat gives off strong, unpleasant odor. Voice becomes hoarse, breathing noisy, swallowing difficult.

2. Membrane Covers Nose

About 5th day, gray membrane may appear on upper lip and nose, and spread up into pharynx. Yellow, bloodstained discharge comes out of nostrils. Glands of neck become enlarged and painful.

3. Schick Test Measures Immunity

All babies should be given anti-diphtheria shots by 9 months of age. Schick tests (tiny injection in forearm) to see whether shots have provided immunity, are given 6 months later and again before child enters school. If oval shaped, mahogany red spot containing rash appears two days after Schick test and reaches peak of color after 4 days, shot has not successfully given immunity.

Drug Abuse: Amphetamines
(Pep pills . . . ups . . . jolly beans . . . meth . . . speed . . .)

the drugs and their effects   Amphetamines are drugs which stimulate the central nervous system. They are sometimes prescribed by doctors to control appetite and aid in reducing diets; to counteract depressed feelings; and to ward off fatigue during dangerous and prolonged tasks.

It is estimated that half the legally manufactured supply of amphetamines finds its way, unfortunately, into illegal channels. Some illegal uses may seem relatively harmless—for example, students may take the drug in order to stay awake and cram during examination periods, or dieters may want the aid of a pill without the bother of a doctor's prescription. A more serious abuser is the one who takes amphetamines to "feel high" at a party or other social occasion. This can lead to repeated, heavy use in order to keep going and not come down from the high.

Another type of abuser is the "speed freak" or "meth head" who gives himself repeated, massive injections intravenously. Some sophisticated drug abusers inject a combination of heroin and amphetamines ("the speed ball") in the hope of getting a more prolonged high.

problems of use/abuse   Unfortunately, amphetamines not only create a dependance, but also the habitual user's tolerance increases rapidly. Consequently, he requires larger and larger doses to obtain the desired effect. The depressed mood into which heavy amphetamine users fall when they come down from their high is extremely severe. Suicide during such moods is a distinct possibility.

efforts to break the habit   On a societal basis, this starts with a drive to eliminate the large-scale illicit sources of amphetamines and with tighter regulation of legitimate producers. Doctors have a responsibility to assess carefully the personality of the patient for whom they are thinking of prescribing amphetamines—and to supervise carefully their prescribed use.

Once a person has been hooked on amphetamines, treatment is very difficult—both medical and psychiatric help may be needed.

Group therapy—in which recovered ex-users join in the group with recent addicts—seems to be getting some results. The ex-user's advice is more likely to be heeded and his example followed by the addict seeking to stop the drug's destructive impact on his life.

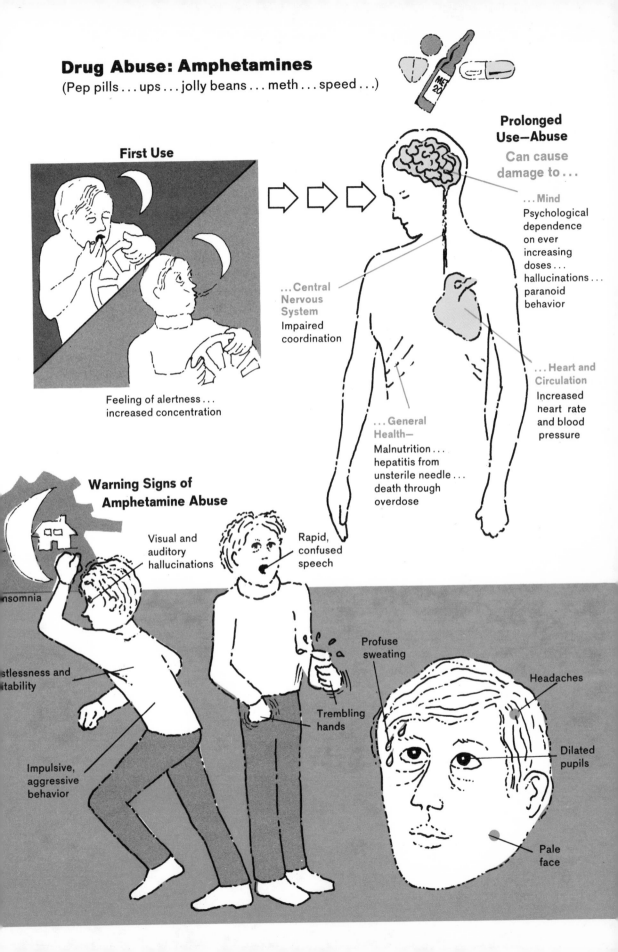

Drug Abuse: Amphetamines

(Pep pills...ups...jolly beans...meth...speed...)

First Use

Feeling of alertness...
increased concentration

Prolonged Use—Abuse

Can cause damage to...

...Mind
Psychological
dependence
on ever
increasing
doses...
hallucinations...
paranoid
behavior

...Central Nervous System
Impaired coordination

...Heart and Circulation
Increased heart rate and blood pressure

...General Health—
Malnutrition...
hepatitis from
unsterile needle...
death through
overdose

Warning Signs of Amphetamine Abuse

Visual and auditory hallucinations

Rapid, confused speech

Insomnia

Restlessness and irritability

Impulsive, aggressive behavior

Profuse sweating

Trembling hands

Headaches

Dilated pupils

Pale face

Drug Abuse: Barbiturates
(Goofballs . . . sleeping pills . . . downers . . . yellow jackets)

the drugs and their effects   Barbiturates are sedative drugs whose effect is to exert a powerful calming action on the central nervous system. Properly prescribed, and taken as directed in small doses, they relieve tension and anxiety. Therefore, doctors sometimes prescribe them for conditions induced by tension like high blood pressure, peptic ulcer, spastic colitis, etc. In larger doses, they are used to produce drowsiness and sleep.

problems of use/abuse   Tense, anxious people—many of them troubled with insomnia—may become overinvolved with barbiturates and dependent on them. These habitual users tend to develop a tolerance to their usual dosage—so that they need to take progressively larger amounts to produce the desired effect. At this stage they are usually getting the drug illegally—without their doctor's knowledge or permission.
Barbiturates are highly dangerous when taken without medical supervision. Accidental deaths, due to mistakenly taking more pills than intended, are not uncommon. Acute barbiturate intoxication is a grave emergency requiring immediate countermeasures. Despite these, it is often fatal. And some 3,000 barbiturate suicides occur each year.
Death can also occur when barbiturates are swallowed by somebody intoxicated with alcohol. The combination of barbiturates and alcohol can prove fatal in doses that would not be disastrous if taken separately at different times.
Formerly, the largest group of persons hooked on barbiturates were adults over 20—principally those in the 40–59 age group. However, barbiturates today are being used more and more frequently by teenagers—who take them by injection as well as orally. "Speed freaks" or heroin addicts frequently inject barbiturates intravenously to help them come off a "high" or tide them over until the next dose.
Some warning signs of abuse of barbiturates are shown in the accompanying illustration.

efforts to break the habit   Quick, unsupervised withdrawal by the chronic user who has become accustomed to taking a large dose of barbiturates daily may result in convulsions, hallucinations, delirium, psychosis, and death. Therefore, withdrawal requires careful medical supervision. After withdrawal, psychiatric help is frequently needed. Since the chronic barbiturate user often suffers from inability to cope with the stress of living and finds reality difficult, he needs considerable psychological and social support if he is to break the drug abuse habit. Group therapy and relating to others who have "kicked the habit" is helpful—as is relocation to a new environment where he can work and live a meaningful life.

Drug Abuse: Barbiturates

(Goofballs . . . sleeping pills . . . downers . . . yellow jackets)

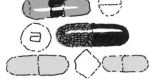

Pentothal . . . . Nembutal
Seconal . . . . . Luminal

First Use

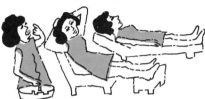

Small dose—
relieves
anxiety

Large dose—
produces
drowsiness
and sleep

Prolonged Use—Abuse
Can cause damage to . . .

. . . Mind
Confusion . . .
depression . . .
suicidal
impulses

. . . Central
Nervous
System
Impaired
coordination . . .
physical
dependence . . .
severe
withdrawal
symptoms
like
D.T.'s

. . . Heart
and Lungs
Can depress
breathing
and heart
activities
to point where
they cease

**Warning Signs of
Barbiturate Abuse**

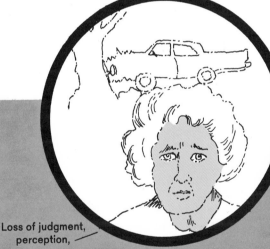

Loss of judgment,
perception,
memory

Drunken behavior
without alcohol
on breath

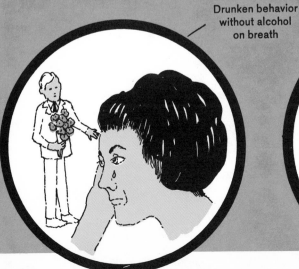

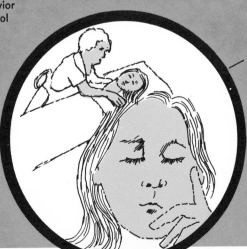

Sluggish,
sleepy,
depressed
behavior

Drug Abuse: Cocaine
(Snow . . . leaf . . . coke . . . flake)

the drug and its effects   Cocaine is a stimulant drug which gives users a temporary sense of well-being, self-confidence, and alertness. Derived from the coca bush, a plant that grows in the uplands of South America, it goes by such street names as snow, leaf, coke, and flake. In the 19th century, cocaine was used by doctors as a local anesthetic. But because of its unfavorable side effects, it has been replaced by effective synthetics. Cocaine is usually taken by sniffing the white powder up the nose. Some users also inject it intravenously, frequently mixing it with heroin.

By taking cocaine, the user stimulates certain areas of the nervous system—which then increase the user's heart, breathing, and metabolic rates. The effect is one of mood elevation, reaching a very exhilarated level.

Cocaine is a potent anti-fatigue agent, and decreases hunger sensations. The user feels superhuman in strength and mental capacity. He frequently overestimates his ability.

problems of use/abuse   As the illustration on the opposite page shows, the use of cocaine can provoke a variety of physical and mental problems. Muscle twitching, high blood pressure, mental impairment, and convulsions may take place. There are also visual and auditory hallucinations. An addict taking cocaine in large doses tends to develop a paranoid state of mind. He is anxious and suspicious, and suffers delusions of persecution. As a result, the cocaine abuser may be a danger to those around him—since his actions are frequently unpredictable.

efforts to break the habit   Since cocaine is not physically addicting, the abuser who tries to break the habit does not suffer any physiological withdrawal symptoms. But heavy use of cocaine often creates a marked psychological dependence—an intense craving for the feelings of increased capability and happiness temporarily acquired.

Therefore, psychological therapy, especially in a group setting, is one of the best ways to help the addict fight the habit. As in the case with alcoholics and other drug addicts, the presence of recovered cocaine addicts in the group gives credibility to the therapy and provides the addict with a model for success in breaking the habit.

Drug Abuse: Cocaine
(Snow . . . leaf . . . coke . . . flake)

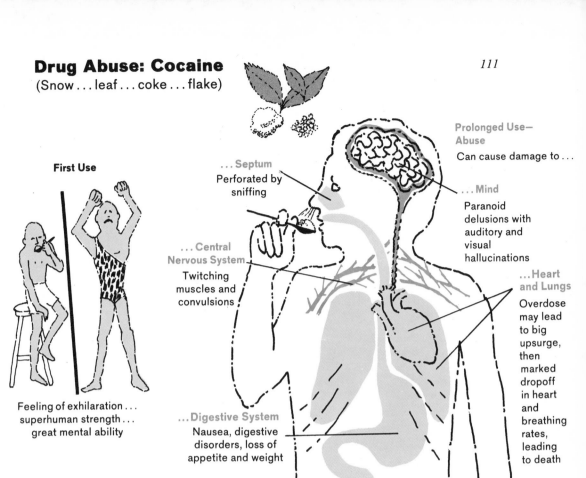

First Use

Feeling of exhilaration . . .
superhuman strength . . .
great mental ability

. . . Septum
Perforated by
sniffing

. . . Central
Nervous System
Twitching
muscles and
convulsions

. . . Digestive System
Nausea, digestive
disorders, loss of
appetite and weight

**Prolonged Use—
Abuse**
Can cause damage to . . .

. . . Mind
Paranoid
delusions with
auditory and
visual
hallucinations

. . . Heart
and Lungs
Overdose
may lead
to big
upsurge,
then
marked
dropoff
in heart
and
breathing
rates,
leading
to death

Warning Signs of Cocaine Abuse

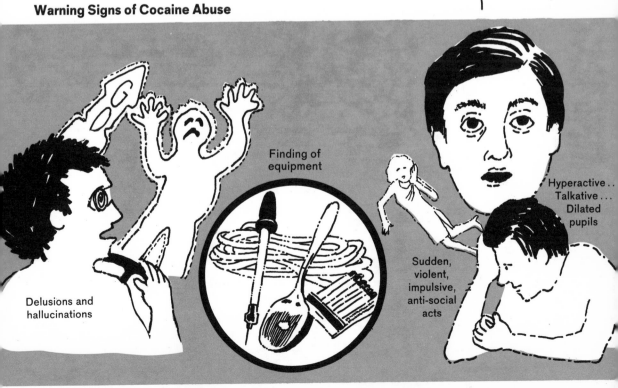

Delusions and
hallucinations

Finding of
equipment

Sudden,
violent,
impulsive,
anti-social
acts

Hyperactive . . .
Talkative . . .
Dilated
pupils

Drug Abuse: Heroin
(Smack . . . horse . . . junk . . . snort . . . scag)

the drug and its effects   Heroin is a narcotic drug—one that relieves pain and reduces tension by depressing the activity of certain areas of the brain. It is derived from opium which is refined into morphine and then chemically altered to become some 3–6 times stronger.

Heroin can be taken in many ways—smoked, inhaled, swallowed, and injected just under the skin (skin popping) or into a vein (mainlining). Almost all users end up as mainliners—since it gives the biggest kick for the smallest dose.

problems of use/abuse   Addiction can develop quickly in the individual who experiments with "just a few bags"—and may end up hooked.

In return for the relief of tension and a sense of well-being, the heroin addict risks the physical and psychological dangers shown in the illustration on the opposite page. This peril is heightened by the fact that heroin is a truly addictive drug. When the addict gets hooked, his body requires repeated and ever larger doses of heroin to produce the same effects. This increases his chances of death through overdosage.

This happens because there is a wide variation in the strength of two seemingly same-sized doses of the drug available from pushers. A dose that may produce a pleasant high on one occasion can be fatal on the next—because the second dose, which appears to be the same strength, is actually much stronger.

efforts to break the habit   Problems of getting off heroin begin with the withdrawal symptoms—as shown in the illustration. If the heroin addict voluntarily or through circumstances is forced to stop heroin abuse, the method may vary from slow withdrawal to "cold turkey" (abrupt cessation), or drug substitution, such as using methadone. With cold turkey, the suffering can be excruciating, and may take as long as 1–2 weeks to subside.

When taken regularly, methadone eliminates the craving for heroin as well as its stimulating effects. In some areas, community clinics are maintaining ex-heroin addicts on methadone by administering daily doses.

As the high rate of relapses shows, the most difficult part of the treatment comes after the addict returns to society. Frequently without job skills and with a poor work record, he needs considerable help to keep from going back to heroin use. Psychological support—particularly through group therapy with other ex-addicts who have succeeded in kicking the habit—seems helpful in many cases.

Drug Abuse: Heroin

(Smack . . . horse . . . junk . . . snort . . . scag)

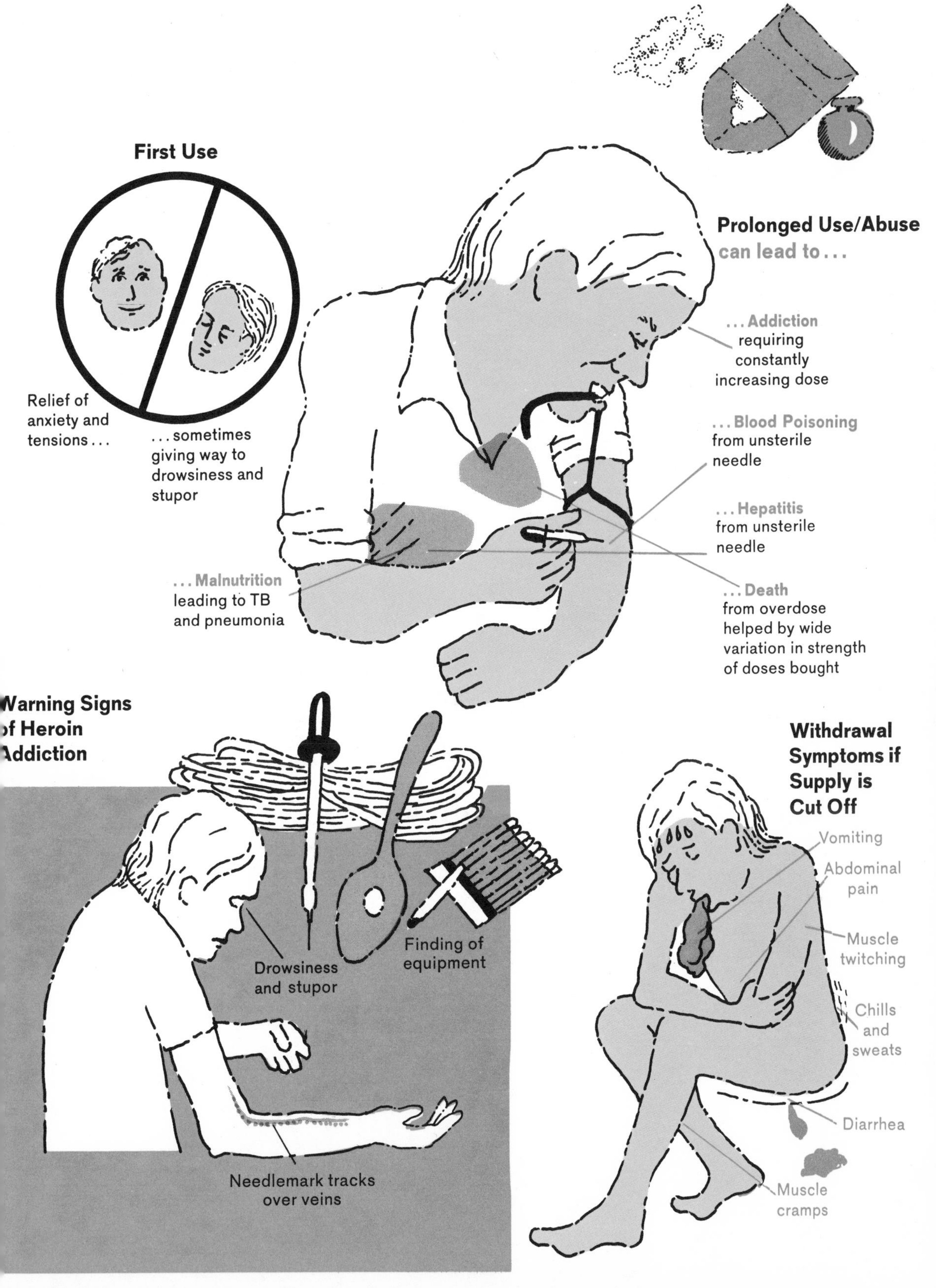

First Use

Relief of anxiety and tensions . . .

. . . sometimes giving way to drowsiness and stupor

Prolonged Use/Abuse
can lead to . . .

. . . Addiction requiring constantly increasing dose

. . . Blood Poisoning from unsterile needle

. . . Hepatitis from unsterile needle

. . . Death from overdose helped by wide variation in strength of doses bought

. . . Malnutrition leading to TB and pneumonia

Warning Signs of Heroin Addiction

Drowsiness and stupor

Finding of equipment

Needlemark tracks over veins

Withdrawal Symptoms if Supply is Cut Off

Vomiting

Abdominal pain

Muscle twitching

Chills and sweats

Diarrhea

Muscle cramps

Drug Abuse: LSD
(Acid . . . Cubes . . . 25 . . . Zen)

the drug and its effects   Lysergic Acid Diethylamide (LSD) is a powerful, man-made chemical which acts as a hallucinogen—a mind-affecting drug. One ounce is enough to provide 300,000 average doses, so controlling its production and spread has proved difficult.

An average dose of LSD amounts to a tiny drop of colorless, tasteless, odorless material which is generally added to a sugar cube and then eaten. The effects come on in about 1 hour, peak in 2, and wear off slowly over about 16 hours.

LSD produces powerful mental reactions in the user and striking distortions in his physical senses—how he sees, touches, smells, and hears. An "acid trip" can be "good"—seeming to be stimulating, mind-expanding, and providing new insights. Or it may be "bad"—a frightening, threatening nightmare. Or there may be a combination of both on the same trip. Unfortunately there is no way to predict who will have a good or bad trip—and the history of having had a good trip is no guarantee that the next drug experience will not be terrifying.

Specific reactions include mood alteration, dream-like feelings, severe hallucinations, detachment or depersonalization. In addition, the user experiences such physical reactions as weakness, dizziness, tingling of the skin, blurred vision, incoherent speech, and alternate laughing and crying.

problems of use/abuse   Any use of LSD can be an abuse, because of the unpredictability of the effect of the drug. As the illustration shows, panic reactions . . . flashback recurrences of negative trips, days or months later, without use of the drug . . . and precipitation of mental illness in susceptible persons are real dangers to the LSD user. There are antidotal drugs to help a user come off a "bad trip," but talking him down by a calm—preferably trained—person is perhaps the best and most effective antidote.

efforts to break the habit   Fortunately LSD is not an addictive drug—so there are no withdrawal symptoms if its use is suddenly discontinued.

Getting LSD users to give up the drug depends in part on the intellectual demonstration that measurable gains in creativity by users have yet to be demonstrated—while the perils of a bad trip are very real. But perhaps more important than logic is an effort to create for the user a stimulating environment where—without drugs—he can get the satisfaction of personal achievement.

Drug Abuse: LSD
(Acid...Cubes...25...Zen)

Good Trip

Bad Trip

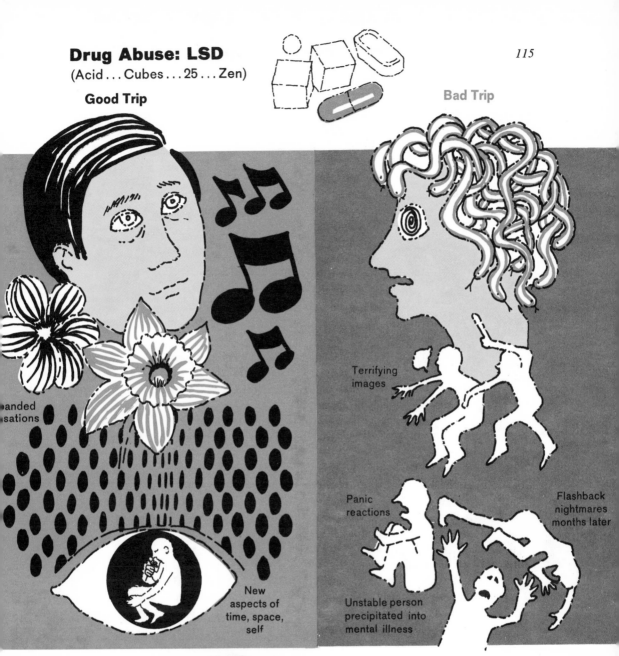

...anded
...sations

New aspects of time, space, self

Terrifying images

Panic reactions

Flashback nightmares months later

Unstable person precipitated into mental illness

Warning Signs of LSD Use

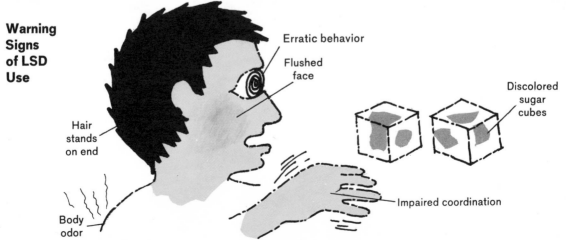

Erratic behavior

Flushed face

Hair stands on end

Body odor

Discolored sugar cubes

Impaired coordination

Drug Abuse: Marijuana and Hashish
(Pot...grass...weed...tea...hash)

the drug and its effects   Marijuana is a mild hallucinogen—altering the user's mood and thinking, and causing dream-like thoughts and illusions. It is derived from the Indian hemp plant (*Cannabis sativa*) which grows wild in many parts of the world.

The leaves of the plant are dried, crushed and (in the western world) usually made into homemade cigarettes called "joints." Marijuana may also be smoked in small pipes, and is occasionally used as snuff or incorporated into food and eaten. The strength of marijuana is extremely variable, depending on the source of the plant and how much it has been adulterated. Hashish (hash) is pure concentrated hemp resin—6–8 times as powerful as marijuana. It is usually smoked in a pipe.

Marijuana quickly enters the bloodstream when smoked, and begins to affect the user's mood and thinking within minutes. Its effect may last from 2–4 hours.

problems of use/abuse   As the illustration on the opposite page shows, any particular use of marijuana may have a wide range of effects. This depends upon the strength of the drug used, the personality of the user, and the social setting in which the use takes place.

Current scientific thinking on marijuana tends to the belief that marijuana is not a narcotic. It does not cause physical dependence, as does heroin.

On the other hand, there is the problem of psychological dependence. The National Institute of Mental Health estimates that there are perhaps 1 million "pot heads" in the U.S. today. They make marijuana a way of life—like the alcoholic who also uses a drug to excess to try to escape from the stresses of daily life.

efforts to break the habit   A social smoker of marijuana is like the social drinker. As long as his pattern consists of only occasional use, it does not usually interfere with his family and economic and social relationships. The chief problem he encounters is the illegality of purchasing and using the drug. The marijuana user who must have a constant supply of "joints" to get through the day is a sick person who needs treatment—both for his present problem and to prevent him from going on to other drug abuse. Challenging work, paid or volunteer, and a stimulating home environment are needed to break dependence upon the drug. Discussion and therapy groups—with people who have conquered this problem—can also prove helpful.

Drug Abuse: Marijuana and Hashish
(Pot...grass...weed...tea...hash)

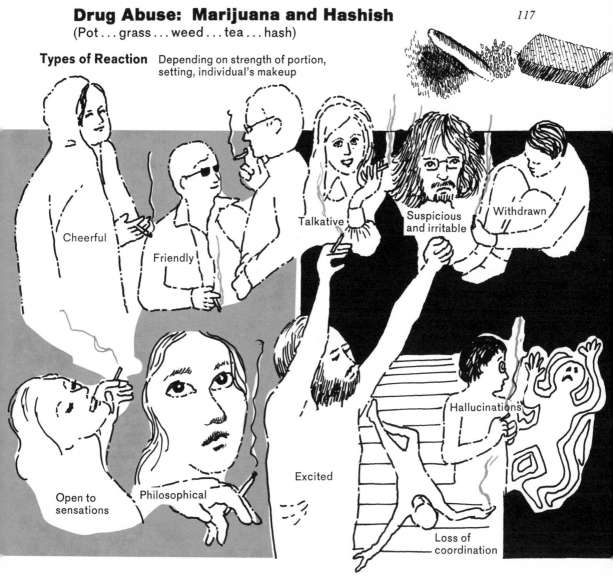

Types of Reaction Depending on strength of portion, setting, individual's makeup

Cheerful

Friendly

Talkative

Suspicious and irritable

Withdrawn

Open to sensations

Philosophical

Excited

Hallucinations

Loss of coordination

Warning Signs of Marijuana Use/Abuse

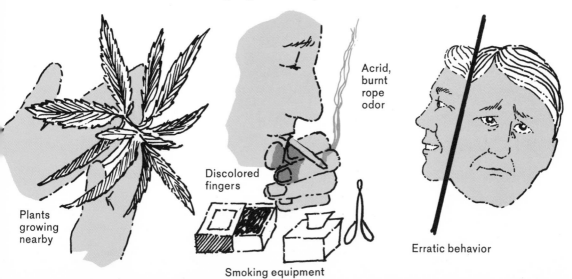

Plants growing nearby

Discolored fingers

Acrid, burnt rope odor

Smoking equipment

Erratic behavior

Drug Abuse: Mescaline and Peyote
(mesc, cactus, button)

the drug and its effects   This hallucinogen is obtained from the peyote cactus which grows in northern Mexico and the southwestern U.S. Mescaline causes a mild anesthesia and colorful hallucinations plus a loss of sense of time.

The drug is made by cutting thick, fleshy slices from the top portion of the cactus plant. These slices are sun-dried, becoming "mescal buttons" or "mescal beans."

It is from these that the active ingredient, mescaline, is obtained. It can be chewed, ground into powder and eaten, or injected under the skin to get the desired effects. Mescaline's effects begin within 30–45 minutes, and reach a peak in 2 hours. These effects usually last from 10–12 hours.

problems of use/abuse   Like other hallucinogens, mescaline is completely unpredictable in its effect. This means the user may have a good trip with pleasurable sensations, a happy mood, and a feeling of reaching profound insights. On the other hand, the user also faces the possibility of a "bad trip": acute anxiety, panic reactions, nausea, vomiting and a depressed mood.

A typical case of mescaline intoxication without severe physical involvement will wear off within a few hours. The only precaution needed is to have a level-headed person in attendance to "talk him down" from the mescaline high and make sure the abuser doesn't succumb to anxiety or irrational acts.

However, a susceptible person taking a large dose of mescaline can suffer from bloody diarrhea, loss of consciousness—and even death by the slowing down of his breathing.

efforts to break the habit   Mescaline is not a drug that produces addiction. That is, the user does not develop a physical need to continue use in increasingly large quantities—or suffer physical withdrawal symptoms when he stops. However, like other drugs, mescaline can become a psychological crutch —luring the user into a mental flight from the problems of everyday living, instead of working to solve them.

So the difficult problem of psychological reorientation comes up, in any effort to break the habit. Since mescaline abusers today tend to come from the intellectual student groups, providing a stimulating and challenging work and home environment, if possible, is very helpful. And regular contacts on a group discussion/therapy basis with people the mescaline user respects—particularly ex-abusers of mescaline and other drugs who have gone on to a more meaningful life without them—can be fruitful.

Drug Abuse: Mescaline and Peyote

(mesc, cactus, button)

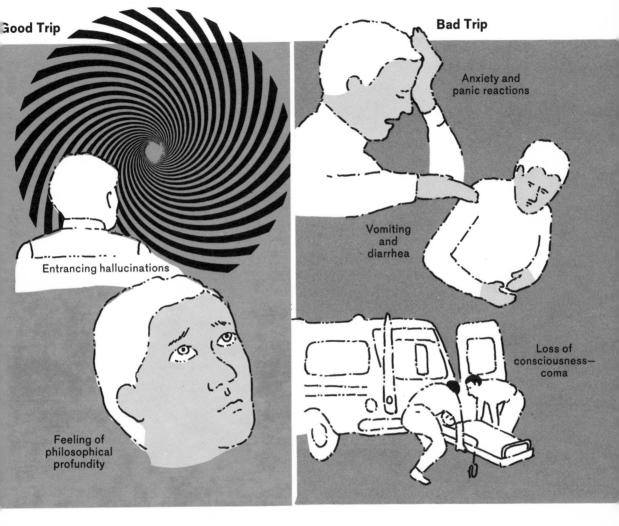

Good Trip

Entrancing hallucinations

Feeling of philosophical profundity

Bad Trip

Anxiety and panic reactions

Vomiting and diarrhea

Loss of consciousness—coma

Symptoms of Abuse of Mescaline/Peyote

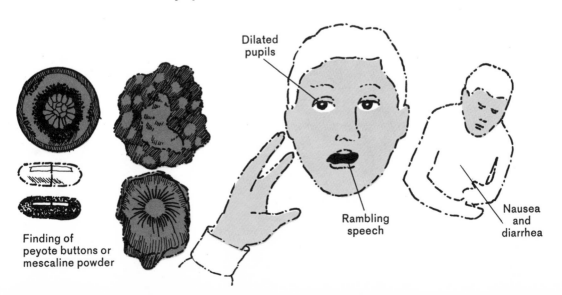

Finding of peyote buttons or mescaline powder

Dilated pupils

Rambling speech

Nausea and diarrhea

Drug Abuse: Sniffing of Glue, Solvents, Aerosols, Anesthetics

(airplane glue ... plastic cement ... paint thinner ... deodorants
and hair spray ... gasoline ... chloroform ... ether)

the drug and its effects   Young children and adolescents in the 8–18 age range have been experimenting in recent years with the sniffing of volatile hydrocarbons. These gases have been called deliriants because of the intoxicated state they produce when inhaled.

Two groups of products, most of them easily available around the house or in stores, provide the sniffing material that distorts the user's consciousness: (1) commercial solvents, such as are found in model airplane glue, plastic cement, paint thinner, gasoline, cleaning fluids, nail polish remover, and cigarette lighter fluid; (2) gases used in aerosol spray cans of insecticides, deodorants, glass chillers, cream whips, and hair sprays. If the sniffing substance used is a liquid, it is poured on a rag or into a plastic bag and the fumes are inhaled. The aerosols are breathed in directly.

The intoxication or delirium from sniffing takes hold almost immediately, and can last from minutes to an hour or two, depending on the dosage. The effects vary from dizziness to giddiness to pleasant "highs." Visual hallucinations and illusions occur.

problems of use/abuse   Accidents, some fatal, have been frequent among sniffers. Unconsciousness, coma, and even death have occurred in cases where users have passed out with the apparatus used still covering their nose and mouth.

The volatile chemicals used in sniffing can cause specific damage to the user's body, as shown in the accompanying illustration. However, there seems little evidence that users become physically dependent on the drugs or suffer withdrawal symptoms. But psychological dependence is a problem.

efforts to break the habit   The pressure of public opinion has caused some chemical countermeasures to be taken—such as the inclusion of nauseating additives like oil of mustard, which has been added to most model airplane glues. Other safe chemical deterrents to misuse can probably be found for some of the other sniffing favorites.

For the individual hooked on sniffing, psychological reorientation is needed to prevent him from continuing, or turning to other drugs. The formula of group therapy or talk sessions with ex-users who have kicked the habit and gone on to a more meaningful life is helpful. Plus an attempt to create a happier, more stimulating home life and a school or work situation in which the ex-user is helped to make progress.

Drug Abuse: Sniffing of Glue, Solvents, Aerosols, Anesthetics

(airplane glue . . . plastic cement . . . paint thinner . . . deodorants
and hair spray . . . gasoline . . . chloroform . . . ether)

First Use

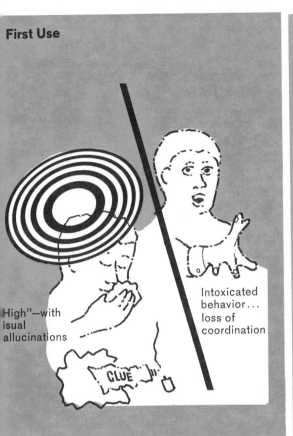

High"—with
isual
allucinations

Intoxicated
behavior . . .
loss of
coordination

GLUE

Prolonged Use/Abuse

Can cause damage to . . .

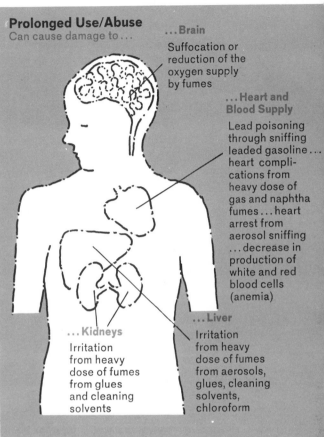

. . . Brain

Suffocation or
reduction of the
oxygen supply
by fumes

**. . . Heart and
Blood Supply**

Lead poisoning
through sniffing
leaded gasoline . . .
heart compli-
cations from
heavy dose of
gas and naphtha
fumes . . . heart
arrest from
aerosol sniffing
. . . decrease in
production of
white and red
blood cells
(anemia)

. . . Kidneys

Irritation
from heavy
dose of fumes
from glues
and cleaning
solvents

. . . Liver

Irritation
from heavy
dose of fumes
from aerosols,
glues, cleaning
solvents,
chloroform

Signs of Abuse

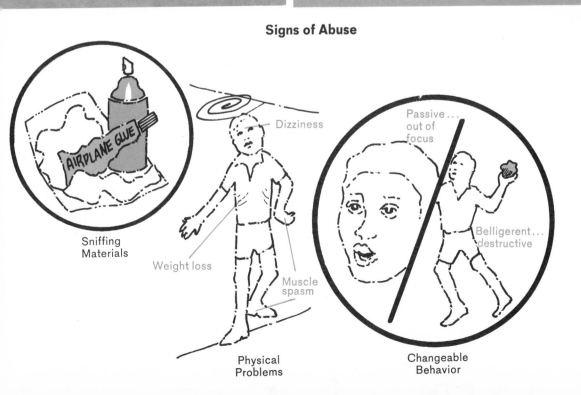

AIRPLANE GLUE

Sniffing
Materials

Dizziness

Weight loss

Muscle
spasm

Physical
Problems

Passive . . .
out of
focus

Belligerent . . .
destructive

Changeable
Behavior

Eclampsia and Preeclampsia
(Toxemia of Pregnancy)

the diseases and their causes   These are very serious complications of pregnancy. Preeclampsia is the early stage of the disorder, while eclampsia is the later, acute toxemic stage. This disorder occurs as often as 1 per 500 pregnancies. It usually appears during the last 3 months of pregnancy— with the curve of cases rising as the mother approaches the date of child-birth. It may appear as late as 24 hours past delivery.

The cause of this toxemia of pregnancy is at present uncertain. It is more frequent in women over 35, in those bearing twins, and in those with a history of high blood pressure or kidney disease.

symptoms   Headache or blurring vision may be the first signs of trouble. High blood pressure and the appearance of protein in the urine follow the headache in the development of preeclampsia. Urine output decreases, resulting in water retention with swelling of the feet and lower part of the body. This swelling can increase greatly and extend up as far as the neck and face.

In severe cases, the flow of urine may cease completely. The headache becomes intense and the blood pressure very high. We have now a full-fledged case of eclampsia, in which chest pains, convulsions, and coma can develop.

complications   If the disease is not diagnosed and treated in time, the baby is almost always stillborn. Heart failure occurs in a significant number of women, due to the development of high blood pressure and kidney disease.

prevention (or lessening of impact)   Periodic medical checks of the mother during pregnancy enable the doctor to check blood pressure, the urine, and other key indicators—and to take any necessary measures to prevent the development of eclampsia. Once the disease is diagnosed, termination of the pregnancy may occur spontaneously—or be brought about by the physician. This is almost always followed by improvement in the mother. Attempts to prolong the pregnancy often result in death for the fetus, and increase the mother's chances of developing heart or kidney complications which could be fatal.

Eclampsia and Preeclampsia
(Toxemia of Pregnancy)

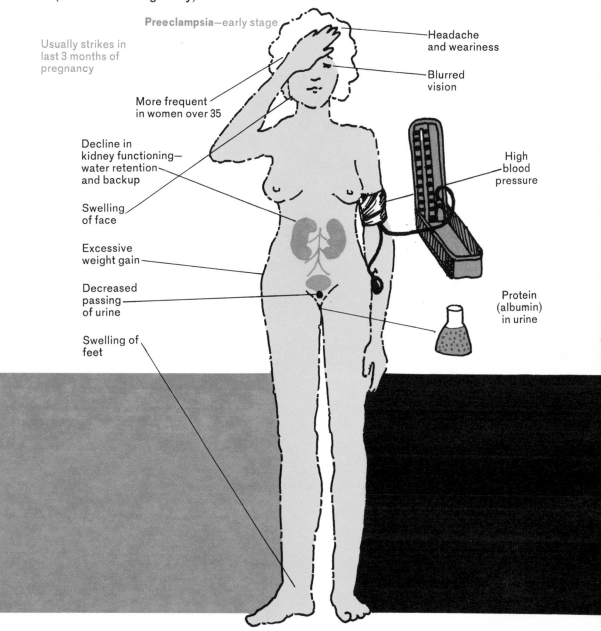

Preeclampsia—early stage

Usually strikes in
last 3 months of
pregnancy

Headache
and weariness

Blurred
vision

More frequent
in women over 35

Decline in
kidney functioning—
water retention
and backup

High
blood
pressure

Swelling
of face

Excessive
weight gain

Decreased
passing
of urine

Protein
(albumin)
in urine

Swelling of
feet

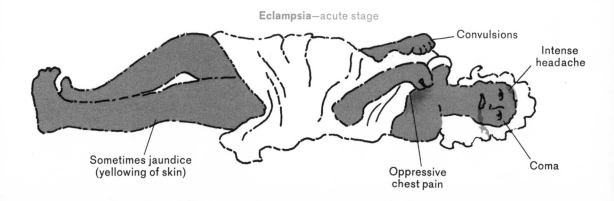

Eclampsia—acute stage

Convulsions

Intense
headache

Sometimes jaundice
(yellowing of skin)

Oppressive
chest pain

Coma

the disease and its cause   This disease covers the abnormal form of pregnancy in which the fertilized egg starts to develop outside of the uterus—the normal area of development.

As the illustration shows, the normal path of the unfertilized egg, after it is released by the ovary, is through the Fallopian tube—which is the area where fertilization by the male's sperm cell ordinarily takes place. Then the fertilized egg moves on to the inside of the uterus wall. There, pregnancy really gets underway, as the egg plants itself and develops. In an ectopic pregnancy, the egg is fertilized and begins to develop in such unsuitable areas as the ovaries, the Fallopian tubes, the outer wall of the uterus, and the abdomen. An ectopic pregnancy occurs as often as 1 in 400 pregnancies, with the ovaries and Fallopian tubes being the areas most often involved.

Our discussion here is based on a pregnancy in the Fallopian tubes. Possible causes of this aberration are partial obstruction of the Fallopian tubes due to an old infection, an abnormal narrowing of the tube preventing the passage of the fertilized egg, or pressure from outside adhesions or tumors which have narrowed the tube.

symptoms   The first symptom is usually delay in menstruation, followed by slight but persistent vaginal bleeding. Pain in the side involved is another symptom—usually mild in the beginning but occasionally sharp and severe.

Normal symptoms of pregnancy, such as morning sickness and enlargement of the breast, may also be present.

complications   Rupture of the Fallopian tube due to the growth of the fetus is possible. This can cause intense pain, weakness, and hemorrhaging.

prevention (or lessening of impact)   Once the doctor's examination has established the presence of ectopic pregnancy, prompt surgery is mandatory to remove the abnormally placed fetus. This saves the mother from further danger. The fetus itself could never develop normally because of its location.

Ectopic Pregnancy

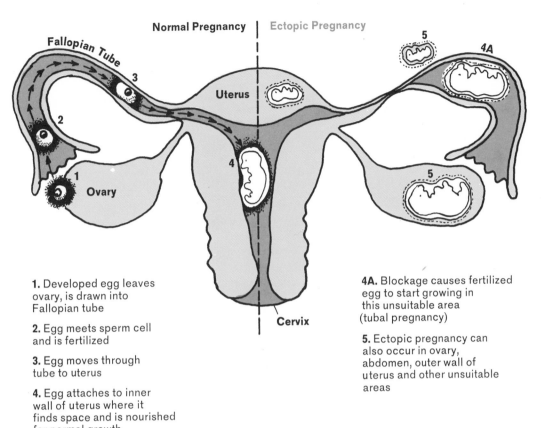

Normal Pregnancy | **Ectopic Pregnancy**

Fallopian Tube

Uterus

Ovary

Cervix

1. Developed egg leaves ovary, is drawn into Fallopian tube

2. Egg meets sperm cell and is fertilized

3. Egg moves through tube to uterus

4. Egg attaches to inner wall of uterus where it finds space and is nourished for normal growth

4A. Blockage causes fertilized egg to start growing in this unsuitable area (tubal pregnancy)

5. Ectopic pregnancy can also occur in ovary, abdomen, outer wall of uterus and other unsuitable areas

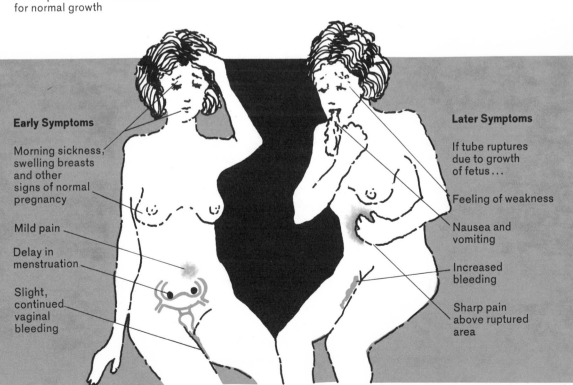

Early Symptoms

Morning sickness, swelling breasts and other signs of normal pregnancy

Mild pain

Delay in menstruation

Slight, continued vaginal bleeding

Later Symptoms

If tube ruptures due to growth of fetus...

Feeling of weakness

Nausea and vomiting

Increased bleeding

Sharp pain above ruptured area

the disease and its causes   A disease of the lungs, emphysema has been increasing with great rapidity as a cause of illness and death. It is now more widespread than lung cancer and TB combined. And it is estimated to disable 1 out of every 14 wage earners over 45 years old in the U.S.

In emphysema, as the MEDIGRAPH illustration shows, the lungs and their air sacs lose elasticity—and so become less efficient in bringing in oxygen and expelling carbon dioxide. Instead of the normal 16 breaths a minute, the emphysema sufferer may breathe 25–30 times a minute and still not get enough oxygen.

The exact cause of emphysema is still unknown. But certain chronic illnesses—such as bronchitis, bronchial asthma, bronchiectasis, silicosis, and other chronic lung problems—are thought to help bring it on. Repeated exposure to lung irritants—such as polluted air, cigarette smoke, and allergenic materials—are also believed to be causes of emphysema. It is about 13 times more prevalent among smokers than non-smokers. The typical sufferer is a male smoker over 40 years of age with a medical history of colds and bronchial troubles.

symptoms   As the MEDIGRAPH illustration shows, one sign is the barrel chest—enlarged because of the inelasticity of the lungs and the difficulty in breathing. The neck muscles of the emphysema victim become overdeveloped in an effort to assist his difficult breathing. Frequent coughing that brings up phlegm, and a history of frequent colds and bronchial troubles are also characteristic.

complications   Untreated, emphysema can lead to repeated and chronic chest infections and breathing problems. As these become progressively more severe, the disease can result in death through heart failure or suffocation.

prevention (or lessening of impact)   Elimination of cigarette smoking and other air pollutants, and prompt medical attention to bronchitis and respiratory infections, are two effective ways to prevent the development of emphysema. Antibiotics are also helpful against bronchitis and other lung infections which can lead to emphysema.

Once the disease is present, treatment is difficult and requires medical supervision. The doctor can prescribe drugs and mechanical breathing aids. He can also recommend draining the lungs of phlegm, breathing exercises, and even surgery to help the patient live with his emphysema and prevent it from worsening.

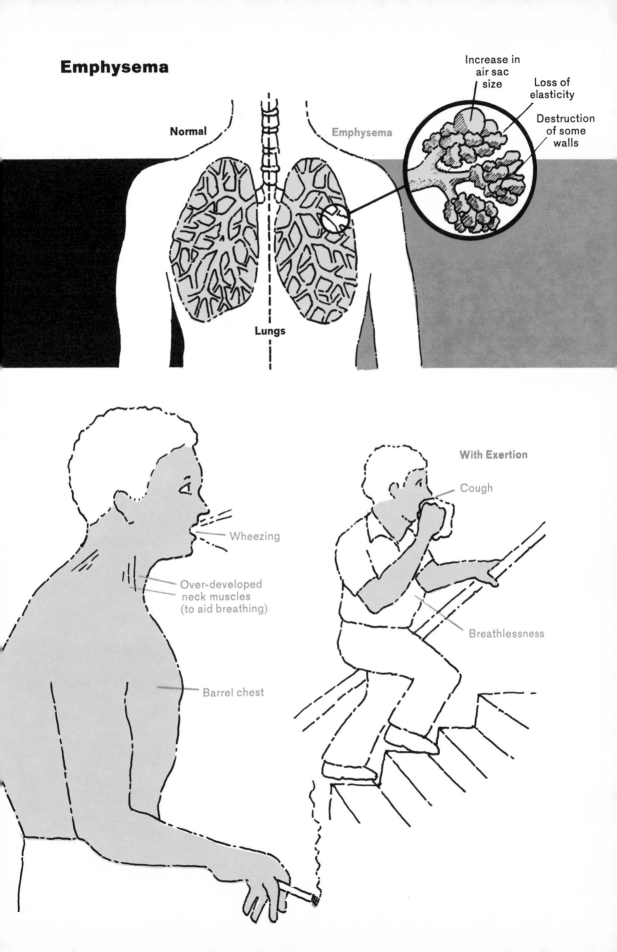

the disease and its causes ENCEPHALITIS—one form of which is commonly called *sleeping sickness* because of such symptoms as drowsiness and slowing down of mental and physical abilities—is an inflammation of the brain, generally produced by a virus.

Among its possible causes are most of the childhood diseases. Sometimes encephalitis breaks out after a vaccination against measles or other diseases such as rabies or smallpox. Influenza, cat scratches and herpes are other illnesses which have led to encephalitis.

One type, EQUINE ENCEPHALITIS, also affects horses, birds, mice, snakes, and possibly other animals, as well as humans. Doctors have also identified types called ST. LOUIS ENCEPHALITIS, AFRICAN ENCEPHALITIS *(sleeping sickness),* JAPANESE B ENCEPHALITIS and many more.

This acute illness has a very varied course—depending on which parts of the brain are involved. It also varies greatly in severity and duration, with death occurring in 5–15% of the cases.

symptoms Various combinations of the following signs and symptoms appear in the victim of encephalitis: coma, stupor, convulsions, confusion, paralysis, dizziness, voice loss, abnormal gait, facial and eye muscle weakness, headache, fever, memory loss.

The illness can last from weeks to months, though the shorter term is more common. A doctor usually makes the diagnosis based on the symptoms, and upon examination of the patient's spinal fluid.

complications An encephalitis attack can range from a mild case with complete recovery to a severe case with long-term disabilities. Weakness, mental deterioration, paralysis, and personality changes are some of the results of a severe case. Coma and death can also occur as a result of a severe attack.

prevention (or lessening of impact) At present, the medical profession has no known vaccine, serum, or drug that will prevent or cure *all* the various forms of encephalitis. There are vaccines that are effective against certain specific types of encephalitis. But since the disease takes so many forms, this treatment can only be used in an outbreak where the cause is known and a vaccine is available against that cause.

In other cases, if the victim and his family will carefully follow the doctor's advice, secondary infections—with their harmful effects—can be prevented. And active physiotherapy under the doctor's supervision can also help to speed the patient's recovery.

Encephalitis

Inflammation of the brain that can be caused by several different viruses

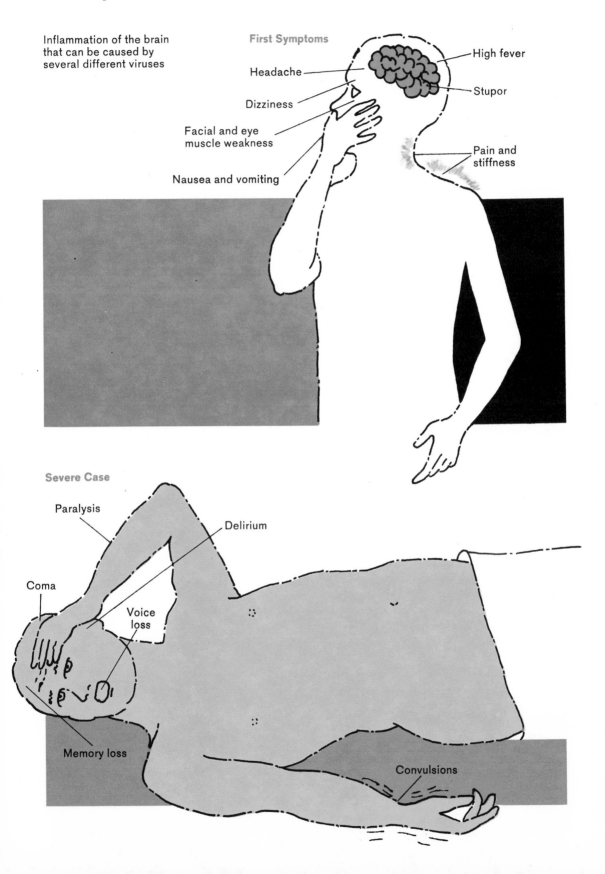

First Symptoms

Headache

Dizziness

Facial and eye muscle weakness

Nausea and vomiting

High fever

Stupor

Pain and stiffness

Severe Case

Paralysis

Delirium

Coma

Voice loss

Memory loss

Convulsions

the disease and its causes   There are many causes of endocarditis, which is an inflammation of the lining membrane within the heart. Subacute bacterial endocarditis, the commonest form, is caused by a bacterial infection—usually the streptococcus viridans—which infects a heart valve previously damaged by rheumatic fever, or infects some congenital heart defect.

Introduced into the body via an infection, the bacteria grow and ultimately reach the heart by way of the bloodstream. Just how the bacteria establish themselves in the heart valve areas involved is still unknown. However, once established, particles composed of bacteria may break off the main clusters around the heart valves, and may be carried as infected emboli (blood clots) into the bloodstream, to all parts of the body. The damage they do depends upon their size, and the organ of the body to which they are carried. Emboli involving the blood vessels of the intestines and the brain are likely to have serious effects.

symptoms   The symptoms are illustrated in the Medi-Graph. In most cases they follow an illness or some minor surgical procedure. There is no typical picture of this disease. The condition of the heart, and the extent of heart damage before the infection is apparent, will determine the effect on the patient. The course of the illness varies also, lasting from as short a time as one month to as long as two years. There was a time when this disease was without hope of cure, but now 70% of the patients respond to antibiotic therapy and survive.

complications   These depend upon the part of the body involved with emboli. Congestive heart failure may appear at any time. A form of nephritis can also develop.

prevention (or lessening of impact)   The underlying disease in bacterial endocarditis is often correctable. Properly diagnosed subacute bacterial endocarditis can be treated with drug therapy and managed in such a way as to minimize or avoid complications.

A patient with a rheumatic or congenital heart condition must make use of antibiotics, as recommended by his physician, whenever he has even a simple infection or is involved with any surgical procedure. He may even be put on preventive doses of antibiotics for life. A patient who has been advised that he has a correctable congenital heart condition should make use of surgery as soon as possible. The maintenance of good health and general well-being are also very important.

Subacute Bacterial Endocarditis

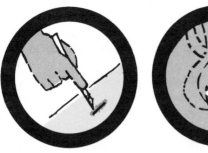
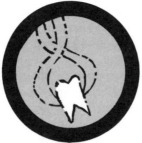

1. Bacteria enter blood stream as aftermath of minor surgery, dental extraction or other infection.

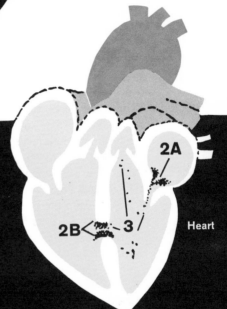

2. Bacteria reach heart and lodge in:
  A. heart valve—usually one previously damaged by illness such as rheumatic fever
  B. birth defect—such as opening in wall between 2 sides of heart

3. Clots (infected emboli) may break off growing bacteria colony and cause damage by blocking circulation or causing infection in other parts of the body.

Heart

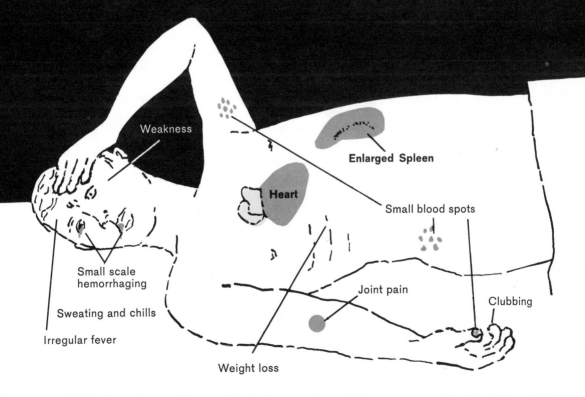

Weakness

Enlarged Spleen

Heart

Small blood spots

Small scale hemorrhaging

Joint pain

Clubbing

Sweating and chills

Irregular fever

Weight loss

the disease and its causes   Epilepsy is a disorder of the central nervous system which makes itself known intermittently. It is an extremely common disease, affecting people of all ages, and attacks can occur once in a lifetime or several times a day.

Epilepsy can occur as a symptom of other well-recognized diseases of the nervous system, such as brain tumor, brain injury, neurosyphilis, or stroke; or its specific cause may be unknown.

There are many theories about what causes epileptic convulsions. The one most generally accepted is that cerebral irritation stimulates some part of the brain. A reaction is triggered which sets up the seizure, and the patient experiences a disturbance of sensation, loss of consciousness, or convulsive movements. These can occur singly or in any combination.

symptoms   There are three types of seizure in epilepsy: Grand Mal, or major attack; Petit Mal, or minor attack; and Psychomotor, or moderate attack (epileptic equivalent). In all of them there is loss of consciousness and loss of memory of the episode. In Grand Mal there are convulsions. The accompanying Medi-Graph illustrates clearly the characteristics of each type.

A patient suffering from one form of epilepsy can also present symptoms of another. Patients suffering frequent attacks may show some mental deterioration. Epilepsy in young children may be accompanied by feeble-mindedness.

complications   As a rule, there are no serious complications in epilepsy, but patients can hurt their heads or severely lacerate themselves when they fall. Or else they can choke to death on food or saliva. In general, however, the life span of the epileptic is not affected.

prevention (or lessening of impact)   The patient with any of the symptoms of epilepsy should undergo careful examination for signs of other diseases of the nervous system. Vascular disturbances within the brain, and even early brain tumors, often can be corrected if they are detected soon enough. A large group of medications are available for patients who have epilepsy from an unknown cause. These can lessen the frequency and even the severity of the attacks. The electroencephalogram or brain wave test has been most helpful in establishing the correct diagnosis.

Once an attack has begun, it is important to keep the patient from injuring himself. His clothing should be loosened, and a gag should be forced between his teeth to keep him from biting his tongue. No other treatment is necessary during an acute attack.

The frequency of attacks can be controlled somewhat if the patient stays on a wholesome, careful diet, avoids constipation, and takes no alcoholic beverages of any kind. His sleep habits should be regular and he should exercise moderately. He should not drive an automobile or operate dangerous machinery. Many communities have vocational rehabilitation centers where epileptics can learn to pursue a normal life.

3 Types of Seizure

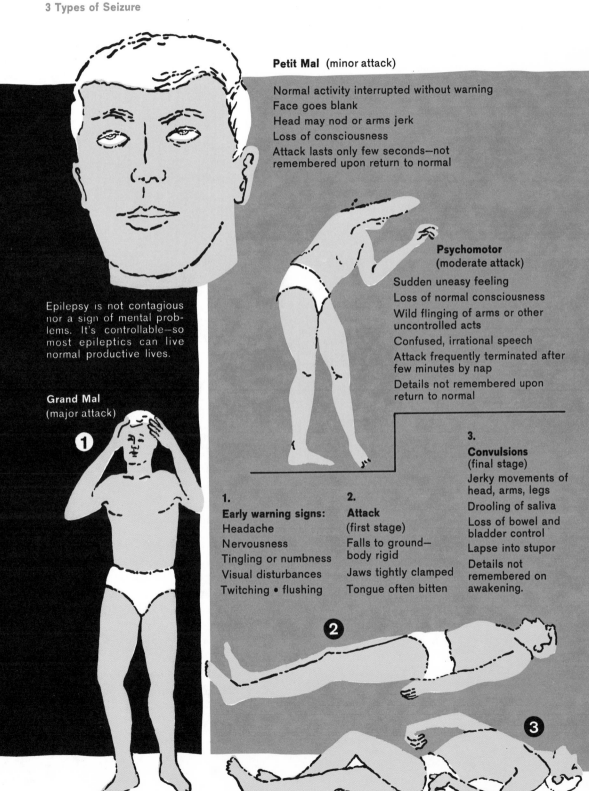

Petit Mal (minor attack)

Normal activity interrupted without warning
Face goes blank
Head may nod or arms jerk
Loss of consciousness
Attack lasts only few seconds—not
remembered upon return to normal

Psychomotor
(moderate attack)
Sudden uneasy feeling
Loss of normal consciousness
Wild flinging of arms or other
uncontrolled acts
Confused, irrational speech
Attack frequently terminated after
few minutes by nap
Details not remembered upon
return to normal

Epilepsy is not contagious
nor a sign of mental problems. It's controllable—so
most epileptics can live
normal productive lives.

Grand Mal
(major attack)

1.
Early warning signs:
Headache
Nervousness
Tingling or numbness
Visual disturbances
Twitching • flushing

2.
Attack
(first stage)
Falls to ground—
body rigid
Jaws tightly clamped
Tongue often bitten

3.
Convulsions
(final stage)
Jerky movements of
head, arms, legs
Drooling of saliva
Loss of bowel and
bladder control
Lapse into stupor
Details not
remembered on
awakening.

the disease and its causes DIVERTICULUM Diverticula are pouches that form off the wall of the esophagus, which is the passage between the throat and the stomach. A patient may have been born with a weakness in the wall of the esophagus, causing it to balloon outward in pouches; or pouches may be the result of an inflammatory disease in the region of the esophagus, which has weakened the wall. These pouches tend to grow larger as time goes on.

CANCER OF THE ESOPHAGUS Cancer of the upper end, middle, and lower end of the esophagus is not uncommon, occurring in about 5% of all patients with cancer. Men over 40 are affected most frequently. The cause is unknown.

symptoms DIVERTICULUM The most noticeable symptoms in diverticulum are difficulty in swallowing, and vomiting undigested food several hours after eating. Pain is not an important factor, although occasionally there may be some pain under the breastbone. The patient often has a feeling of fullness beneath the breastbone and is relieved only after vomiting.

CANCER OF THE ESOPHAGUS As the cancer grows, it obstructs the food passage, and so the first symptom is difficulty in swallowing, progressing to vomiting. This may begin with solids, extend to soft foods, and eventually even liquids are brought up. Occasionally the matter brought up is bloody. Pain is a rare symptom. The diagnosis is usually made by X ray.

complications DIVERTICULUM A patient with diverticulum can live for years without any real difficulties unless the vomiting is so severe that he is unable to tolerate food and suffers from malnutrition. Rupture of the pouches is a rare but serious complication. Ulceration and hemorrhage can also develop.

CANCER OF THE ESOPHAGUS The progressive obstruction of the food passage can result in actual starvation. Sometimes the cancer can rupture into the windpipe and allow food to pass into the lungs at the site of the rupture and cause pneumonia. Complications from the spread of the cancer to other parts of the body inevitably result in death.

prevention (or lessening of impact) DIVERTICULUM There is no way a condition such as this can be prevented. The only treatment when the diagnosis has been established would be one of surgical correction. The need for this type of surgery would be as a life-saving measure only.

CANCER OF THE ESOPHAGUS There is no way the cancer can be prevented. When it becomes a matter of saving the patient's life, surgical correction is attempted. This is resorted to only if the obstruction becomes so large that it effectively prevents the digestion of food.

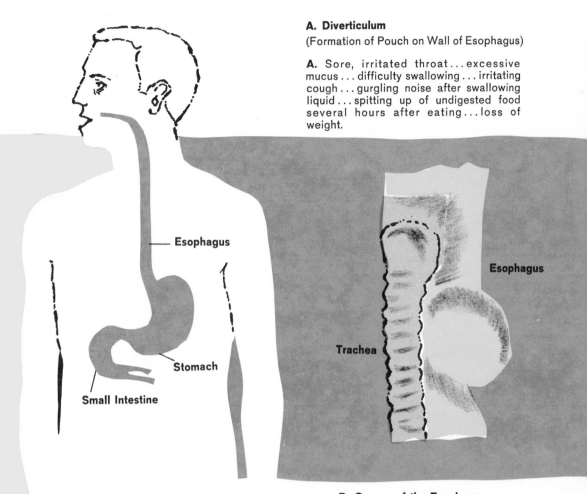

A. Diverticulum
(Formation of Pouch on Wall of Esophagus)

A. Sore, irritated throat...excessive mucus...difficulty swallowing...irritating cough...gurgling noise after swallowing liquid...spitting up of undigested food several hours after eating...loss of weight.

Esophagus

Stomach

Small Intestine

Esophagus

Trachea

B. Cancer of the Esophagus

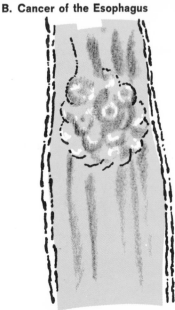

B. Difficulty swallowing...spitting up of undigested food...excessive saliva...feeling of fullness, pressure or pain high in chest...eventual obstruction.

the disease and its causes   The most frequently found tumors in the female are fibroids, which are swellings that can appear in all parts of the uterine wall, extending to the outer surface as well as toward the uterine cavity. The cause is thought to be some kind of imbalance in the production of hormones by the ovaries. This theory is based on the fact that in all instances fibroid tumors shrink and rarely cause symptoms after menopause when the ovarian hormones cease to appear.

symptoms   Many fibroids have no symptoms at all and are found only on routine examination. When symptoms do appear, they are usually related to the size and location of the tumor. When a fibroid tumor is near the region of the urinary bladder and exerts pressure on it, the patient needs to urinate frequently. When one exerts pressure on the rectum, constipation can result.

Bleeding is probably the most common symptom. It can either occur between normal menstrual cycles, or cause an unusually heavy menstrual flow, or extend the duration of the flow.

Fibroid tumors may degenerate, or calcify, or twist on a pedicle—which is a stalklike extension of the uterine wall. In the latter case, severe pain is the result.

Back pain is not unusual. When a tumor is unusually large, the patient herself can feel it easily through the lower abdominal wall. Or, it may even protrude in this area.

complications   There are no serious complications to fibroid tumors and they almost never become malignant. However, bleeding during menstruation can become so profuse that treatment is necessary. Fibroids present a problem during pregnancy since, depending on their size and location, they can interfere with the development of the fetus and cause a miscarriage. They are also thought to be related to sterility in some women, but this probably applies to those cases where the tumors are multiple or very large.

prevention (or lessening of impact)   There is no known method of preventing the development of fibroid tumors. Their presence is no cause for alarm unless there is severe bleeding, or the patient becomes pregnant.

When the fibroid tumors are detected they should be watched carefully to note how rapidly they are growing and their effects on the bladder or bowel. When nothing unusual is found, a woman close to menopause can wait safely for her fibroid tumors to shrink.

Surgery is indicated only in special cases and only on the advice of a trained gynecologist.

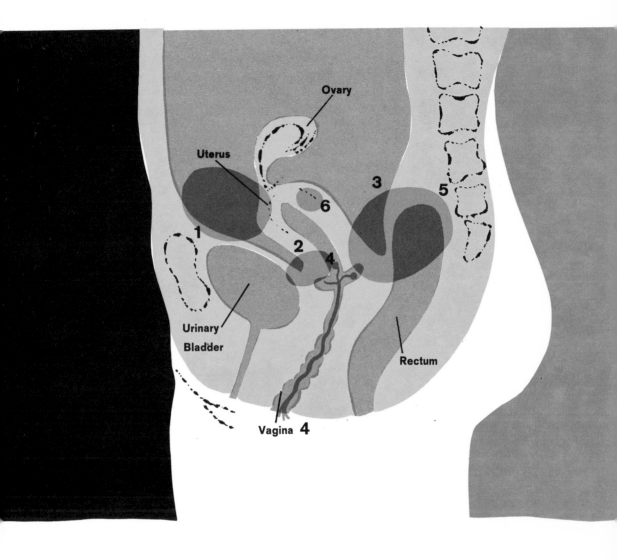

1. Large size tumors may be felt through abdominal wall
2. Tumor exerts pressure on bladder — increases frequency of urination
3. Tumor exerts pressure on rectum — constipation develops
4. Increased bleeding at menstrual period or between periods
5. Unusual pressure on nerves may result in back pain
6. But many fibroid tumors produce no symptoms

Fibroid tumors almost never become malignant. They shrink after menopause—and cease to cause symptoms

the disease and its cause   This disease is an inflammation of the fibrous or connective tissues of the muscles. It can be caused by exposure to cold or dampness, or by local injury or strain. It can also occur without any apparent cause. One medical theory holds that poisonous toxins from infected teeth or throat or another infected area are the underlying cause. When the pain and the inflammation of fibromyositis strike the shoulders, neck, and scalp, this condition is popularly called "rheumatism." Causing trouble lower down in the ribs or lower back, it is usually known as "lumbago."

symptoms   The most apparent symptom is pain in a specific muscle or group of muscles—particularly when pressure is applied or upon motion. The pain may be localized in small "trigger" areas. The pain may increase in intensity for a while, and last from a few days to a few weeks. During an acute attack, an affected muscle will feel worse when it is put to use after a period of inactivity.

complications   No serious complications result from fibromyositis—although muscular pain can herald a more serious underlying cause. So when the condition persists, a search should be made for the possible presence of another disease.

prevention (or lessening of impact)   Temporary relief can usually be had through moderate exercise, massage, heat, and the use of mild analgesics (pain killers). Avoidance of strain or draft on the affected area usually bring the incident to a close in a few days.

Fibromyositis

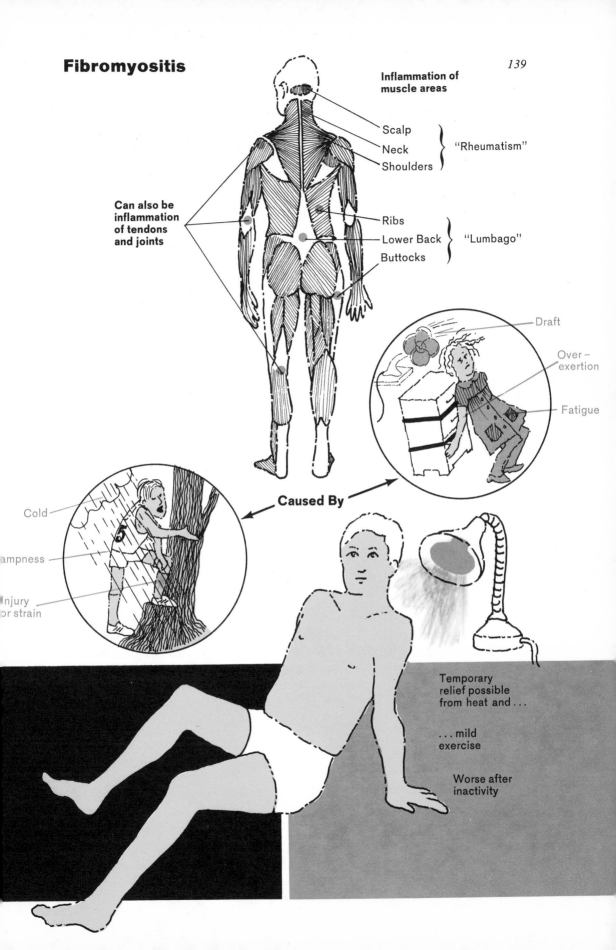

Inflammation of muscle areas

Scalp
Neck   } "Rheumatism"
Shoulders

Can also be inflammation of tendons and joints

Ribs
Lower Back } "Lumbago"
Buttocks

Draft
Over-exertion
Fatigue

Caused By

Cold
Dampness
Injury or strain

Temporary relief possible from heat and...

...mild exercise

Worse after inactivity

the disease and its causes Influenza, popularly called flu, is an acute, highly
contagious respiratory infection caused by a specific virus. It occurs
most often during the late winter months and is spread by direct contact with secretions of the respiratory tract—the nose and the mouth.
The patient is contagious as long as the cold symptoms persist; the incubation period is short. Young infants generally have natural immunity.
Because the virus is so readily airborne, it spreads easily and epidemics
are common throughout the world. The disease itself is not serious, but
patients are susceptible to secondary infections of the lungs and these
can be quite serious.

Grippe, which is caused by a different virus, has similar symptoms, as
shown in the Medi-Graph, but is milder and shorter in duration. There
are usually 1 to 3 days of low-grade temperature; aches and pains are
less severe; and the patient is less subject to complications.

symptoms The onset of flu is sudden, with chills, severe muscle aches, joint pains,
and headache. It may also start with loss of appetite, vomiting, and
diarrhea. Occasionally, bloody stools are seen. There are severe cold
symptoms, with heavy nasal discharge and a persistent cough. Temperature may go up to 104°-105°. The patient feels weak and depressed,
especially if he becomes active too soon.

complications Tonsillitis, bronchitis, pneumonia, and meningitis are possible
complications.

Special care should be taken during pregnancy since an attack of flu
at this time can lead to miscarriage or have fatal results.

prevention (or lessening of impact) During epidemics it is advisable to take
advantage of an influenza vaccine which gives quick immunity and lasts
6 to 8 months. Elderly people and patients with any serious illness
should be immunized just before the winter season.

The disease is known as a self-limiting one because it runs a definite
course within a short specific time. Unless complications develop, nursing care concentrating on the symptoms is all that is required. Bed rest
is important as soon as there is some sign of illness. It should be continued until convalescence is well along. Throughout the period of high
fever the patient should be sponged down with warm water and given
plenty of liquids. Complications are treated by the doctor as they
develop.

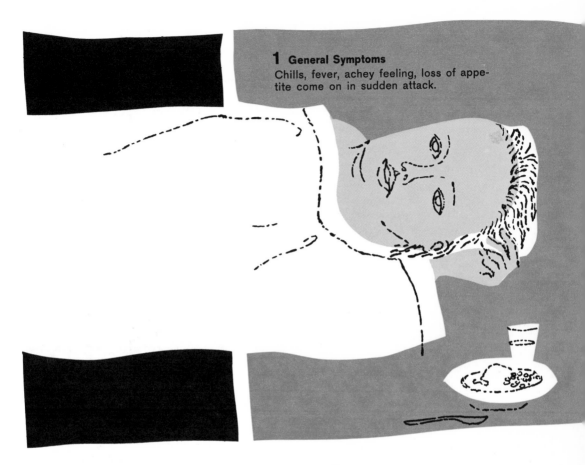

1 General Symptoms
Chills, fever, achey feeling, loss of appetite come on in sudden attack.

2 Respiratory Flu
Severe cold in head with nasal discharge, inflamed throat and tonsils, cough, pain in chest.

3 Intestinal Grippe
Abdominal pain, diarrhea, stools containing mucus and sometimes blood.

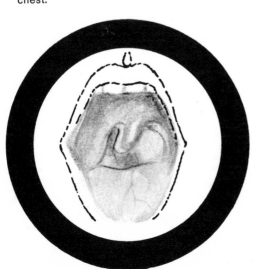

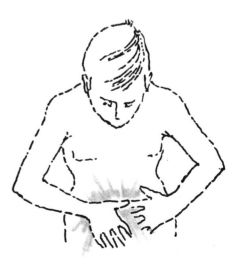

the injury and its causes   An injury is described as a fracture when there is any break in the continuous line of the bone. It may be a complete fracture, which means right through the bone, or an incomplete one in which the break is partial. When the ligament tears a small piece of bone at the point where it is attached, it is called a chip or sprain fracture. A compound fracture is one in which the broken bone protrudes through the skin. Other fractures are identified by the direction of the break and the position of the fragments.

A fracture is usually the result of violence to the part involved and occurs most often to the young age group exposed to accidents, and older people subject to falls. However, it also can be caused by weakness of the bone structure, local bone disease, rickets, and old age.

A dislocation of a bone always occurs at a joint. This, too, may be complete or partial. The patient cannot move the part involved, and there is deformity which disappears when the dislocation is corrected.

symptoms   Most often the patient is involved in some kind of accident and feels a sharp pain at the point of the fracture as it happens. He may even hear the snap of the bone. There is swelling, pain, and tenderness along with bruise marks. The bone moves at some point where it should not, in a direction different from its normal one. There can be deformity of the part, and the patient will not be able to use it freely. Sometimes a grating sound is heard at the site of the fracture. In severe cases there is shock.

The symptoms of a dislocation are similar, except that there is no grating sound, and the deformity is usually much more obvious.

complications   "Fracture fever" may develop, a condition which begins a day after the injury and can last several days. Infection is not an unusual development in cases of compound fracture. Other complications depend on how well the fracture heals. It is not unusual to have destruction of the local blood vessels and nerves when there is poor healing, and this may result in serious vascular and nerve disorders.

Dislocations can result in neuritis or palsy of the affected part. Or else the joint can become so loose that it dislocates at the slightest provocation.

prevention (or lessening of impact)   Obviously, there is no way to prevent development of a traumatic fracture. Patients with bone disorders can only exert extreme care so they are not placed in a position where they are more susceptible to injury. Once the fracture has occurred, adequate and careful medical management is necessary to prevent poor healing and future problems. The diagnosis and the course of healing are followed by X Ray.

These same factors also apply to the prevention or lessening of impact of dislocations.

Fractures and Dislocations

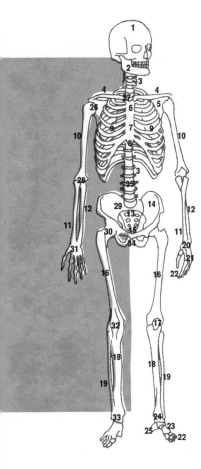

Principal Bones, Ligaments and Joints

BONES

1. Skull
2. Mandible
3. Vertebrae
4. Clavicle
5. Scapula
6. Manubrium
7. Body of sternum
8. Xiphoid process
9. Ribs
10. Humerus
11. Radius
12. Ulna
13. Sacrum
14. Ilium
15. Coccyx
16. Femur
17. Patella
18. Tibia
19. Fibula
20. Carpals
21. Metacarpals
22. Phalanges
23. Metatarsals
24. Tarsals
25. Heel

LIGAMENTS AND JOINTS

26. Capsule of shoulder
27. Sternoclavicular
28. Capsule of elbow
29. Sacroiliac
30. Iliofemoral
31. Wrist
32. Capsule of knee
33. Ankle
34. Pubic symphysis
35. Intervertebral discs

Example: Fracture of Upper Arm

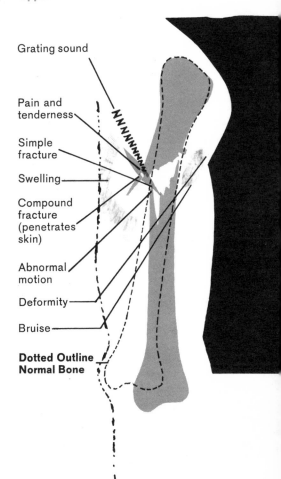

Grating sound

Pain and tenderness

Simple fracture

Swelling

Compound fracture (penetrates skin)

Abnormal motion

Deformity

Bruise

Dotted Outline Normal Bone

Example: Dislocated elbow

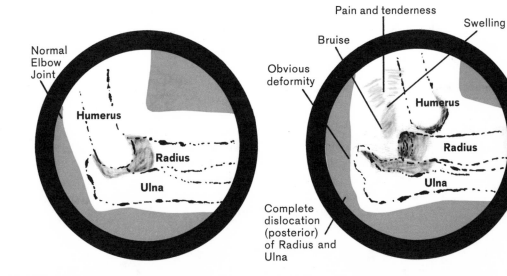

Normal Elbow Joint

Humerus

Radius

Ulna

Obvious deformity

Bruise

Pain and tenderness

Swelling

Humerus

Radius

Ulna

Complete dislocation (posterior) of Radius and Ulna

Fungus Infections of the Skin (Athlete's Foot, Ringworm, Jock Itch)

the disease and its causes Fungi are responsible for many types of common skin disorders. These include athlete's foot, ringworm, and so-called jock itch or rash. They are contagious, although the individual reaction varies greatly. Perspiration, irritation from clothing, generalized illness, and skin sensitivity or allergy all play a role.

symptoms ATHLETE'S FOOT This type of fungus infection begins with the formation of small, watery blisters on the hands or feet. Itching is usually quite intense. The blisters dry and go through the peeling stage, but new areas of fresh lesions usually appear at nearby sites. Scratching or rubbing causes a spread of the infection, local irritation, and occasionally secondary infections. The areas between the toes are most frequently involved, and deep cracks or fissures frequently develop. It is not unusual to have athlete's foot spread to the soles and top of the feet. Allergic reactions to medications used in treatment are not unusual and may make the diagnosis and treatment more difficult.

RINGWORM OF THE BODY This is characterized by the development of a lesion which is usually round or ringlike in nature, has a scaly surface, and spreads from its red outer margin. The inside portion frequently appears clear. Again perspiration, with the increase of skin moisture and heat, appears to be an important factor.

Ringworm may involve any part of the body, and it differs somewhat in appearance depending upon the area affected. In men the beard area is a common site, and the lesion, while still round in appearance, frequently includes watery and pussy blisters. On the head it is associated with hair loss in the area involved, and the patches are usually grayish in color. The early stage of infection may be overlooked until a bald spot appears. The hair is found to be broken off near the skin, and the latter gives the impression of being coated with cigar ashes. The lesions are usually bean sized, but may involve larger or smaller areas. It is frequently difficult to see areas involved with the naked eye, but they are apparent under examination with a specific fluorescent light.

JOCK ITCH This eruption appears on the upper, inner surface of the thighs, extending almost to the buttocks. It also occurs in the armpits and beneath the breasts in women. The skin is inflamed, usually brownish red in color, with a deeper red toward the edge. Excessive perspiration can give it a very raw appearance. It is common during the hot weather.

complications The only complications are secondary infections. But the unsightly effect, when the head or face is included, can also be distressing.

prevention (or lessening of impact) Fungus infections are contagious and spread from human to human and animal to human. Contact with infected people or animals should be avoided and good hygiene practiced. Unsterilized barber tools should be avoided, and clothing should not be exchanged. Patients with athlete's foot should avoid group showers, wear protective slippers, and bathe their feet frequently.

Fungus Infections of the Skin (Athlete's Foot, Ringworm, Jock Itch)

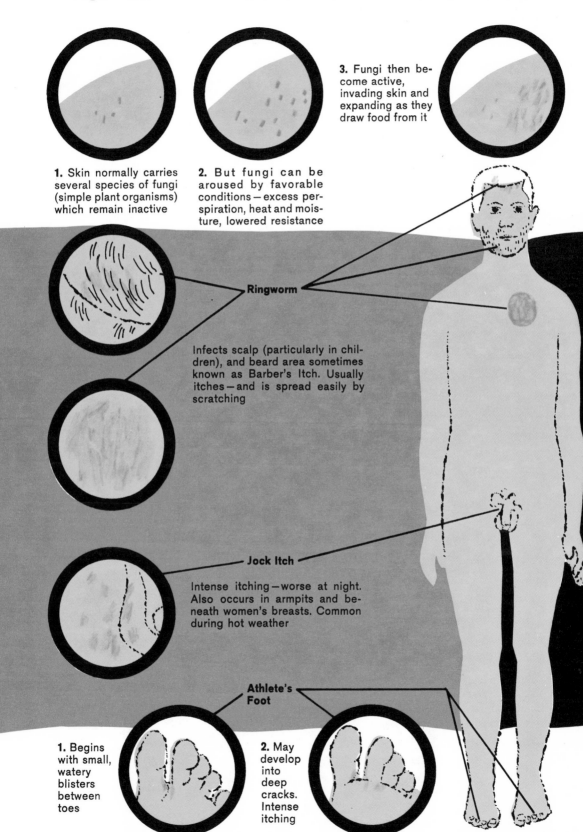

3. Fungi then become active, invading skin and expanding as they draw food from it

1. Skin normally carries several species of fungi (simple plant organisms) which remain inactive

2. But fungi can be aroused by favorable conditions — excess perspiration, heat and moisture, lowered resistance

Ringworm

Infects scalp (particularly in children), and beard area sometimes known as Barber's Itch. Usually itches — and is spread easily by scratching

Jock Itch

Intense itching — worse at night. Also occurs in armpits and beneath women's breasts. Common during hot weather

Athlete's Foot

1. Begins with small, watery blisters between toes

2. May develop into deep cracks. Intense itching

the disease and its causes   It is not yet known what causes stones to form in the gallbladder. Chemically, gallstones are made up of a combination of bile pigment (bilirubin), cholesterol and calcium, although occasionally pure stones of a single chemical are found.

Gallstones are very common, occurring in up to 25% of the older age group. Stones, varying widely in size and number, are seen more in women than in men, particularly among those who are overweight.

symptoms   Many people with gallstones have no symptoms whatsoever. But there can be a variety of symptoms, including belching, bloating, and attacks of abdominal pain. The abdominal pain is severe and knife-like, radiating from the right upper abdomen to the back. It is caused by the movement of a stone into the duct carrying bile to the intestine. A gallstone attack may follow a fatty meal, or it may have nothing to do with what the patient has eaten that day. At its peak there is severe nausea and vomiting, and the patient may find it difficult to breathe. The upper abdominal wall is tender and tense. Medication may help stop the attack, or it may stop of its own accord. Between attacks the patient may be in excellent health. Some patients may have some difficulty in digesting fatty or fried foods. When a gallstone attack does not subside or respond to medication, surgery may be necessary.

complications   Inflammation and gangrene of the gallbladder are the most common complications. Others are related to the blocking of the drainage duct of the gallbladder and liver by gallstones. This can cause liver infection, abscess, a form of cirrhosis, or yellow jaundice. Cancer of the gallbladder is another complication.

prevention (or lessening of impact)   There is no way known to prevent the development of gallstones, and no medications are available that will dissolve them. The effects of low-cholesterol diets and weight control are hard to evaluate, but it would be worthwhile to follow these practices where there is a strong family history of gallstones. A patient who knows he cannot tolerate fatty or other foods should stick to a diet that excludes them.

When a routine examination reveals the presence of gallstones, although the patient has had no discomfort, the doctor will consider the advisability of preventive surgery in the light of many factors, including the patient's age and general health.

Gallstones

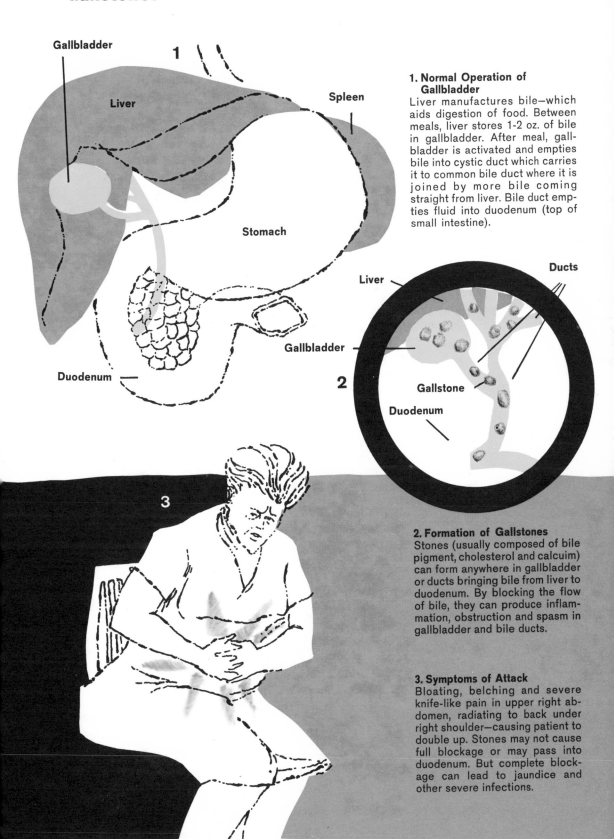

Gallbladder

1

Liver

Spleen

Stomach

Duodenum

Liver

Ducts

Gallbladder

2

Gallstone

Duodenum

3

1. Normal Operation of Gallbladder

Liver manufactures bile—which aids digestion of food. Between meals, liver stores 1-2 oz. of bile in gallbladder. After meal, gallbladder is activated and empties bile into cystic duct which carries it to common bile duct where it is joined by more bile coming straight from liver. Bile duct empties fluid into duodenum (top of small intestine).

2. Formation of Gallstones

Stones (usually composed of bile pigment, cholesterol and calcuim) can form anywhere in gallbladder or ducts bringing bile from liver to duodenum. By blocking the flow of bile, they can produce inflammation, obstruction and spasm in gallbladder and bile ducts.

3. Symptoms of Attack

Bloating, belching and severe knife-like pain in upper right abdomen, radiating to back under right shoulder—causing patient to double up. Stones may not cause full blockage or may pass into duodenum. But complete blockage can lead to jaundice and other severe infections.

Gastritis
(Inflammation and Irritation
of Stomach Lining)

the disease and its causes   Gastritis is the term used for inflammation of the stomach lining—a very common medical problem. When irritated or infected, the stomach lining becomes red and swollen, and in some cases may even bleed.

There are two types of gastritis: chronic and acute. Acute cases (a sudden attack) may be caused by food poisoning, drugs, alcohol, metal poisoning, and certain acute illnesses. Chronic forms (developing and persisting for considerable periods of time) are associated with diabetes, cancer, ulcers, gastric juice deficiencies, and a large variety of wasting diseases such as pernicious anemia.

symptoms   For the sudden, acute attack, these include nausea, loss of appetite, and upper abdominal pain. Vomiting brings some relief.

In chronic gastritis, the symptoms are similar—but persist over long periods of time. The nausea is constant—frequently made worse by seeing or smelling food. The victim feels full quickly, after eating only a small amount. He is bothered by abdominal pain, which may radiate into the back. Bleeding is a common problem in both types of gastritis—and may be heavy and persistent.

This may be a difficult disease for the doctor to diagnose, with the normal GI series often revealing nothing significant. A biopsy or gastroscopy may be needed to diagnose the disease with absolute certainty.

complications   A serious complication is the tendency to hemorrhage and lose a vital amount of blood. In the case of an acute attack brought on by swallowing chemical poison, quick action by a doctor is needed to remove the substance—or the stomach wall may become perforated and acute peritonitis set in.

Chronic cases of gastritis can create social and economic problems, due to the prolonged disability which prevents the sufferer from leading a normal, vigorous life.

prevention (or lessening of impact)   The doctor usually prescribes a diet of antacids, diet supplements to correct anemia if present, and elimination of all gastric irritants, including cigarettes and alcohol. Acute cases will usually respond quickly to this formula.

Chronic cases require more prolonged care. Small meals of easily digestible foods, taken at frequent intervals, are frequently recommended by the doctor. But effective results depend upon careful diagnosis and correction of any underlying contributing illness.

Gastritis
(Inflammation and Irritation of Stomach Lining)

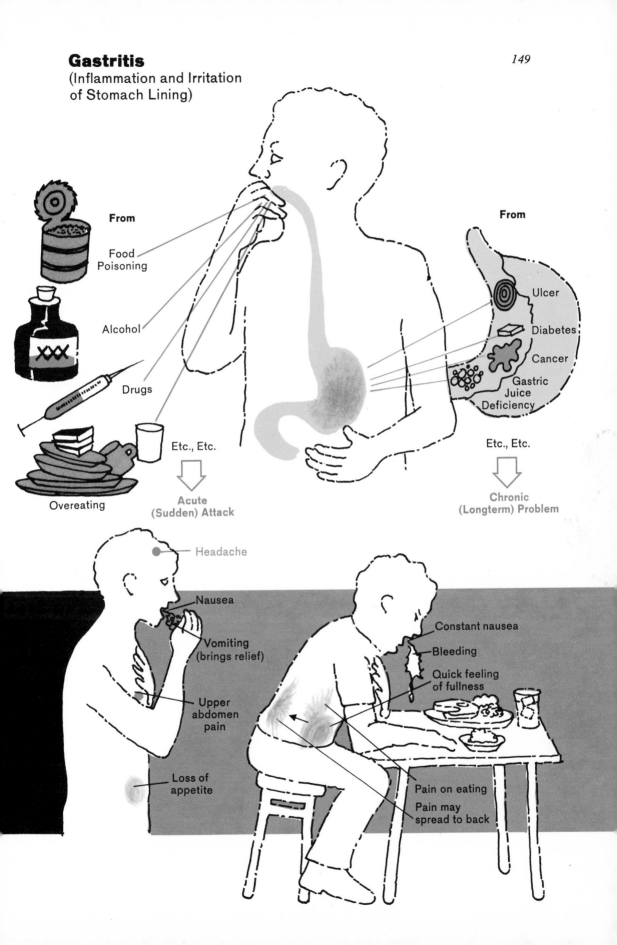

From

Food Poisoning

Alcohol

Drugs

Etc., Etc.

Overeating

Acute (Sudden) Attack

From

Ulcer

Diabetes

Cancer

Gastric Juice Deficiency

Etc., Etc.

Chronic (Longterm) Problem

Headache

Nausea

Vomiting (brings relief)

Upper abdomen pain

Loss of appetite

Constant nausea

Bleeding

Quick feeling of fullness

Pain on eating

Pain may spread to back

the disease and its causes   German measles is a mild but highly contagious disease caused by a virus present in secretions such as nasal discharge and saliva. It is spread by direct contact and almost never through objects or a third person. One attack usually give lifelong immunity. It occurs most often in winter and early spring, and follows a pattern of epidemics every three to four years. The incubation period is 2 to 3 weeks. The disease is most contagious from a day or two before the rash appears until the rash leaves. It is rare to find it in anyone over 40. Infants under six months are probably immune if their mothers are immune.

symptoms   The symptoms are mild, and the whole disease is usually over in 2 to 4 days. There may be a low fever, mild aches and pains, a running or stuffed nose, red running eyes, and swelling of the glands, as shown in the accompanying Medi-Graph. The throat may be sore. But often the symptoms are so mild that the patient doesn't know he has German measles until the rash breaks out. The rash starts with individual rose-red spots on the face or neck, then spreads onto the head, arms, trunk and, in small amounts, onto the legs. It disappears in the same order in which it began. The glands remain swollen 5 to 7 days after the rash clears.

complications   These are very rare, although during severe epidemics, cases of ear and kidney infections, arthritis, and encephalitis are occasionally reported. However, a serious complication of German measles can occur when a woman contracts it during the first three months of her pregnancy. The virus may attack many parts of the unborn child, such as the eyes, heart, ears, or brain; and serious defects occur in as many as 50% of such births. When a pregnant woman learns she has been exposed to this disease, she should notify her doctor immediately.

prevention (or lessening of impact)   A vaccine is now available which, when in general use, should eliminate this disease. In the absence of the vaccine, very little treatment is required. There is generally no itching and the patient is comfortable with bed care for a day or two.

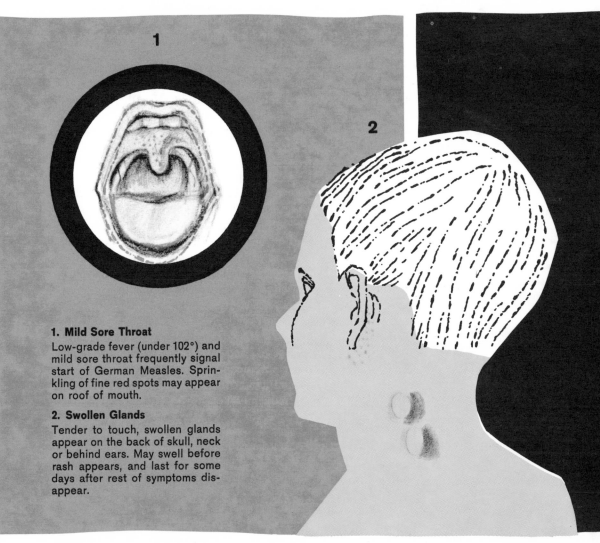

1. Mild Sore Throat

Low-grade fever (under 102°) and mild sore throat frequently signal start of German Measles. Sprinkling of fine red spots may appear on roof of mouth.

2. Swollen Glands

Tender to touch, swollen glands appear on the back of skull, neck or behind ears. May swell before rash appears, and last for some days after rest of symptoms disappear.

3. Rash

Faint, blotchy rash appears—first on face or neck, then spreading to rest of body. Usually fades within 2 days in children, takes a day or two longer in adults.

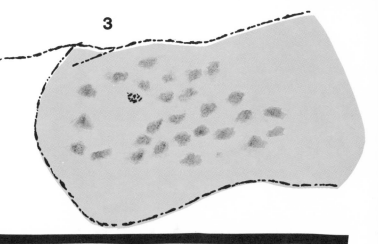

the disease and its causes   Glaucoma is a disease of the eye brought about by an increase in the pressure of the vitreous fluid within the eyeball. This pressure against the retina of the eyeball begins to crush nerves that control side vision and, if unchecked, goes on to destroy nerves controlling frontal vision. The disease affects both sexes equally and occurs in middle and advanced age, often between 40 and 70. Usually it involves both eyes.

The exact cause of glaucoma is unknown, but there are a number of conditions which predispose a patient to the disease—age, heredity, arteriosclerosis, and farsightedness.

symptoms   There are many types of glaucoma. Symptoms vary with the rapidity with which the eyeball pressure rises and the height to which the pressure goes. As shown on the Medi-Graph, early symptoms include a slight fogging of vision and dull pain in the eye. The patient sees colored halos around lights. The pupil may appear somewhat larger than normal, and the eye may appear slightly congested (bloodshot).

These symptoms may occur in attacks that are weeks, months, or even years apart. Between the attacks vision is normal until severe, acute glaucoma develops. This comes on rapidly, with decreasing vision and severe, constant pain all over the head. There may be nausea and vomiting. The eye becomes congested and hard to the touch. The pupil appears steamy and usually remains open and sluggish in its reaction to light. The patient see less and less at the sides of one or both eyes. Glasses have to be changed frequently because of the patient's constantly decreasing vision.

complications   The usual complication of untreated glaucoma is blindness.

prevention (or lessening of impact)   Eye drops and proper medications can prevent acute attacks of glaucoma. These are prescribed by an ophthalmologist (eye specialist), who should be seen as soon as any of the symptoms noted appear. If possible, the patient should avoid tension, insomnia, or sudden shock, because they can precipitate an attack. A patient with any symptom suggesting glaucoma should strenuously avoid taking any medicines or using any eye drops likely to cause widening of the pupils, because this can precipitate an attack. The family physician can give him a list of drugs to avoid.

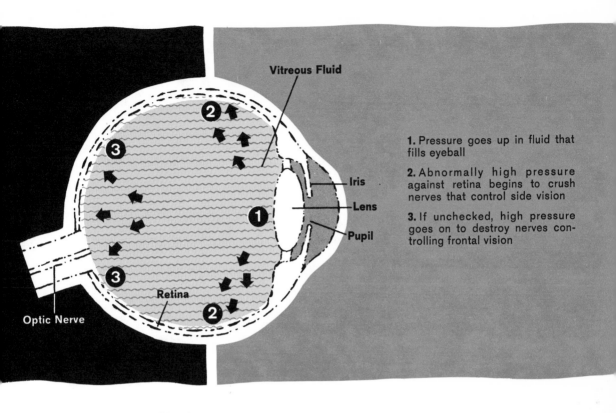

Vitreous Fluid

Iris

Lens

Pupil

Retina

Optic Nerve

1. Pressure goes up in fluid that fills eyeball

2. Abnormally high pressure against retina begins to crush nerves that control side vision

3. If unchecked, high pressure goes on to destroy nerves controlling frontal vision

Glaucoma's Danger Signals

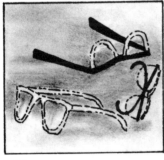

Glasses—even new ones—don't give satisfactory sight

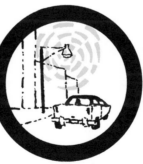

Rainbow colored rings appear around lights

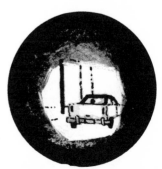

Difficulty with darkened rooms—like movie theatre

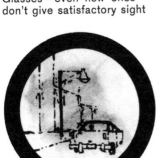

Spells of blurred or foggy eyesight

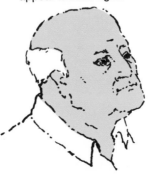

Loss of vision at sides of one or both eyes

the disease and its causes   Gonorrhea is one of the most common of the venereal diseases. It is caused by a specific type of bacteria which lodge in the genito-urinary tract of both sexes. Most often it is seen in adults who become infected during sexual intercourse. The eyes may also become involved as a result of a person handling infected material and then rubbing his eyes. Young girls sometimes get this gonorrheal eye infection from contact with infected toys or household articles.

The incubation period is rapid, usually within 72 hours of exposure. The disease occurs in all races, at all times of the year, in the age group of sexual activity.

symptoms   Generally, the first symptoms in men are itching and burning at the tip of the penis. This is accompanied by a slight pussy discharge which daily becomes more copious and yellow. Urination is painful and frequent, and the urine may be cloudy. There may be low-grade fever and a general feeling of illness. The lymph nodes in the groin may become enlarged, swollen, and painful.

In the female, where the pelvic organs are involved, there is pain in the lower abdomen and it is sensitive to touch. Frequently, because of the pain in this area, it is mistaken for acute appendicitis.

complications   An infant born of an infected mother can suffer serious eye infections. Many are born blind as a result. In women, the fallopian tubes and ovaries can be involved, with destruction of those organs, followed by sterility. In men, there may be destruction of the testicles and involvement of the prostate gland or the seminal vesicles. A painful complication is a narrowing of the urethra, which interferes with the passage of urine. Arthritis is a rare complication of gonorrhea.

prevention (or lessening of impact)   The only sure preventive is to avoid casual sexual contacts. However, there are protective measures which are reasonably effective in preventing this disease. Both men and women should take pains to keep the genital areas clean and follow recommended prophylactic procedures.

When the bacteria respond to drugs, the course of the disease may be quite short and the complications avoided or lessened. As more resistant strains of the bacteria develop, complications are likely to be more severe.

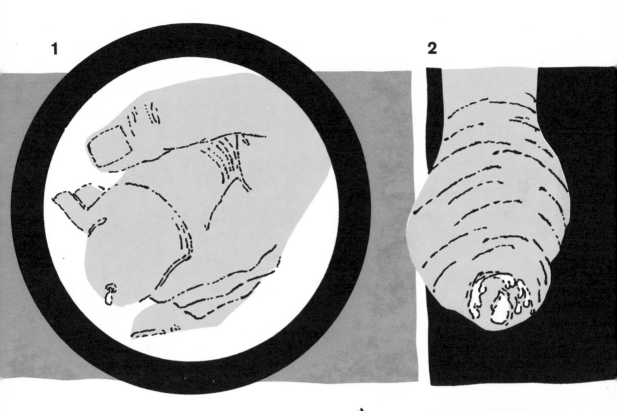

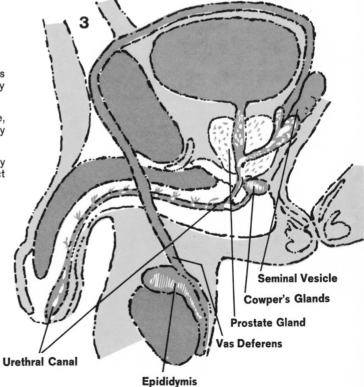

1. Yellow discharge from tip of penis varies in quantity of flow with severity of case.

2. In severe case in uncircumcised male, swelling of foreskin (Phimosis) may shut off flow of urine.

3. If untreated, gonorrhea bacteria may spread up urethral canal and infect other organs connected to it.

Seminal Vesicle

Cowper's Glands

Prostate Gland

Vas Deferens

Urethral Canal

Epididymis

the disease and its causes   Uric acid is one of the many chemicals produced by the body in the course of digestion. Normally it is disposed of, but if there is a disturbance in the protein metabolism of a patient, it collects in his joints and kidneys and results in a condition called gout. The disease tends to run in families, in a wide age group from 20 to 60, affecting mostly men. Attacks can be brought on by excesses in eating or drinking, or by certain acute medical or surgical problems. In such an attack the patient suffers from acute arthritic pain involving any of his joints, particularly those of the large toes.

symptoms   In most cases the first sign of gout is the sudden appearance of pain in one or several joints. These become swollen, red, shiny, and tender to the touch. As the attack subsides, the skin usually peels. During the attack, temperature may be high and there is weakness and headache. The Medi-Graph gives a more detailed picture of the symptoms. Gout may also begin with the sudden appearance of kidney stones. Crystalline deposits (tophi) may be found in the skin—particularly in the ear lobes.

The severity and length of a gout attack depend upon how quickly a diagnosis is made and treatment begun. In the early stages of the disease the joints recover from an acute attack without permanent injury. Months or years elapse between attacks, during which time the patient is quite comfortable. However, as the disease progresses, these intervals become shorter—and chronic, gouty arthritis, resembling rheumatoid arthritis, is likely to develop.

complications   The most serious complication is a slow, progressive kidney involvement which can lead to uremia and death. Younger patients with gout frequently develop high blood pressure and generalized hardening of the arteries. A gout patient can become virtually crippled from the deformation, stiffening, and impaired motion of the involved joints.

prevention (or lessening of impact)   In a family where there is gout, men should routinely be given a blood test for uric acid. A diet may be suggested to delay the onset of gouty symptoms, since there are foods which are thought to predispose to the formation of uric acid. However, it should be noted that while patients are usually given a specific diet to follow, it has not been established that this approach is effective.

A wide range of medication is available which tends to delay the formation of kidney stones and the development of serious joint problems. Patients who are overweight are put on a weight-losing program. Oddly enough, attacks of gout are not unusual during this very program.

Gout

1. During digestion of protein, uric acid produced is easily disposed of by normal person. However, gout victim retains it in blood, and it is deposited in joints to produce inflammation and swelling

2. Joint of big toe is most frequent site of attack. However, ankle, knee, wrist, elbow and other joints sometimes affected. First attacks last 3-14 days. Tenderness persists for two weeks. Generally full recovery from early attacks. But if not treated, attacks recur with increased frequency and may result in crippling impairment

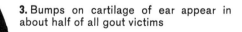

Uric Acid

Kidneys

Bladder

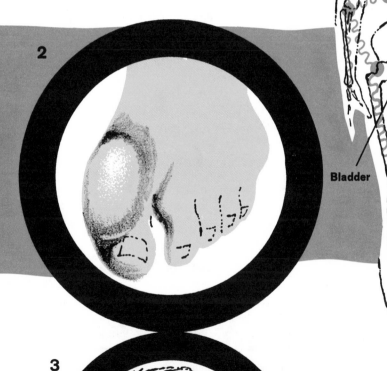

3. Bumps on cartilage of ear appear in about half of all gout victims

4. Most gout victims are men. Disease tends to run in family. Kidney stones are also frequently formed as result of gout attack

the disease and its causes   HANSEN'S DISEASE (or *leprosy,* as it is commonly called) occurs almost exclusively in very warm (tropical or subtropical) climates. Long feared as a highly contagious disease, leprosy is actually only moderately infectious. Its incubation period is uncertain, but it is thought to be long (up to 15–20 years). Contracting the disease also requires prolonged contact with an infected individual.

Hansen's disease is caused by specific bacteria *(Myobacterium lepeae)* that affect the skin, peripheral nervous system, and mucous membranes of the body. It is thought that these bacteria get into the body through a break in the skin.

symptoms   The first sign of Hansen's disease is usually the development of hard patches of skin. These can appear anywhere on the body. These patches lose all sensitivity to heat, cold or pain. As the disease progresses, larger areas become involved.

The skin on the forehead and face becomes thickened, resulting in the so-called "lion face." The eyebrows disappear and the ear lobes become elongated. If the disease is allowed to go unchecked, the nose can become eroded and may collapse.

There is a possibility of losing fingers and toes. The eyes, testicles and heart also may become involved.

complications   Tuberculosis may occur as well as a form of nephrosis (kidney degeneration)—both of which can lead to death. Cataracts, glaucoma and other eye problems resulting from the disease can lead to blindness. Another complication, if the disease is untreated, is widespread ulceration of the victim's body. This can lead to death through secondary infections.

prevention (or lessening of impact)   Fortunately, drugs are now available which appear to be effective in curing as well as arresting the progress of Hansen's disease. However, it is important that the diagnosis be made early. This involves disregarding the old stigma against the disease and seeking help for the patient as early as possible. With modern medical treatment, the patient can frequently be returned to his home environment without danger to family or others with whom he comes into daily contact.

Hansen's Disease
(Leprosy)

Early Symptoms

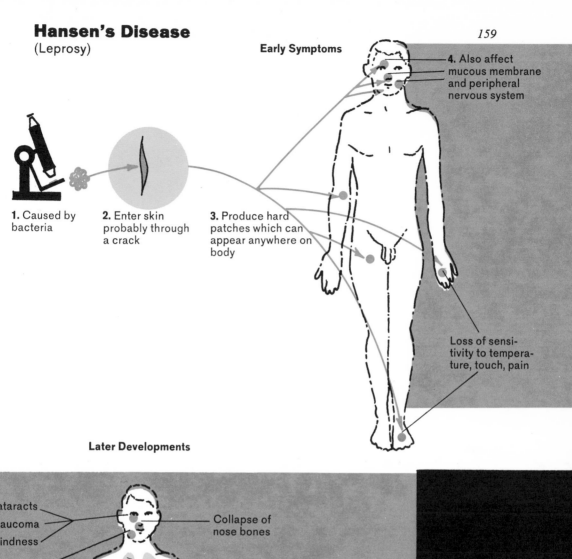

1. Caused by bacteria

2. Enter skin probably through a crack

3. Produce hard patches which can appear anywhere on body

4. Also affect mucous membrane and peripheral nervous system

Loss of sensitivity to temperature, touch, pain

Later Developments

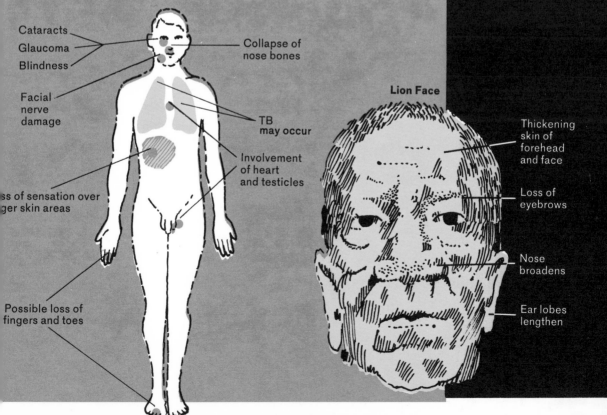

Cataracts
Glaucoma
Blindness

Facial nerve damage

ss of sensation over ger skin areas

Possible loss of fingers and toes

Collapse of nose bones

TB may occur

Involvement of heart and testicles

Lion Face

Thickening skin of forehead and face

Loss of eyebrows

Nose broadens

Ear lobes lengthen

the disease and its causes   These allergic diseases, frequently inherited (50% have a family history), are caused most often by airborne pollen, dust, and dander (dust from animals). Of these, pollen is the most frequent offender. Hence, the disease is usually seasonal.

This type of hay fever begins at an early age, during the season of most active spread of the allergy-producing pollen. In general, hay fever in early spring is due to tree pollens; in late spring and early summer to grain pollens; in August to October, to weed pollens. Because a patient may react to several of these pollens, his symptoms may overlap these time periods.

For non-seasonal hay fever there is rarely a family history, and it is usually associated with some infection of the upper respiratory system. Sinusitis is frequently the cause. Growths inside the nose, called nasal polyps, are often an incidental finding.

symptoms   Hay fever is characterized by bouts of sneezing, nasal discharge of thin, watery mucus, itching and tearing of the eyes. The eyes also become sensitive to light, and become reddened. Itching of the nose, throat, and roof of mouth is also very common. Frequently there is difficulty in breathing through the nose because of the swollen mucous membrane. Fatigue and loss of appetite are often related to the general discomfort.

complications   Secondary respiratory infection is the most common complication. Occasionally there is the development of bronchial asthma because of allergy to the same offending agent.

prevention (or lessening of impact)   Elimination of the offending agent, if possible, is the best means of preventing hay fever. This is not always easy. If dander from dogs or cats is implicated, those animals should be removed from contact. Foam rubber bedding may be used where feathers are a cause. Air conditioning may help by filtering the offending pollens.

For the acute attack there are many medications available which are quite effective. This subject is best handled by the family physician.

In those cases where treating the attack is unsuccessful, desensitization may be tried. This consists of injecting the individual with gradually increasing doses of the offending agent. In this way it is hoped he will become immune and free of reaction. This form of therapy should always be done under supervision of a physician, since severe reactions may occur.

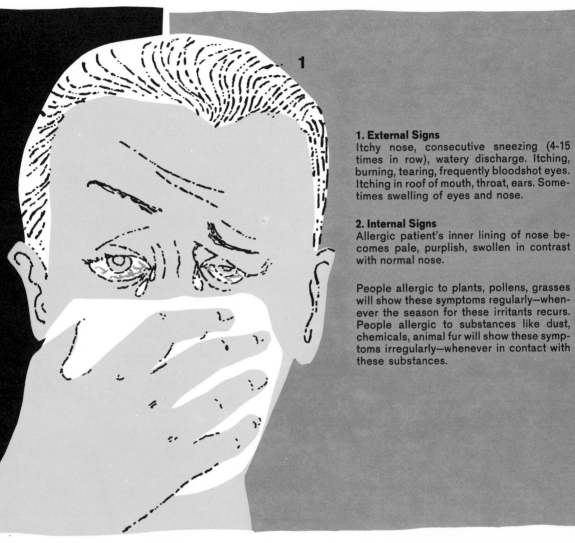

1. External Signs
Itchy nose, consecutive sneezing (4-15 times in row), watery discharge. Itching, burning, tearing, frequently bloodshot eyes. Itching in roof of mouth, throat, ears. Sometimes swelling of eyes and nose.

2. Internal Signs
Allergic patient's inner lining of nose becomes pale, purplish, swollen in contrast with normal nose.

People allergic to plants, pollens, grasses will show these symptoms regularly—whenever the season for these irritants recurs. People allergic to substances like dust, chemicals, animal fur will show these symptoms irregularly—whenever in contact with these substances.

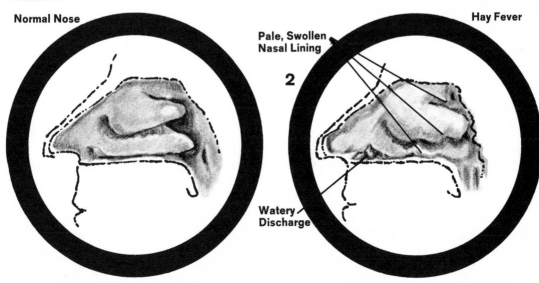

Normal Nose

Hay Fever

Pale, Swollen Nasal Lining

Watery Discharge

the disease and its causes Congenital heart disease is the name given to structural defects present in the heart at birth. These include abnormal septae, changes of the heart valves, persistence of fetal circulation, narrowing of the aorta artery, and abnormal positions of the great blood vessels of the heart. The cause of these defects is not known, although there are many theories about why the heart fails to develop beyond a certain stage in the fetus, or a portion of the heart develops abnormally. Among these theories are poor oxygen supply to the fetus, inflammation of the lining membrane of the fetal heart, deficiencies of certain vitamins, certain inherited abnormalities, and exposure to some form of irradiation. There also seems to be a definite relationship between congenital heart defects and a mother who has had German measles during the first three months of her pregnancy.

The disease is usually discovered early in life. Mortality is high in infants with severe and unusual defects.

symptoms The more common symptoms are illustrated in the accompanying Medi-Graph. Specific symptoms depend upon the type of defect and its effect upon the circulation.

Children with congenital heart disease are subject to frequent respiratory infections and there may be interference with growth and development.

complications A common complication is an inflammation of the lining membrane of the heart, called bacterial endocarditis. It can occur at any age, but is seen most often in young adults.

Clotting within blood vessels (thrombosis) is another serious complication. This can diminish or cut off circulation of blood and oxygen to the brain, in particular, and thus cause sudden paralysis, convulsions, or coma.

Brain abscess early in life, and congestive heart failure (which is the result of constant strain on the circulation) are other complications of this disease.

prevention (or lessening of impact) Cardiac surgery has changed the entire approach to congenital heart disease. More and more defects are being corrected each year, and the outlook is brighter with each passing day. However, every case must be individually evaluated after thorough, comprehensive examination.

The goal of the family and the physician caring for a patient with congenital heart disease is to guard against complications. Infections should be treated promptly. The patient's general health must be maintained at the same time that he is given a program of activity geared to his capacity. There should be regular follow-up care and periodic review of his condition.

Congenital Heart Disease

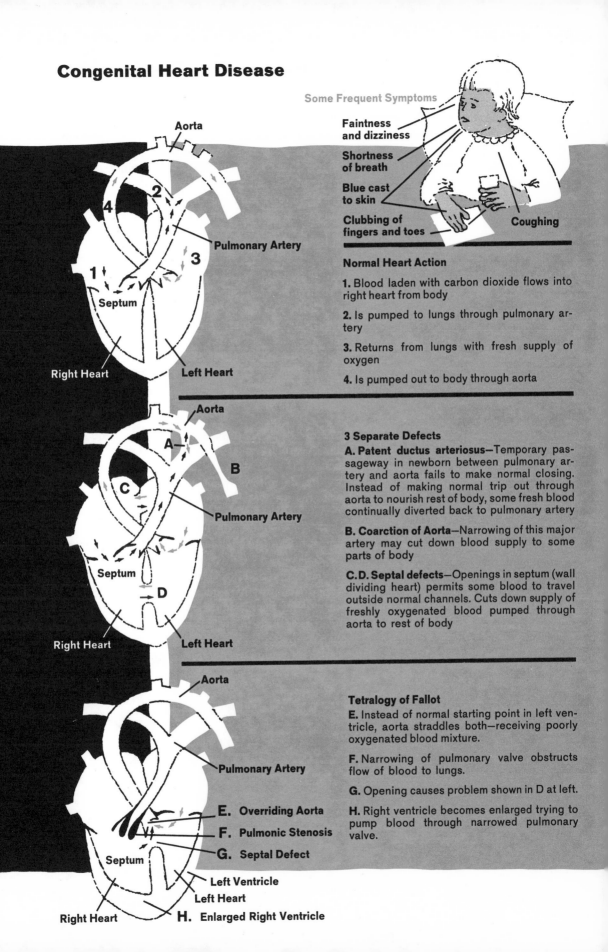

Aorta

2

4

3

Pulmonary Artery

1

Septum

Right Heart

Left Heart

Some Frequent Symptoms

Faintness and dizziness

Shortness of breath

Blue cast to skin

Clubbing of fingers and toes

Coughing

Normal Heart Action

1. Blood laden with carbon dioxide flows into right heart from body

2. Is pumped to lungs through pulmonary artery

3. Returns from lungs with fresh supply of oxygen

4. Is pumped out to body through aorta

Aorta

A

B

C

Pulmonary Artery

Septum

D

Right Heart

Left Heart

3 Separate Defects

A. Patent ductus arteriosus—Temporary passageway in newborn between pulmonary artery and aorta fails to make normal closing. Instead of making normal trip out through aorta to nourish rest of body, some fresh blood continually diverted back to pulmonary artery

B. Coarction of Aorta—Narrowing of this major artery may cut down blood supply to some parts of body

C.D. Septal defects—Openings in septum (wall dividing heart) permits some blood to travel outside normal channels. Cuts down supply of freshly oxygenated blood pumped through aorta to rest of body

---

Aorta

Pulmonary Artery

E. Overriding Aorta

F. Pulmonic Stenosis

G. Septal Defect

Septum

Left Ventricle

Left Heart

Right Heart

H. Enlarged Right Ventricle

Tetralogy of Fallot

E. Instead of normal starting point in left ventricle, aorta straddles both—receiving poorly oxygenated blood mixture.

F. Narrowing of pulmonary valve obstructs flow of blood to lungs.

G. Opening causes problem shown in D at left.

H. Right ventricle becomes enlarged trying to pump blood through narrowed pulmonary valve.

the disease and its causes High blood pressure, which is discussed in another section of this book, results when the heart has to pump harder to force blood through arterial openings that have narrowed for a variety of reasons. The effect on the heart is to enlarge it, particularly the left ventricle. And as a result of this enlargement, heart failure can result. Generally this heart disease affects both men and women over the age of 40. The age is significant because it is about this time when hypertension is more common. The disease is associated with a tense, driving personality.

symptoms The symptoms of this disease are detailed and illustrated in the accompanying Medi-Graph. It includes headache, dizzy spells, and constricted arterioles of the retina of the eye on doctor's examination. There is shortness of breath, mid-chest pain, occasional palpitations of the heart, and swelling of the feet.

It should be noted that prolonged hypertensive heart disease usually ends with congestive heart failure. Older patients are more prone to coronary thrombosis, which is a blocking by a blood clot of one of the blood vessels that nourish the heart.

complications Whenever and wherever the heart fails to function adequately, complications can occur. A stroke results when the blood pressure is so high that it causes rupture of one of the blood vessels of the brain (cerebral hemorrhage). Uremia follows when not enough blood circulates through the kidney to remove waste products.

prevention (or lessening of impact) In dealing with hypertensive heart disease the doctor directs treatment toward the high blood pressure itself. Associated complications are dealt with as they develop. Heart failure especially requires the prompt attention of a physician.

There are effective drugs to control hypertension. Treatment can be prescribed by the doctor to delay the progression of the illness and allow the patient to function. It is well to follow the physician's instructions regarding rest, maintenance of good health and well-being, lessening of tension, and the elimination or cutting down of smoking.

Hypertensive Heart Disease

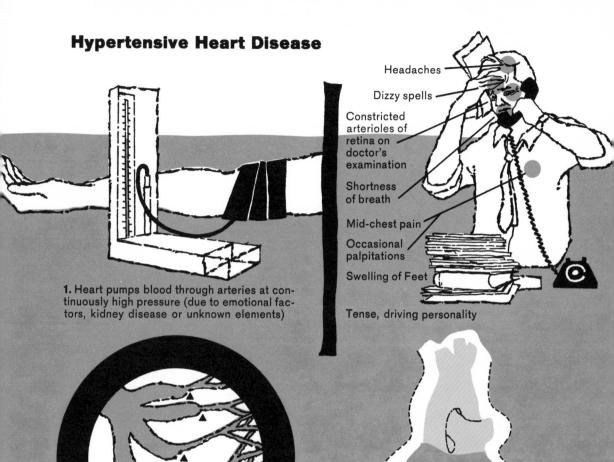

1. Heart pumps blood through arteries at continuously high pressure (due to emotional factors, kidney disease or unknown elements)

Headaches

Dizzy spells

Constricted arterioles of retina on doctor's examination

Shortness of breath

Mid-chest pain

Occasional palpitations

Swelling of Feet

Tense, driving personality

2. Continuously high pressure on arterioles (small branches of arteries) causes them to tighten and shrink

3. Heart enlarges to force blood through narrowed arterial openings

Continued strain of hypertensive heart disease may lead to:

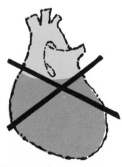

Heart Failure
Heart unable to continue to move blood through narrowing arterial system

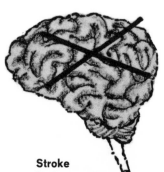

Stroke
Brain fails because of insufficient supply of fresh oxygen-carrying blood

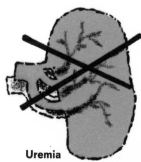

Uremia
Insufficient circulation of blood through kidneys means waste products accumulate instead of passing out in urine

the disease and its causes This type of heart disease, one of many, sometimes develops as a result of a chronic lung infection, such as emphysema, asthma, and bronchiectasis, or a combination of these infections. Often there is also an association between pulmonary heart disease and silicosis, anthracosis, Boeck's sarcoid, or any other condition producing scarring of the lungs. The disease develops when there is an interruption in the normal circulatory flow between the heart and lungs, which creates a strain that eventually causes the right side of the heart to become enlarged.

An acute form of pulmonary heart disease can occur in the presence of a blood clot (pulmonary embolism) large enough to interfere seriously with circulation of blood in the lungs.

Less frequently, rapidly spreading lung cancer can cause this disease. Any other rapidly progressing infection of the lungs, such as tuberculosis and certain bacterial and fungus infections, can also play a role.

symptoms As shown on the Medi-Graph, there is a blue tinge to the face, and the patient is short of breath, and coughs. The liver and heart become enlarged. The abdomen and feet swell and the fingers become clubbed. In addition, some patients complain of pain in the middle of the chest. On other occasions, when a patient exerts himself, there is dizziness and weakness.

complications Congestive heart failure is the main complication of this disease, and it is serious because it responds poorly to treatment. In this state, as the Medi-Graph indicates, the right side of the heart enlarges, trying to overcome resistance to normal blood flow between the heart and lungs. Heart failure follows.

prevention (or lessening of impact) Whatever is causing the interruption of normal circulatory flow between the heart and lungs must be dealt with first. Infections must be treated before they get beyond control.

In the case of heart failure, there is still hope for the patient if he is treated in accordance with the specific instructions of the physician.

Pulmonary Heart Disease

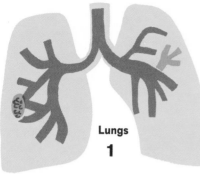

Lungs

1

1. . . . Serious Lung Disease . . .

Blood clot (embolus)

Bronchiectasis

Asthma, other chronic conditions

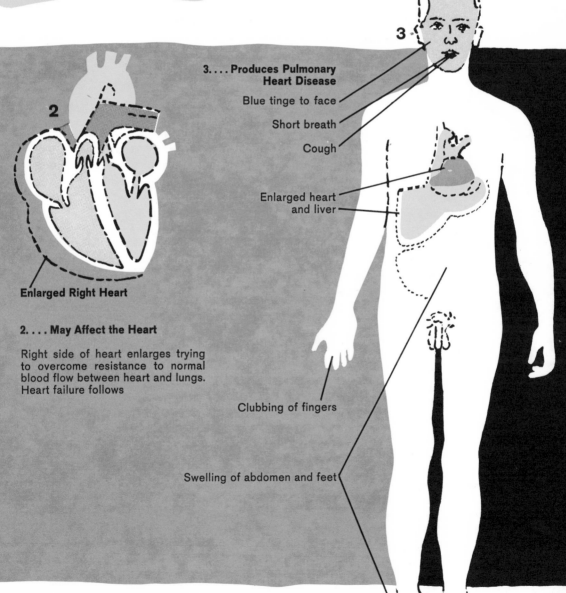

3

**3. . . . Produces Pulmonary
Heart Disease**

Blue tinge to face

Short breath

Cough

Enlarged heart
and liver

2

Enlarged Right Heart

2. . . . May Affect the Heart

Right side of heart enlarges trying
to overcome resistance to normal
blood flow between heart and lungs.
Heart failure follows

Clubbing of fingers

Swelling of abdomen and feet

the disease and its causes   Some two-thirds of the known cases of rheumatic heart disease have a history of rheumatic fever, and it is generally accepted that acute rheumatic fever invariably involves the heart. In the course of such an attack the heart valves (most often the mitral and aortic) become scarred, usually quite rigid and contracted, and sometimes calcified. The accompanying Medi-Graph illustrates how the valves are affected.

In rheumatic heart disease the entire heart is involved—the pericardium, the myocardium, and the endocardium. There are often irregular heart rhythms which patients describe as a jumping sensation in the chest, or a sensation of having the heart skip a beat. Most so-called palpitations are of no consequence, but when they occur in an organically damaged heart, the doctor will want to study them carefully.

symptoms   Symptoms depend upon several factors, including the presence of active rheumatic infection and associated heart failure. After the first attack of rheumatic fever there may be no symptoms for years. An adult may learn he has a heart murmur in a routine physical examination years after he has recovered uneventfully from a rheumatic fever siege. If the patient has had only minor heart valve damage he will probably have been living a normal, functioning life without signs of discomfort or disability.

The diagnosis is made by examination, electrocardiographic studies, and heart X rays.

complications   It is the complications which are usually the clue to the presence of rheumatic heart disease. A serious one is the recurrence of rheumatic fever infection and further involvement of the heart and heart valves. Recurrence increases the destructive changes in the valve previously involved and puts additional strain on an already weakened heart muscle.

Despite the availability of antibiotic drugs, a not infrequent and serious complication is bacterial endocarditis—an infection of the lining membrane of the heart. Congestive heart failure and pericarditis, discussed elsewhere in this book, are other serious complications.

Emboli or blood clots discharged from the heart to distant parts of the body can often cause a condition that resembles stroke, if the brain is involved, or cause certain gangrenous changes when the lower extremities are involved.

prevention (or lessening of impact)   As described in the section on rheumatic fever, it is important for a patient who has had this disease to take special care of himself. If the heart is not involved after rheumatic fever, a patient can in time do just about what he pleases. But appropriate antibiotics should be taken, as prescribed, when he undergoes minor surgical procedures or has dental extractions. If rheumatic heart disease symptoms develop, the doctor will decide upon a suitable program of activity.

Rheumatic Heart Disease

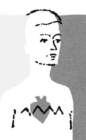

Most rheumatic heart disease develops between ages of 5-20

Rheumatic fever predisposes toward development of rheumatic heart disease — but many cases develop without history of rheumatic fever

Palpitations or jumping sensation in chest are sometimes sign of rheumatic heart disease

Normal Heart Action

1. Blood from body comes to heart through veins

2. Right heart pumps blood to lungs to get rid of carbon dioxide

3. Blood returns to heart after picking up oxygen supply in lungs

4. Freshened blood pumped out to body through Great Artery (aorta)

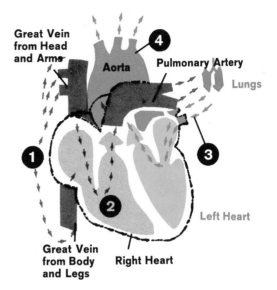

Mitral Valve Affected

1. Scar tissue from Rheumatic Fever obstructs mitral valve or prevents it from closing properly

2. Blood backs up putting increased pressure on left auricle

3. Pressure feeds back through pulmonary veins and arteries to right ventricle. It may eventually become enlarged and fail

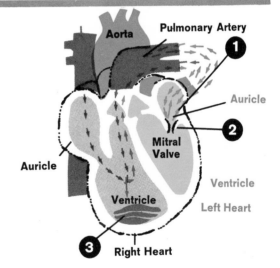

Aortic Valve Affected

1. Scar tissue from Rheumatic Fever obstructs aortic valve or prevents it from closing properly

2. Instead of pumping through aorta to rest of body, blood backs up, putting increased strain on left ventricle

3. Left ventricle may eventually become enlarged and fail

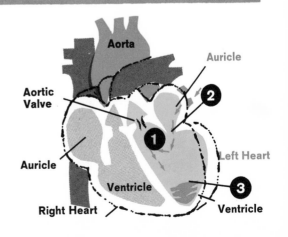

the disease and its causes　This disease, which is the result of an overactive thyroid, is a less common form of chronic heart disease. The thyroid secretes an excess amount of hormone and causes other organs and tissues of the body to speed up beyond their normal pace. The heart attempts to keep up with the demands placed on it and pumps faster. The result is a change in the normal rhythm of the heart beat, and ultimately congestive heart failure. The age group affected is 35 to 50. Women are more susceptible than men.

symptoms　Sometimes the overactive thyroid is overlooked because symptoms of the heart condition are more prominent. There is weakness, nervousness, and loss of weight. The patient may sweat profusely and always feel warm. Sometimes there are heart palpitations. The pulse is usually very rapid, even at rest, or else it is irregular. Blood pressure may or may not be higher than normal, but the heart is enlarged because of the heavier demands made on it. Usually there is some shortness of breath and swelling of the feet.

In addition, there are the symptoms of congestive heart failure, such as blue lips and fingernails, swollen neck veins, cough and breathing difficulty, fluid in the lungs and abdomen. As the condition worsens, it takes less and less exertion to produce these symptoms.

complications　The usual complication of hyperthyroid heart disease is heart failure plus the abnormal rhythm previously mentioned.

prevention (or lessening of impact)　Since the underlying cause of this disease is an overactive thyroid, measures must be taken to correct this. Surgical and medical treatment are both quite satisfactory, as well as radioactive iodine given orally. Every case must be considered individually and the most advisable approach used. Thyroid heart disease is a form of heart disease which may be cured permanently if it is recognized promptly and treated before excessive damage is done.

Thyroid Heart Disease

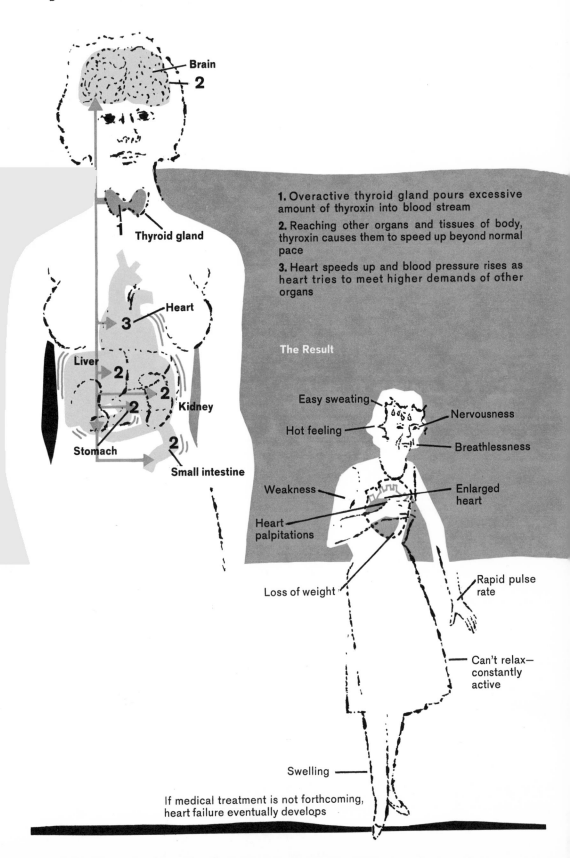

Brain

2

1. Overactive thyroid gland pours excessive amount of thyroxin into blood stream

2. Reaching other organs and tissues of body, thyroxin causes them to speed up beyond normal pace

3. Heart speeds up and blood pressure rises as heart tries to meet higher demands of other organs

1

Thyroid gland

Heart

3

Liver

2

2

2

Kidney

2

Stomach

Small intestine

The Result

Easy sweating

Nervousness

Hot feeling

Breathlessness

Weakness

Enlarged heart

Heart palpitations

Loss of weight

Rapid pulse rate

Can't relax— constantly active

Swelling

If medical treatment is not forthcoming, heart failure eventually develops

the disease and its causes   The heart is like a delicate pump which supplies the body with a given amount of blood at certain pressures. This pressure is not the same on the right and left sides of the heart, but it is this very difference in pressure which must be maintained at a precise balance if the heart is to function properly. When some disease or malformation alters the balance, normal intake and outgo of blood is interrupted and the heart is not able to supply essential organs with the amount and quality of blood necessary. The resulting condition is called heart failure.

symptoms   Regardless of the underlying heart disease responsible, the symptoms of heart failure are the same in all cases. These are described and illustrated in the accompanying Medi-Graph.

An early symptom of heart failure is the inability of the kidneys to excrete salt properly. While the mechanism is not fully understood, it is believed that this kidney failure results, in part, from the diminished blood supply it receives.

A patient with heart failure is sometimes subject to a sudden onset of lung congestion known as acute pulmonary edema. He becomes very short of breath, or else he brings up frothy, pinkish sputum which is the sudden fluid accumulation in his lungs.

As the illness progresses, the heart failure patient will become more limited in his activities and will require more and more rest to avoid discomfort. Eventually he may have heart failure even when his body is completely at rest.

complications   When the heart failure is caused by a condition that responds to medical or surgical treatment, much can be expected. For other patients, the outlook is chronic invalidism. These patients are susceptible to generalized and respiratory infections, lung infarcts (areas of the lung for which circulation is blocked and not functioning), and loss of kidney function.

prevention (or lessening of impact)   If the underlying cause is responsive to treatment, heart failure can be postponed or alleviated. When surgery is indicated, it should be done before heart failure develops. Patients with a history of endocarditis or a rheumatic heart should be on a preventive, antibiotic drug program to help them avoid recurrent infections. Patients with coronary artery disease will be guided by the physician and may be put on anti-coagulant therapy. Thyroid heart disease responds to treatment and should be corrected.

Most cases of heart failure can be controlled for years with proper care by the patient under the guidance of the physician.

Heart Failure

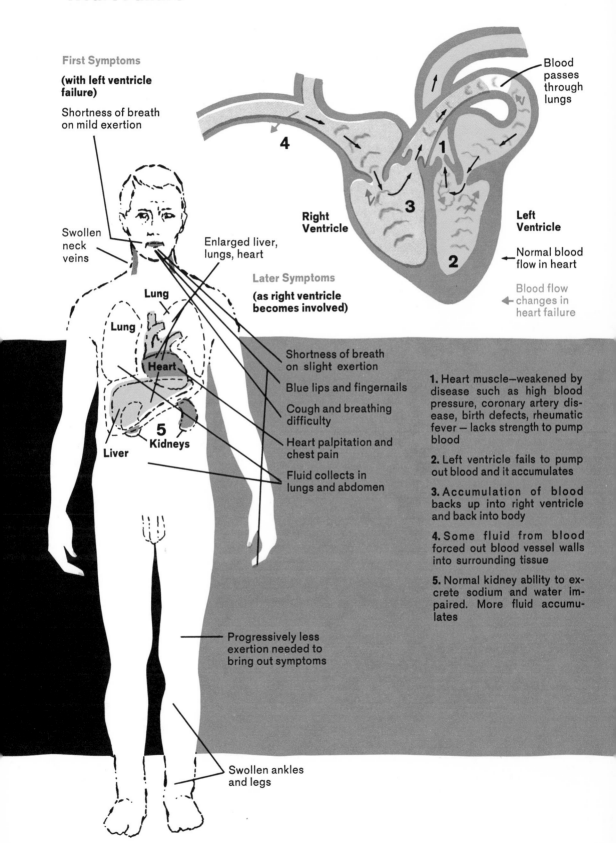

First Symptoms

(with left ventricle failure)

Shortness of breath on mild exertion

Swollen neck veins

Enlarged liver, lungs, heart

Later Symptoms

(as right ventricle becomes involved)

Blood passes through lungs

Right Ventricle

Left Ventricle

Normal blood flow in heart

Blood flow changes in heart failure

Lung

Lung

Heart

Liver

Kidneys

Shortness of breath on slight exertion

Blue lips and fingernails

Cough and breathing difficulty

Heart palpitation and chest pain

Fluid collects in lungs and abdomen

1. Heart muscle—weakened by disease such as high blood pressure, coronary artery disease, birth defects, rheumatic fever — lacks strength to pump blood

2. Left ventricle fails to pump out blood and it accumulates

3. Accumulation of blood backs up into right ventricle and back into body

4. Some fluid from blood forced out blood vessel walls into surrounding tissue

5. Normal kidney ability to excrete sodium and water impaired. More fluid accumulates

Progressively less exertion needed to bring out symptoms

Swollen ankles and legs

the condition and its cause   Heat stroke is a serious condition that can result from prolonged exposure to high temperature and high humidity. Among the people most susceptible to heat stroke are young children, old people, alcoholics, extremely overweight persons, and people weakened by illness. Sunstroke is the most common form of heat stroke. It is most likely to occur during the early days of a heat wave, before the body has a chance to acclimatize.

Sweating is the body's chief defense against heat disorders—and heavy sweating removes a large amount of the normal salt in the body's fluids. A primary cause of heat sickness is this loss of salt. As long as the body replaces the salt and water it has lost through sweating, it can stand very hot temperatures.

symptoms   A noticeable decrease in sweating—indicating that the body is not bringing its natural cooling system into play—is an important sign of heat stroke. Headache, dizziness, faintness, and abnormal distress follow. The skin becomes hot and dry, and the body temperature may reach 105°–110° F. A rapid pulse, evidence of circulatory collapse, is present.

complications   Damage to all internal organs of the body due to the exposure to high temperature can occur. In untreated cases, heart failure, kidney failure, and brain damage may result. These severe problems occur most often when the body temperature is 106° or more. Unconsciousness can develop rapidly, and about one-fourth of all serious cases end fatally.

prevention (or lessening of impact)   Wearing light, loose clothing and a hat to protect oneself against the sun are helpful. Strenuous activity should be kept to a minimum during heat spells or in areas of high temperature. Salt pills should be taken, and frequent rest periods observed. To maintain proper sweat production, a person working in high temperatures should drink about 12 glasses of water a day. A light diet that includes lots of fruits, juices and vegetables, and only limited amounts of fat foods and alcoholic beverages, is helpful.

If a case of heat stroke develops, hospital care is mandatory.

Heat Stroke (Sunstroke)

Caused by exposure to high temperature and high humidity

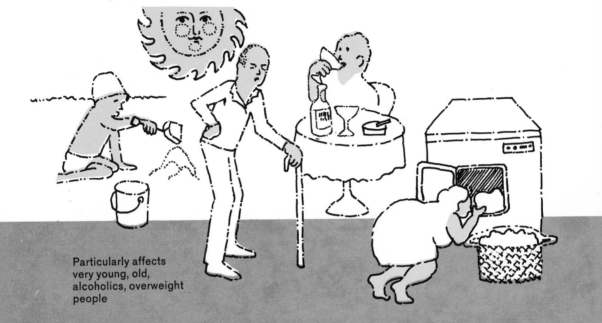

Particularly affects
very young, old,
alcoholics, overweight
people

Signs of Heat Stroke

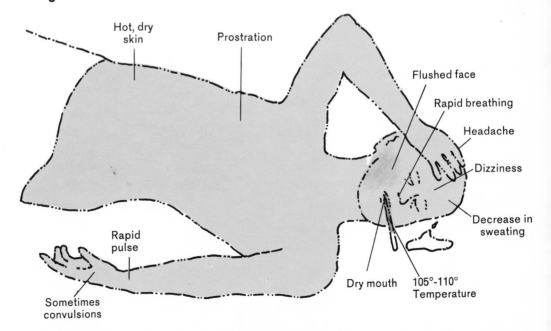

Hot, dry
skin

Prostration

Flushed face

Rapid breathing

Headache

Dizziness

Decrease in
sweating

Rapid
pulse

Sometimes
convulsions

Dry mouth

105°-110°
Temperature

the disease and its causes   HEMOPHILIA is sometimes popularly referred to as *Bleeder's disease*. The blood of victims of the disease is very slow in clotting or coagulating when their skin has been punctured or they have received other types of wounds. As a result, they suffer from excessive bleeding. The defect of the blood is generally thought to be a deficiency in Factor VIII, which is essential in the formation of blood clotting elements.

This is a hereditary disease which strikes only males. However, it is transmitted from generation to generation by females—the daughters of male hemophiliacs—who pass the disease on to their own male offspring. The disease usually becomes apparent in early childhood.

symptoms   The main symptom is excessive bleeding. This usually occurs after injury—but occasionally occurs without any apparent cause. The bleeding is prolonged, out of all proportion to the injury, and lasts from days to weeks.

In addition to bleeding from skin punctures, hemophilia victims may also suffer nosebleeds, hemorrhaging upon loss of a tooth, and bleeding from the gums. Swollen, painful joints are another symptom of hemophilia. And black and blue marks (hematomas) may appear where bleeding has taken place under the skin.

Different families of hemophiliac victims have different levels of severity of the disease—levels which are usually constant for a given family.

The doctor diagnoses the disease from the prolonged coagulation time of the blood, and the deficiency in the amount of Factor VIII he finds on examination of the blood.

complications   A patient with severe hemophilia is in constant danger of bleeding episodes. This prolonged loss of blood may result from internal bleeding or from a wound or puncture that will not clot. If uncontrolled, death may result.

If the joints are involved, swelling may develop which will interfere with the use of the joints—leading to muscle atrophy.

prevention (or lessening of impact)   At the present time, prevention of spread of the disease is possible only if male hemophiliac victims do not reproduce. Males already suffering from the disease must be protected as much as possible from an injury that would cause bleeding. Any medical, surgical or dental procedure should be done under hospital conditions with adequate blood that has just been donated available for transfusions.

Joints that become swollen because of hemorrhaging should be immobilized. Starting physiotherapy early in this situation can prevent deformities from developing. Drugs have been developed that promote the clotting of blood around wounds, so the doctor will apply them when indicated.

A drug that will replace the deficient clotting factor and can be taken daily has been developed and is available at high cost.

Hemophilia

A blood deficiency disease which occurs only
in males and usually appears at an early age

Normal Person

Hemophiliac

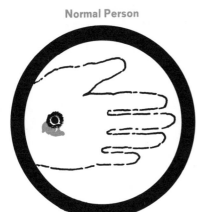

Within 5-6 minutes
after skin is punctured,
blood begins to clot, forms
scab, and seals off wound

Blood doesn't clot properly, so bleeding
may continue for days or weeks

Typical Hemophiliac Problems

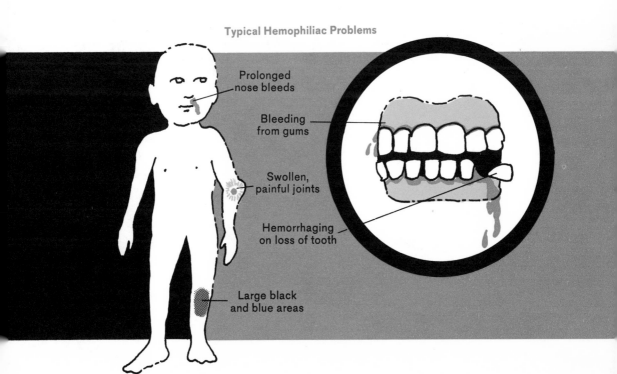

Prolonged
nose bleeds

Bleeding
from gums

Swollen,
painful joints

Hemorrhaging
on loss of tooth

Large black
and blue areas

the disease and its causes   HEMORRHOIDS   Hemorrhoids are really varicose veins that develop in the rectum. There are two kinds: external hemorrhoids, which occur at the lower end of the rectum at the area of the anus, covered with skin; internal hemorrhoids, which occur inside the rectum above the skin area, and are covered with mucous membrane.

There are many causes or factors that contribute to the development of hemorrhoids. Among them are straining at stool, prolonged diarrhea, constipation, heavy lifting or over-exertion, pregnancy, and tumors of the bowel.

FISSURES   A fissure is a tear of the anal canal which results at the time of a forceful bowel movement. There is severe, acute pain, and sometimes some bleeding. While a fissure can occur at any age, it appears more often in middle life—and somewhat more frequently in women.

symptoms   HEMORRHOIDS   There may be itching, burning, or a firm but tender swelling around the rectal area. Bright red blood may coat the outer surface of the stool.

FISSURES   There is usually severe pain with the sudden development of a fissure. Multiple fissures, also more frequent in women, are not unusual.

complications   HEMORRHOIDS   The only serious complication of hemorrhoids results from prolonged bleeding. The blood loss can result in anemia and weakness. Frequently there is gangrene of a strangulated hemorrhoid, a correctable condition which sounds more serious than it is.

FISSURES   There are no serious complications in fissures other than the discomfort and the possibility of infection.

prevention (or lessening of impact)   Steps should be taken to correct the constipation or diarrhea or the straining at stool which causes hemorrhoids. Stool-softening drugs such as mineral oil may help to prevent flare-ups where hemorrhoids or fissures already exist. However, the prolonged use of mineral oil depletes the body of certain vitamins.

In both cases, surgery may be necessary where the previously mentioned measures have not proved effective. This surgery usually proves effective—though hemorrhoids may recur if toilet habits and attitudes are not changed.

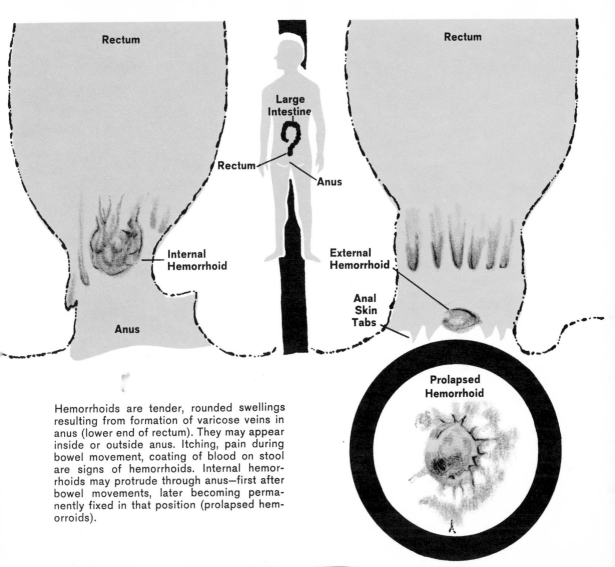

Rectum

Large Intestine

Rectum

Anus

Internal Hemorrhoid

External Hemorrhoid

Anal Skin Tabs

Anus

Prolapsed Hemorrhoid

Hemorrhoids are tender, rounded swellings resulting from formation of varicose veins in anus (lower end of rectum). They may appear inside or outside anus. Itching, pain during bowel movement, coating of blood on stool are signs of hemorrhoids. Internal hemorrhoids may protrude through anus—first after bowel movements, later becoming permanently fixed in that position (prolapsed hemorroids).

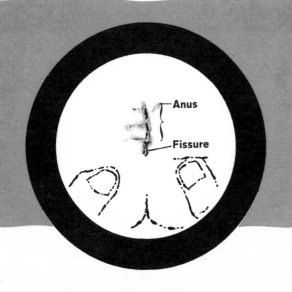

Anus

Fissure

Fissure is painful tear or split in anal canal lining. Results in bleeding and painful bowel movement.

the disease and its causes Hepatitis—an acute viral infection affecting the liver—occurs in two forms. One type, infectious hepatitis (IH), can be transmitted to man through injection or through the mouth. It is seen in epidemic form under conditions of poor sanitation, and is spread by close contact with people passing virus in their stools. Food and water, if contaminated, become excellent agents for the transmission of the disease. The incubation period is 2 to 6 weeks.

The other type, serum hepatitis (SH), is transmitted only through injection via contaminated syringes or through blood transfusions from unwitting carriers. The incubation period of SH is from 6 weeks to as long as 6 months. An attack of one form of hepatitis gives immunity for that form only.

symptoms Both types of hepatitis produce essentially the same symptoms. The disease may begin with what appears to be a respiratory or intestinal infection. Symptoms then develop along the lines shown in the accompanying Medi-Graph.

The jaundice stage reaches its peak in 5 to 15 days and can indicate the severity of the liver involvement. It takes from 1 to 6 weeks to get relief from the jaundice and the accompanying symptoms. Once the jaundice has subsided, it may take another 2 to 6 weeks for the liver to heal. Specific blood tests are made to check on this.

complications Chronic hepatitis is a form in which the course of the disease is prolonged for many months, with persistent jaundice and other symptoms. The most common complication here is the development of liver cirrhosis. Occasionally massive infections may cause a rapid, destructive type of hepatitis which can lead to death.

prevention (or lessening of impact) An injection of gamma globulin to anyone exposed to IH hepatitis is very effective in preventing the disease. There is no preventive against SH hepatitis, but the use of disposable needles and syringes by physicians and dentists does much to prevent the spread of both types. Proper hygiene and sanitation in restaurants and among food handlers is important. Recent evidence reveals that gamma globulin given in very large doses a month apart may be effective in minimizing SH hepatitis. However, the study is not conclusive.

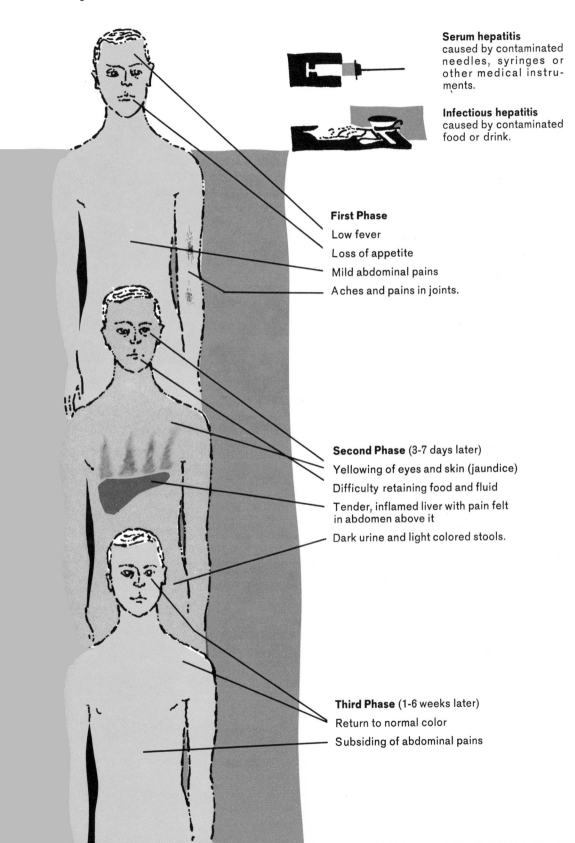

Serum hepatitis
caused by contaminated needles, syringes or other medical instruments.

Infectious hepatitis
caused by contaminated food or drink.

First Phase

Low fever

Loss of appetite

Mild abdominal pains

Aches and pains in joints.

Second Phase (3-7 days later)

Yellowing of eyes and skin (jaundice)

Difficulty retaining food and fluid

Tender, inflamed liver with pain felt in abdomen above it

Dark urine and light colored stools.

Third Phase (1-6 weeks later)

Return to normal color

Subsiding of abdominal pains

the disease and its causes   Any hernia is a protrusion through an abnormal opening. In hiatus hernia varying portions of an abdominal organ—most
frequently the stomach—protrude into the chest cavity through an opening in the diaphragm. The opening may be one the patient was born
with, or it may be the result of an injury such as can occur in an automobile accident when the steering wheel is forced into the driver's
chest. In rare instances the entire stomach protrudes into the chest
cavity, badly crowding and interfering with the heart and lungs.
Most hiatus hernias slide and vary in the amount of organ protruding
into the chest. In cases of associated esophageal inflammations this canal
to the stomach appears to shorten, pulling the stomach into a permanent
chest location.
Hiatus hernia occurs quite frequently, more often in women than in
men, and generally in the older age group.

symptoms   Often a heart condition is incorrectly thought to be the source of the
patient's discomfort. Actually it is the functions of the stomach which
are disturbed in hiatus hernia and the symptoms reflect that disturbance.
There is heartburn, indigestion, sour regurgitation, and the feeling of
a lump under the breastbone after eating. All of these symptoms seem
worse after meals or when the patient is lying down. There may be
shortness of breath. Gurgling sounds are often heard in the chest. The
most common complaint is pain high in the abdomen, sometimes radiating under the left ribs to the shoulders and down the left arm. Belching
and hiccoughing are not unusual.

complications   A serious, common complication is bleeding either from the walls
of the hernia itself or from an associated esophageal ulcer. Inflammation
of the esophagus (esophagitis) can be another complication.

prevention (or lessening of impact)   There is no known way of preventing the
development of hiatus hernia. However, most patients can be made
more comfortable by following a program in which they eat frequent
small meals and do not eat at all within three hours of bedtime. Sometimes a patient finds relief in sleeping with two or three pillows which
raise the upper half of his body.
Specific medicines are available which are of some benefit. Surgery is
used cautiously—being generally reserved for those cases where the
herniation is tremendous and is interfering with heart and lung functions.
When there is ulceration, it is treated like an ulcer anywhere in the
digestive system.

Hiatus (Diaphragmatic) Hernia

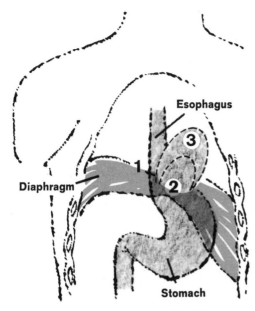

Esophagus

3

1

2

Diaphragm

Stomach

Common Type

1. Weakness develops in diaphragm muscle around opening where esophagus passes through to connect with stomach

2. Stomach or other abdominal organ pushes up into chest cavity through weak spot in diaphragm

3. Heart and lungs may be crowded and hampered in functioning if large hiatus hernia develops

May have such symptoms as

Belching and hiccups

Breathlessness and blue face if breathing hampered

Heartburn and indigestion

May be vomiting — sometimes blood from friction on stomach or esophagus

Sharp, stabbing pain which radiates

Discomfort increases after meals or when lying down

the disease and its causes By definition a hernia is a protrusion or bulging of an organ, or part of an organ, through the containing wall in which it is located. An inguinal hernia or rupture is a weakness of the abdominal wall in the area of the groin, with protrusion of the abdominal wall contents through this weakened area. Inguinal hernias are very common and are responsible for 80% of all hernias. Infant males under a year are the most frequent victims, but they occur in men in all age groups. Inguinal hernias are less frequently seen in women, and sometimes result from pregnancy.

Inguinal hernia is caused by sudden strains, coughing, heavy manual labor, lifting, or by a condition present at birth, or any combination of these. While sudden strain may cause actual tearing of the ligaments that normally prevent herniation, the more common cause is related to continuous increase in pressure gradually stretching these ligaments.

symptoms There may be few or no symptoms in the beginning. The first sign is likely to be an abnormal swelling in the area of the groin. There may be occasional nagging pain. The swelling may get worse. In acute cases the patient feels a sudden severe tearing pain following some sort of exertion and comments on the appearance of a protruding mass. When he lies down, the swelling and the mass disappear. Male patients report that in time the swelling gets worse and the scrotum (sac holding the testicles) becomes enlarged. There may be some interference with normal bowel movements, and there can be occasional sharp pains in the lower groin.

complications Two serious complications can develop in inguinal hernia. First, a condition may develop where the protruding mass cannot be replaced in the abdominal cavity. Second, strangulation can occur when the protruding mass twists or swells and cuts off the blood supply. Then gangrene threatens the affected area. Both of these conditions must be corrected surgically.

prevention (or lessening of impact) When an infant is born with a hernia nothing can be done to prevent its development. Occasionally the abdominal wall weakness or opening will strengthen and close up as the child matures. More frequently surgery is the most feasible course.

People who develop signs of an abdominal weakness should take care to avoid uncontrolled lifting and unusual exertions. If, for one reason or another, surgery is not advisable when a hernia is revealed, supporting trusses are available and helpful.

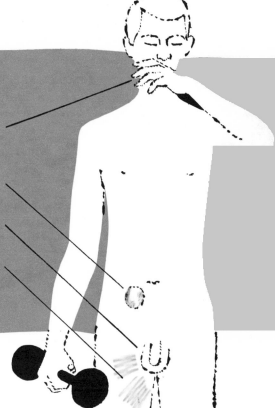

1. Inherited physical makeup, coughing, lifting, sudden strain or combination weakens abdominal wall

2. Abnormal swelling appears. May disappear again, particularly when lying down

3. After time, swelling may enlarge and spread to scrotum (sac holding testicles)

4. May be sharp pains and interference with bowel movements

Common Sites of Abdominal Hernias

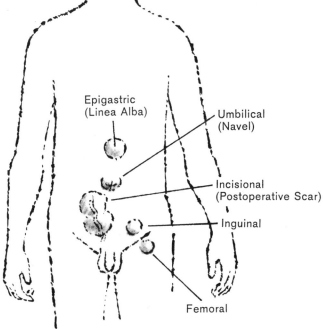

Epigastric
(Linea Alba)

Umbilical
(Navel)

Incisional
(Postoperative Scar)

Inguinal

Femoral

Cross-Section View (from above)

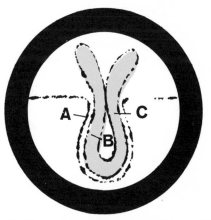

A. Weakened abdominal wall has bulged out...

B. ...under pressure of intestines, which spill into sac that has formed

C. Twisting or swelling of intestine may cut off blood supply to loop of intestine in sac (strangulation). Gangrene sets in unless promptly attended to

the disease and its causes   Blood pressure readings are taken to learn the force
with which blood is pressing on artery walls. The heart exerts the highest pressure (systole phase) when it is pumping a fresh supply of blood,
and the lowest pressure (diastole phase) when it pauses between beats
to fill with blood. When readings are repeatedly above 150 systolic and
100 diastolic, they indicate that the blood circulation of the patient is
impaired, and he is said to have high blood pressure, or hypertension.
Factors within the blood vessels, such as the elasticity and resistance of
the circulatory system, play a major role. The amount of blood within
the circulatory system, the thickness of that blood, and the amount of
blood put out by the heart with each beat are other considerations.
Known causes of high blood pressure include anemia, hyperthyroid
disease, chronic kidney diseases, certain endocrine disorders, brain
tumors, and congenital defects in the aorta. However, in most patients
suffering from high blood pressure, the cause is unknown.

symptoms   Elevated or high blood pressure itself rarely produces any significant
symptoms.
There can be complaints of dull, pounding headaches over the back of
the head, which start in the morning and wear off during the day. There
can be nervousness, dizziness, palpitations, and weakness. Nosebleed
is sometimes a symptom.
With kidney disease there may be blood in the urine.
When there is cerebral arteriosclerosis or coronary heart disease, the
symptoms are as described in this book under those headings. When
hypertensive heart disease develops, heart failure and its symptoms can
follow. On rare occasions, hypertension will develop rapidly and progressively—with acute attacks marked by headaches, visual disturbances,
vomiting, coma, and convulsions.

complications   Again, these depend upon the organ involved. With the kidneys,
kidney failure with uremia can develop. With coronary artery disease,
myocardial infarction, in which there is death of some of the tissues of
the heart muscle, can develop. If hypertensive heart disease develops,
a common follow-up is congestive heart failure. When there is involvement of blood vessels of the brain, complications include cerebral vascular accidents such as strokes.

prevention (or lessening of impact)   The cause should be established, if possible.
If one kidney is involved, surgery very often can either cure the condition or delay the onset of serious symptoms. If tumors of the endocrine
system are the cause, surgery may be the cure. If a patient is badly
overweight, that condition should be corrected.
The emotional state of a patient could be a factor and should be investigated and treated, if possible.
When no cause is found, the doctor will prescribe a program of diet and
medication to make the patient more comfortable.

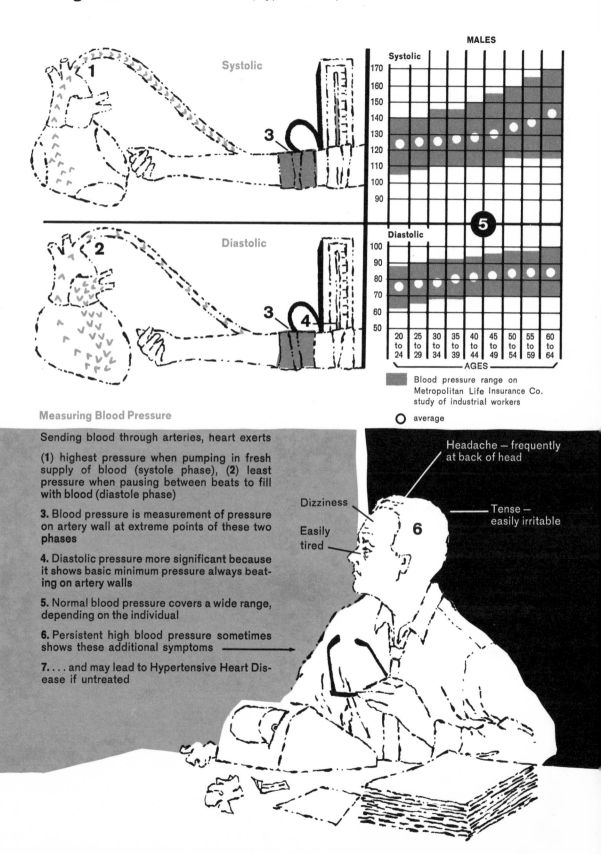

MALES

Systolic

170 160 150 140 130 120 110 100 90

Diastolic

100 90 80 70 60 50

AGES: 20 to 24 | 25 to 29 | 30 to 34 | 35 to 39 | 40 to 44 | 45 to 49 | 50 to 54 | 55 to 59 | 60 to 64

Blood pressure range on Metropolitan Life Insurance Co. study of industrial workers

○ average

Measuring Blood Pressure

Sending blood through arteries, heart exerts

(**1**) highest pressure when pumping in fresh supply of blood (systole phase), (**2**) least pressure when pausing between beats to fill with blood (diastole phase)

3. Blood pressure is measurement of pressure on artery wall at extreme points of these two **phases**

4. Diastolic pressure more significant because it shows basic minimum pressure always beating on artery walls

5. Normal blood pressure covers a wide range, depending on the individual

6. Persistent high blood pressure sometimes shows these additional symptoms ———→

7. . . . and may lead to Hypertensive Heart Disease if untreated

Headache — frequently at back of head

Dizziness

Easily tired

Tense — easily irritable

the disease and its causes   This disease is caused by a spore of the fungus
Histoplasma capsulatum. (A fungus is a simple plant lacking chlorophyll
—like mushrooms, molds, and mildews. A spore is a one-celled form
by which the fungus reproduces. Microscopically small, spores float in
the air all around us.)
The fungus for histoplasmosis grows mainly in moist soil—in areas fre-
quented by chickens, bats, and birds. But even the soil of some urban
areas has been found to be infected.
Various forms of the disease have affected many thousands of people
living in the central portion of the U.S., principally around the Missis-
sippi, Missouri and Ohio river valleys.
The disease is usually contracted by inhaling air bearing spores. However, the disease can also be caught by eating contaminated food or
drinking contaminated liquids. It may be localized in the lungs, but in
severe cases it can spread throughout the body—affecting the lymph
system, liver, spleen, bowel, adrenal glands, bones, and nervous system.
Histoplasmosis makes its most severe attacks on infants and older people.
It strikes men more frequently than women.

symptoms   These may range from mild to severe. In the former case, the patient
suffers a mild form of pneumonia or grippe which is over in 7–10 days.
Among the symptoms that appear are mild fever, cough, scratchy throat,
and chills. In cases caused by eating contaminated food, ulceration
(pitting) of the tongue, mouth, gums and larynx may occur. A severe
case of histoplasmosis may result in cough, chest pain, high fever, and
enlargement of the liver and spleen.
A wide variety of other symptoms can be present, depending on the
organs involved. The disease may cause cavities in the lungs which heal
by calcification of the lesion, as in tuberculosis. Therefore, histoplamosis
is sometimes confused on a chest X ray with tuberculosis.
A doctor is able to identify this disease by isolating the fungus in cultures
taken from sites of infection in the patient. Skin tests and blood tests are
also helpful.

complications   Complications occur in severe cases where the disease has spread
through the body. These complications can include endocarditis, meningitis, adrenal shock, and death.

prevention (or lessening of impact)   Prevention can best be accomplished by avoiding exposure to soil and dust in areas known to be infected. People
working around chickens in disease-prone areas should, if possible, wear
gauze masks to prevent inhalation of the spores. It is also important to
observe strict sanitary precautions, such as always washing the hands
before eating.
Specific drugs are available for treatment. But in the severe form, histoplasmosis may take several months of medical attention to clear up.

Histoplasmosis

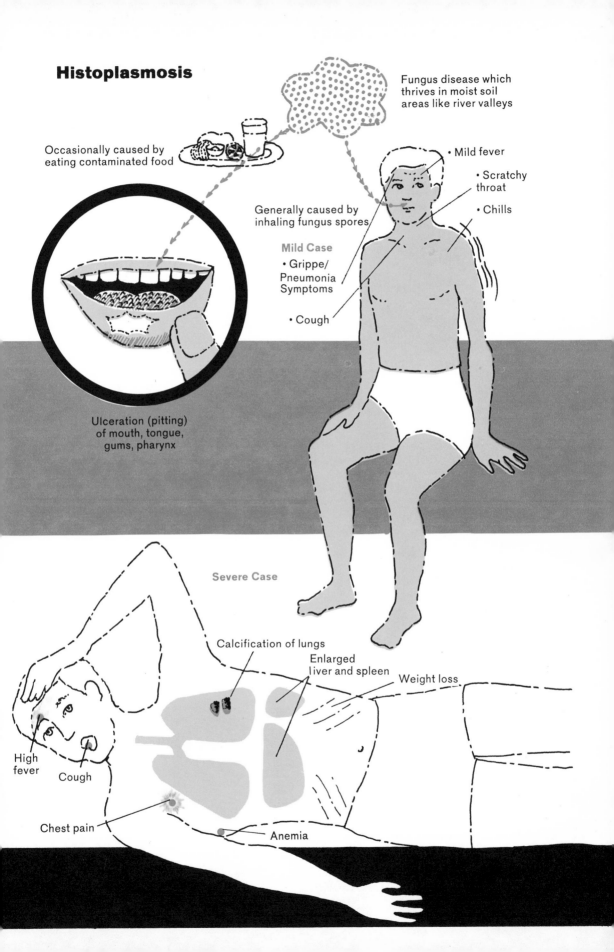

Fungus disease which thrives in moist soil areas like river valleys

Occasionally caused by eating contaminated food

Generally caused by inhaling fungus spores

• Mild fever

• Scratchy throat

• Chills

Mild Case
• Grippe/ Pneumonia Symptoms

• Cough

Ulceration (pitting) of mouth, tongue, gums, pharynx

Severe Case

Calcification of lungs

Enlarged liver and spleen

Weight loss

High fever

Cough

Chest pain

Anemia

the disease and its causes   Hives are most often a reaction to foods or drugs. The most common foods responsible for hives include shellfish, chocolate, strawberries, nuts, citrus fruits, and eggs. In the drug group, the most common causes include penicillin, iodides, and the aspirin group. Often the cause cannot be determined. Frequently hives can be related to some form of emotional distress. There can be a relationship between hives and intestinal parasites. And hives can result from a focus of infection elsewhere in the body.

symptoms   The onset is usually sudden, although it is preceded as a rule by severe itching in the areas involved. When the hives appear, the skin is raised, the lesions are of various sizes and of various shades of color ranging from white to red. Within only a few minutes, hives can develop. Often they grow together to form one large hive or lesion.

Sometimes they come and go within a period of a few hours. Or they can remain as long as several days. In rare cases the hives are topped by watery blisters. Any part of the body can be involved, including the mouth and rectum. With some patients, even stroking the skin can produce a hive.

The itching can vary from mild to intense. The areas most commonly involved are those where there is some form of body pressure. In severe cases, the swelling can be tremendous, and the face or part of the body involved can become considerably disfigured.

complications   A serious complication can result when the throat becomes involved. Breathing can become difficult and there can be shortness of breath. In very acute cases the patient suffocates.

prevention (or lessening of impact)   Every effort should be made to avoid foods or drugs known to cause hives, or situations that precipitate them. Drugs are available to give relief to patients with hives. Where they are not effective, desensitization may be recommended to minimize reaction to agents which bring on hives.

An allergic disease of skin commonly caused by . . .

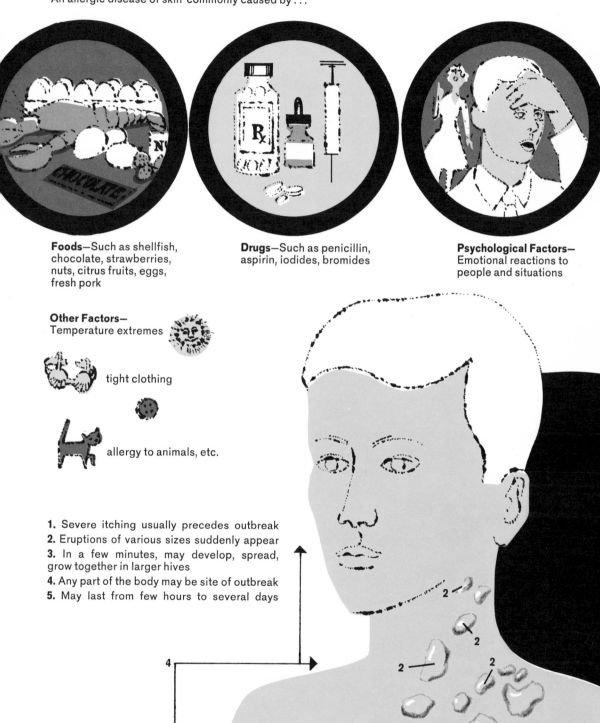

Foods—Such as shellfish, chocolate, strawberries, nuts, citrus fruits, eggs, fresh pork

Drugs—Such as penicillin, aspirin, iodides, bromides

Psychological Factors— Emotional reactions to people and situations

Other Factors— Temperature extremes

tight clothing

allergy to animals, etc.

1. Severe itching usually precedes outbreak
2. Eruptions of various sizes suddenly appear
3. In a few minutes, may develop, spread, grow together in larger hives
4. Any part of the body may be site of outbreak
5. May last from few hours to several days

Hodgkin's Disease
(Form of cancer that affects lymph glands)

the disease and its causes   This illness is a form of cancer which—like all cancers —is of unknown origin. It attacks the lymphoid system vital in the formation of blood. As a result, the body is unable to produce sufficient quantities of a type of blood cell which acts to combat disease.

Hodgkin's disease strikes more men than women—and generally between the ages of 25–35. Considered incurable ten years ago, it is now being successfully treated in a high percentage of cases in some large medical centers.

symptoms   Swelling of the lymph glands of the neck or chest are the most common early symptoms. These swellings are not painful or tender, and are freely movable in the early stages. Occasionally the glands in the armpits and groin are the first to enlarge. But in any case, all the glands of the body may eventually enlarge. Cough and voice changes are common when the glands in the chest enlarge.

Intermittent fever and sweating are also common symptoms of Hodgkin's disease. Often the liver and spleen enlarge.

complications   These depend on the severity of the disease—and what organs of the patient's body may have been invaded. If not diagnosed in time, the disease can reach the liver, spleen and bone marrow. The result can be severe anemia, secondary infections, and death. The doctor is able to diagnose by a biopsy (cutting out a piece of the tissue and examining it) of an affected lymph gland and, occasionally, by studies of the bone marrow.

prevention (or lessening of impact)   As with other cancers, there is no known method of preventing Hodgkin's disease. However, early diagnosis and treatment of the disease now hold out good hope for the victim.

Broadly speaking, when the disease is discovered early, treatment consists of surgical removal of the involved glands where possible, and X ray therapy to prevent spread or regrowth. Chemotherapy, using combinations of some of the new anti-cancer drugs, is also used—especially when the disease has spread to vital organs and surgery or radiation therapy would be harmful to them.

Hodgkin's Disease

(Form of cancer that affects lymph glands)

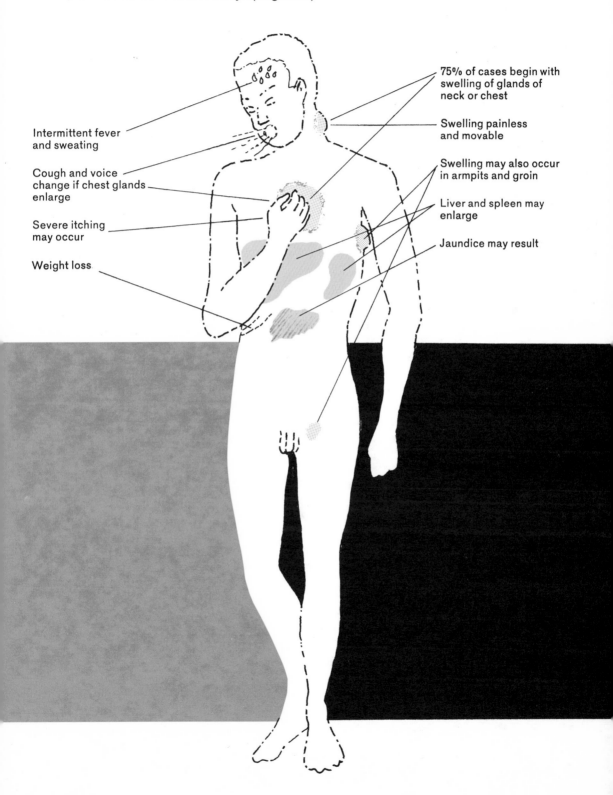

Intermittent fever and sweating

Cough and voice change if chest glands enlarge

Severe itching may occur

Weight loss

75% of cases begin with swelling of glands of neck or chest

Swelling painless and movable

Swelling may also occur in armpits and groin

Liver and spleen may enlarge

Jaundice may result

the disease and its causes Hookworm is a form of worm infection that can be a
severe problem because of the damaging nature of the worm *(Necator
americanus)* involved. This parasite was named the hookworm because
it attaches itself by prominent hook-like teeth to the victim's intestinal
wall where it sucks his blood.

As in other worm invasions, this disease spreads through the presence
of worms in the feces of infected individuals. The usual route for hookworm is for the feces of an infected individual to pollute the ground in
areas of poor sanitation. The larval form of hookworm penetrate a new
victim's bare feet and work their way via his bloodstream to his lungs
and back down to his digestive tract—where they attach themselves and
complete their life cycle.

A person may also be infected by the direct ingestion of the eggs, but
this is uncommon.

The worm develops to approximately half an inch in length. It is widely
found in the warmer parts of the western hemisphere—the southern
U.S., the West Indies, Central America, and northern South America.

symptoms Since the hookworm usually invades through the feet, primarily between
the toes, the victim develops red, inflamed, itching feet. This is called
ground itch.

During the migration of the parasite through the lungs, coughing and
fever may develop. Vomiting, diarrhea, and abdominal pain are possible
when the worms return to establish themselves in the intestines. If the
infection is a large one, the patient loses much blood and can become
anemic with resultant weakness.

A doctor can diagnose the disease rather easily by finding the eggs in
the patient's stool.

complications A severe case of hookworm in older people can lead to heart
problems. Among younger patients, physical and mental retardation can
result. If left untreated, a severe case can lead to severe loss of blood,
anemia and death.

prevention (or lessening of impact) Proper disposal of human feces is essential to
avoid soil pollution and the danger of hookworm. In most urban areas,
with adequate sewage disposal and flush toilets, this is no problem. But
in rural areas where hookworm is prevalent, it is important to wear
shoes at all times and avoid contacting the soil with bare feet.

If a diagnosis of hookworm is established, the doctor has effective ways
to combat the disease. Several drugs, such as *tetra chlorethyline,* can
eradicate the worms from the digestive tract. In addition, the doctor will
probably prescribe a proper diet and methods for replenishing the iron
that has been lost from the blood.

Hookworm

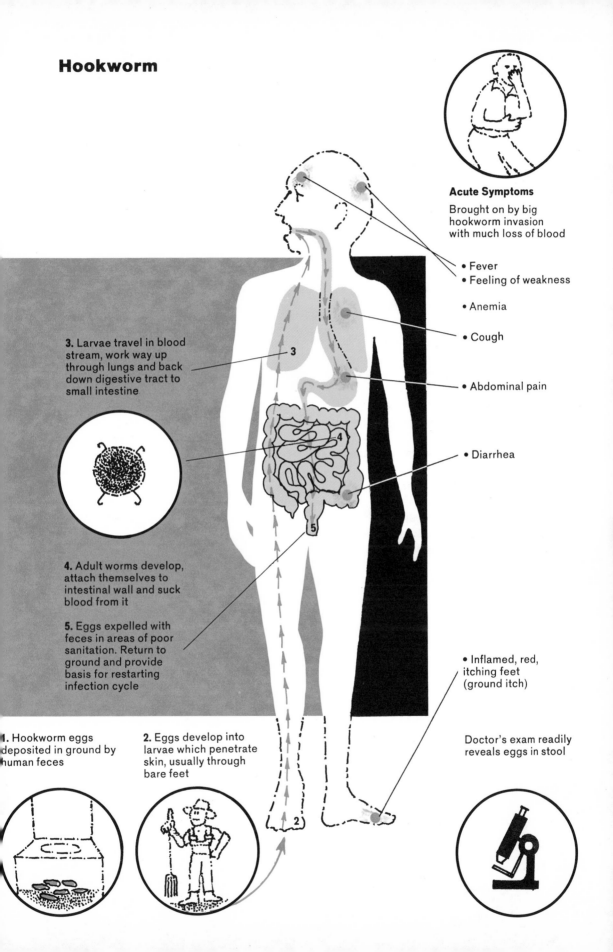

Acute Symptoms
Brought on by big hookworm invasion with much loss of blood

- Fever
- Feeling of weakness

- Anemia

- Cough

- Abdominal pain

- Diarrhea

3. Larvae travel in blood stream, work way up through lungs and back down digestive tract to small intestine

4. Adult worms develop, attach themselves to intestinal wall and suck blood from it

5. Eggs expelled with feces in areas of poor sanitation. Return to ground and provide basis for restarting infection cycle

- Inflamed, red, itching feet (ground itch)

Doctor's exam readily reveals eggs in stool

1. Hookworm eggs deposited in ground by human feces

2. Eggs develop into larvae which penetrate skin, usually through bare feet

the diseases and their causes   These are abnormalities that appear within the scrotum—the bag of flesh that surrounds the testicles. The causes are unknown. However, hydrocele may occur after the testicle has suffered an
inflammatory disease.
Varicocele usually develops after the onset of puberty (in the early
teens). Hydrocele may develop at any age. While not serious, they may
become disabling due to the size the abnormality attains or the symptoms
produced.

symptoms   In the case of hydrocele, the scrotal sac begins to increase in size. It
may get so large that the penis becomes completely hidden. The scrotum
then resembles a bag filled with water. It creates a heavy, dragging sensation. During a medical examination by the doctor, the sac transmits
light, indicating that there is no tumor or hernia to block the ray of light.
A varicocele consists of varicose veins along the spermatic cord, as
shown in the accompanying illustration. An extremely large development of these may cause the patient to feel—and complain of—heaviness
or actual pain in the groin. Varicoceles have been described as feeling
like a "bag of worms." They usually occur on the left side. However,
varicoceles are usually small, and frequently disappear.

complications   Neither of these conditions presents a serious threat to the sufferer's
health. But the size of the hydrocele may create an obstacle to leading
an active, normal daily life.

prevention (or lessening of impact)   Hydroceles may be drained or surgically removed. In either case, future prospects are excellent.
Treatment is rarely undertaken for varicoceles, since they frequently disappear by themselves. In extreme cases, the varicose vein may be surgically removed with little risk.

Hydrocele and Varicocele

Hydrocele

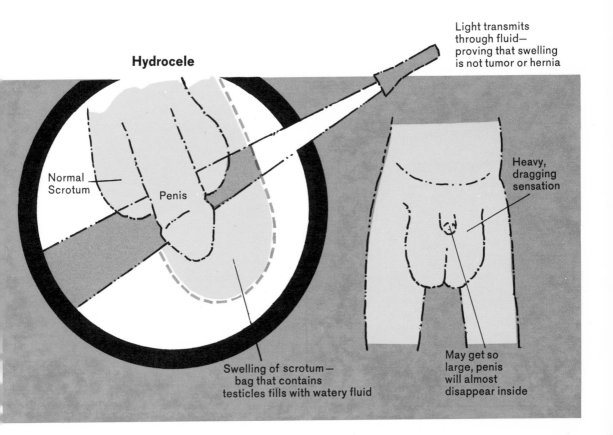

Light transmits through fluid— proving that swelling is not tumor or hernia

Normal Scrotum

Penis

Heavy, dragging sensation

Swelling of scrotum— bag that contains testicles fills with watery fluid

May get so large, penis will almost disappear inside

Varicocele

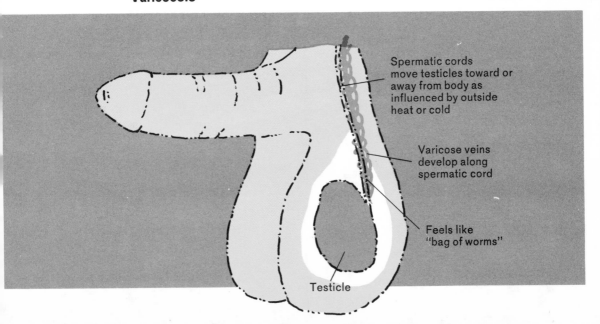

Spermatic cords move testicles toward or away from body as influenced by outside heat or cold

Varicose veins develop along spermatic cord

Feels like "bag of worms"

Testicle

the disease and its causes   A benign or malignant tumor of the parathyroid, or simple overstimulation of one of the four parathyroid glands, can cause an abnormal increase in their activity and the amount of parathyroid hormone they secrete. The result is a disease called hyperparathyroidism. It is seen more often in women than in men, and most often in middle age.

The disease is important because it is frequently an unrecognized cause of kidney stones. These are formed when the excessive secretion of parathyroid hormone causes calcium to be withdrawn from the bones and excreted by the kidneys. This calcium depletion can also result in a cystic disease of the bone (a hole in a bone caused by the disappearance of calcium). And excess calcium is often deposited in other organ systems.

Since calcium is excreted primarily by the kidneys, the greatest harm is done to the urinary system. Renal insufficiency, which is an inadequate functioning of the kidneys, is a frequent end result.

Symptoms   Generally, the earliest symptoms are the result of the depletion of bone calcium and increased calcium in the blood. These include constipation, nausea, muscle weakness, and appetite loss. The patient has to urinate frequently and heavily because of the extra calcium excreted in the urine, and complains of excessive thirst.

There may be anemia, deafness, bone pain, unusual tingling of the hands or feet, and weight loss. Peptic ulcer often develops as an associated illness. Most often the earliest symptom is the appearance of kidney stones or a bone fracture.

Body deformities often result from fractures or vertebral collapse. X ray examination reveals characteristic cystic bone changes, most often in the long bones, vertebrae, skull, and jaw. Blood calcium studies help to make the diagnosis.

complications   These include spontaneous bone fractures (fractures without sufficient cause), inadequate kidney function resulting from kidney destruction, deafness, and the disability that results from repeated passage of kidney stones.

prevention (or lessening of impact)   Once the diagnosis is made, the cure is to remove the offending parathyroid gland. The bones then heal. If the deformities are not great, the cure can be complete. The bones recalcify normally, the blood level of calcium becomes normal, kidney stones are no longer formed, and all symptoms disappear.

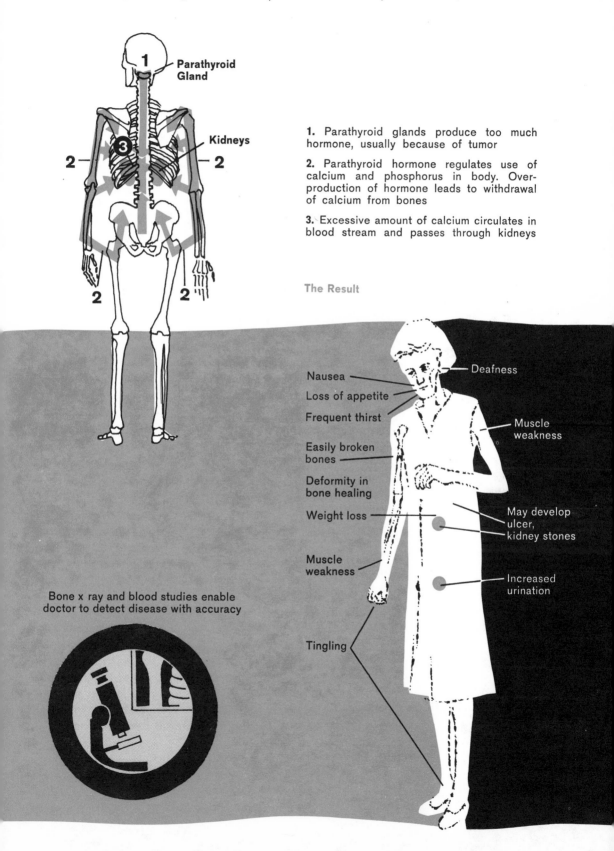

Parathyroid Gland

Kidneys

1. Parathyroid glands produce too much hormone, usually because of tumor

2. Parathyroid hormone regulates use of calcium and phosphorus in body. Overproduction of hormone leads to withdrawal of calcium from bones

3. Excessive amount of calcium circulates in blood stream and passes through kidneys

The Result

Deafness

Nausea

Loss of appetite

Frequent thirst

Muscle weakness

Easily broken bones

Deformity in bone healing

Weight loss

May develop ulcer, kidney stones

Muscle weakness

Increased urination

Tingling

Bone x ray and blood studies enable doctor to detect disease with accuracy

the disease and its causes In these conditions there is an overproduction of thyroid hormone by the thyroid gland. Goiter, which is the name given to any thyroid enlargement, is not the same as hyperthyroidism, although in some cases it is associated. While hyperthyroidism can be seen at any age, it occurs most frequently from 20 to 40 years, and occurs more in females—especially during puberty, pregnancy, and menopause—than in males. The disease appears to run in families.
The cause is completely unknown, but there may be some relationship to overstimulation by the pituitary gland. In some cases it seems to be correlated with infections, stresses, or psychic trauma, but the relationship is unclear.

symptoms As illustrated in the Medi-Graph, the classical patient with an overactive thyroid has protruding, staring eyes, tremors of the fingers when they are extended, increased nervousness, and profuse sweating. Hot weather bothers her. Her breath is short and she has palpitations or associated findings which may be related to the effects on the heart. Menstruation may cease. Enlargement of the thyroid gland may become apparent to the eye or touch. Muscle weakness is common. The patient complains she cannot climb stairs as she did previously. She has a marked stare and blinks infrequently. Her skin appears reddened and sweaty. The nails' shape changes and becomes concave, like a shallow spoon. On examination the doctor may find a change in the heart rate and rhythm, and in the blood pressure.
As the disease advances there is very evident weight loss. The patient becomes almost intolerably irritable. A basal metabolism test, specific blood studies, and radioactive iodine studies are used by the doctor to establish a diagnosis.

complications A serious complication is thyroid storm which occurs in debilitated patients or those exposed to unusual stress or strain. There is high fever, delirium, and abnormal racing of the heart. Shock, and even death, can occur. Thyroid heart disease (more fully described elsewhere in this book) is not unusual and can end in heart failure.
Another complication has to do with the unfavorable appearance caused by the protruding eyes characteristic of this condition. Unfortunately, this may or may not change—even after treatment.

prevention (or lessening of impact) There is no known way of preventing hyperthyroidism. In areas where iodine is lacking in the diet, it is recommended that iodized foods be used to prevent the development of simple goiter. If treated early enough and before complications develop, hyperthyroidism responds to treatment by drugs, surgery, or radioactive chemicals. Early recognition is usually not too difficult and prompt therapy, simple in nature, may be enough to control all symptoms and any disability.

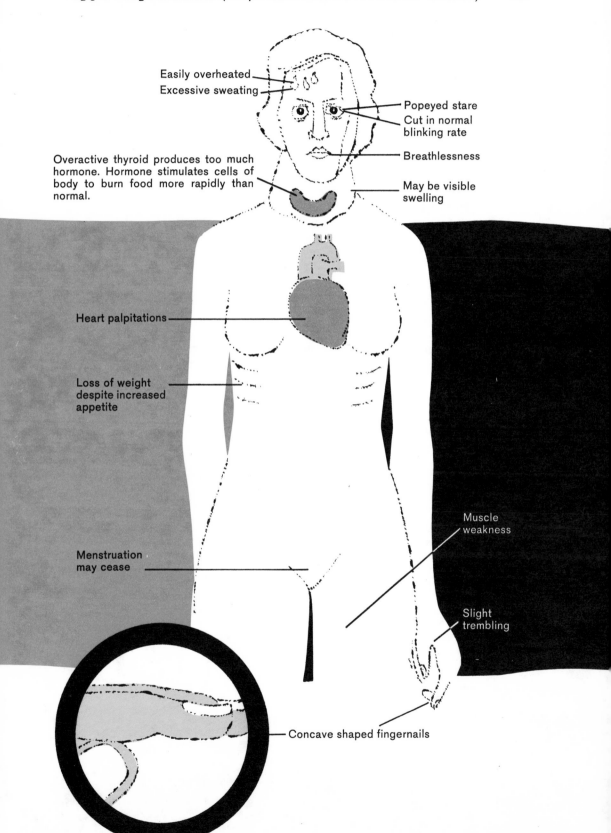

Easily overheated

Excessive sweating

Popeyed stare

Cut in normal blinking rate

Breathlessness

Overactive thyroid produces too much hormone. Hormone stimulates cells of body to burn food more rapidly than normal.

May be visible swelling

Heart palpitations

Loss of weight despite increased appetite

Muscle weakness

Menstruation may cease

Slight trembling

Concave shaped fingernails

Hypoglycemia (Low Blood Sugar)

the disease and its causes   This is a disease in which the amount of sugar in the blood falls to abnormally low levels. Without a normal fuel supply, the hypoglycemia sufferer feels weak and tired—and in extreme cases goes into a coma or convulsions.

The condition is due to overproduction of insulin (which regulates blood sugar levels) by the pancreas (which manufactures insulin for the body). A wide variety of factors can cause this illness. These include tumors of the pancreas, inadequate functioning of the pituitary or adrenal glands, and certain liver diseases. Diabetics taking insulin to remedy their condition can suffer hypoglycemia attacks because of mistakenly taking too large a dose—or because of their exceptional reactions to the drug.

In some cases of hypoglycemia, the cause is emotional. One type of person seems to overreact to stress by producing too much insulin, thereby driving his blood sugar down.

symptoms   As the accompanying illustration shows, the symptoms vary, depending on whether there is a sudden and rapid decline of blood sugar in an acute attack of hypoglycemia or whether the blood sugar drops slowly over a long period of time.

Symptoms developing because of pancreatic tumors or other physical problems usually cause a slow drop in blood sugar with those associated symptoms. Attacks caused by emotional problems usually exhibit the symptoms associated with a rapid drop in blood sugar. These symptoms usually occur 2–4 hours after eating, usually are mild, and subside in about 30 minutes.

The doctor diagnoses the illness by a glucose tolerance test.

complications   Hypoglycemia sufferers who also have cerebral or coronary arteriosclerosis can suffer a stroke or heart attack because of a sudden drop in blood sugar. Prolonged hypoglycemia can result in death.

prevention (or lessening of impact)   When pancreatic tumors are the cause of hypoglycemia, surgery is effective.

When the disease is caused by emotional reactions, it is helpful if the sufferer switches to a high-protein, high-fat, and low-carbohydrate diet, eaten in small quantities on a 6 meal a day basis, and tries to eat these meals under relaxed circumstances.

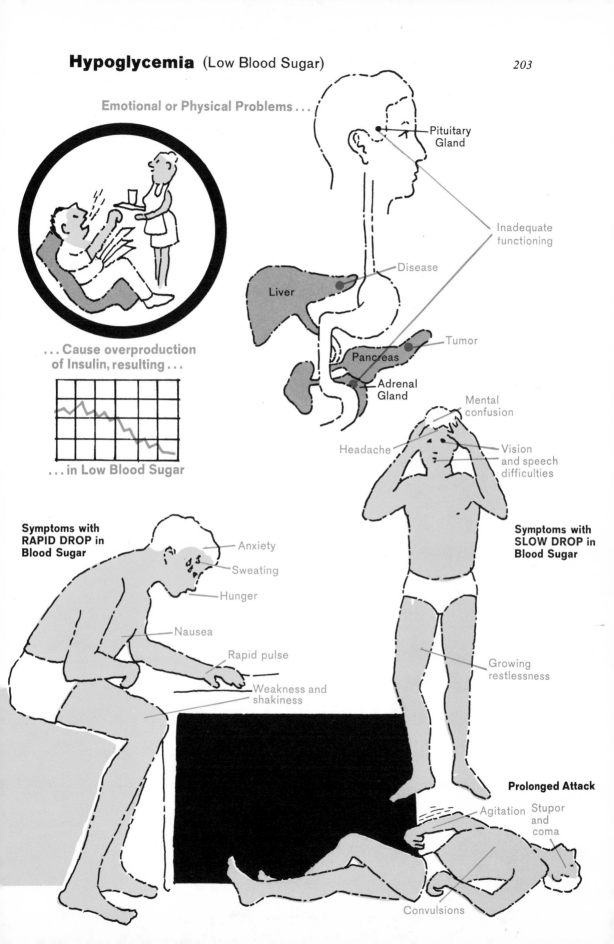

Hypoglycemia (Low Blood Sugar)

Emotional or Physical Problems...

... Cause overproduction of Insulin, resulting ...

... in Low Blood Sugar

Pituitary Gland

Inadequate functioning

Disease

Liver

Tumor

Pancreas

Adrenal Gland

Mental confusion

Headache

Vision and speech difficulties

Symptoms with SLOW DROP in Blood Sugar

Symptoms with RAPID DROP in Blood Sugar

Anxiety

Sweating

Hunger

Nausea

Rapid pulse

Weakness and shakiness

Growing restlessness

Prolonged Attack

Agitation

Stupor and coma

Convulsions

Hypogonadism and Simmonds' Disease

(Underactive Pituitary Gland Disorders)

the disease and its causes   The anterior, or forward part, of the pituitary gland affects the working of a variety of other glands such as the thyroid, ovary and testicle, adrenal, breast, and pancreas. In addition, the anterior pituitary hormone is responsible for body growth.

When any condition prevents the pituitary gland from functioning properly, the body is profoundly affected and suffers from a variety of disorders grouped under the heading of hypopituitarism, which means underactivity of the pituitary gland. Most often this interference with the pituitary gland is the result of the destructive effects of a tumor, or some inflammatory disease, or a vascular disturbance. The age at which the disease develops determines to some extent the symptoms and end result.

symptoms   When there is destruction or change in the pituitary gland *before* the onset of puberty (the age at which boys and girls mature sexually— usually in the early or middle teens), the disease is marked by dwarfism and subnormal sexual development. There is little change in other glandular functions. The patient's mentality is unaffected. He is a well-proportioned dwarf who remains sexually immature. Such cases are quite rare and are usually caused by the destructive effects of a tumor upon the anterior pituitary gland.

In cases of hypopituitarism which occur *after* the onset of puberty, there are deficiencies in most of the glands affected by the pituitary. These glands may become inactive at various times, but it may take years for the negative effects to become clear.

Symptoms of hypogonadism and Simmonds' disease—two disorders resulting from underactivity of the pituitary gland—are detailed in the accompanying Medi-Graph.

complications   These depend on the cause. When a malignant tumor is responsible, one complication, of course, can be a spread of the malignancy. If it attacks the nearby optic nerves, the patient can become blind. Eventually, since there is interference with all glandular functions, the patient can die from secondary infections as well as from general loss of strength.

prevention (or lessening of impact)   Nothing can be done to prevent this disease, but early recognition can help to stop its progression before secondary effects seriously affect body functions.

X ray or surgery may be effective in removing tumors. If the body metabolism is not thrown off balance too severely, treatment to replace lost hormones can be effective and give the patient a remarkable degree of recovery of lost functions.

The subject of glandular malfunction is a complicated one. This form, as well as most others, requires expert care and evaluation.

Hypogonadism and Simmonds' Disease
(Underactive Pituitary Gland Disorders)

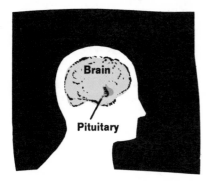

Front part of pituitary gland is attacked by tumor, impairment of blood supply or inflammation. Result may be under-production of sex—and other—hormones.

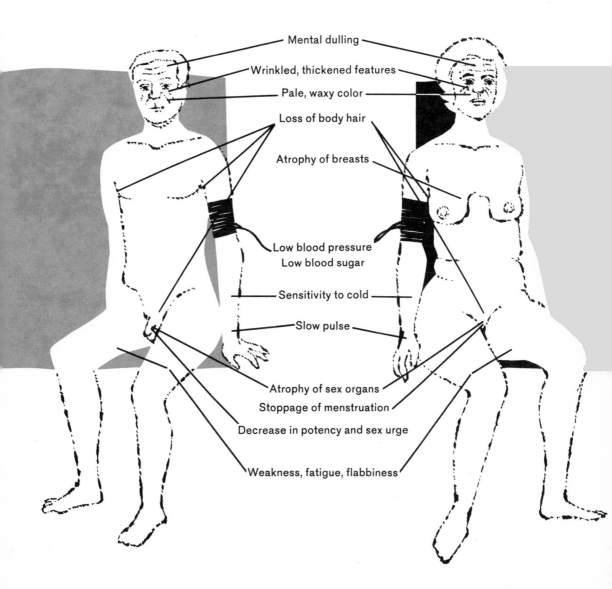

Mental dulling

Wrinkled, thickened features

Pale, waxy color

Loss of body hair

Atrophy of breasts

Low blood pressure
Low blood sugar

Sensitivity to cold

Slow pulse

Atrophy of sex organs

Stoppage of menstruation

Decrease in potency and sex urge

Weakness, fatigue, flabbiness

the disease and its causes   Regional ileitis, also known as enteritis, is an inflammatory disease of the ileum—the lower portion of the small intestine lying at a point close to the appendix. Sometimes it extends the full length of the small intestine and even into the large bowel. The cause is uncertain, but it is believed that emotional stress and anxiety play a large part. Both sexes are affected, generally between the ages of 35 and 50. The course of the disease is marked by periods of apparent cure, unfortunately followed frequently by relapses.

symptoms   Ileitis is often confused with acute appendicitis because the symptoms and the region of pain are much the same. There may be a history of mild nausea, continuous or intermittent, over a long period of time. Frequently there is crampy pain over the right lower part of the abdomen. The abdomen swells. The patient may have a low-grade fever. Occasionally there is severe, bloody diarrhea. As the scar tissue builds up and the obstruction becomes more severe, there is constipation and conspicuous abdominal bloating.

Sometimes fistulas develop. These are narrow, curved passages or openings which cannot close up because they are infected. In this situation they develop between loops of the intestine or from the ileum through to the skin.

As the disease progresses, the patient shows signs of weight loss, malnutrition, and swelling of the feet.

complications   The constant inflammation can result in a perforation or piercing through the intestines. This, in turn, can lead to abscess or peritonitis (a severe infection). Other complications include intestinal obstruction, arthritis, and occasionally severe intestinal hemorrhage.

prevention (or lessening of impact)   There is no way of preventing ileitis, but if it is diagnosed soon enough the progress of the disease can be halted. In addition to a program of medicine and diet, steps may be taken to help the patient deal with some of his emotional problems. Ileitis can and does recur, but it is not unusual for a patient to recover after a single attack.

Where the disease has progressed too far and the complications are threatening, surgery is required to correct the condition.

Inflammation of Intestine

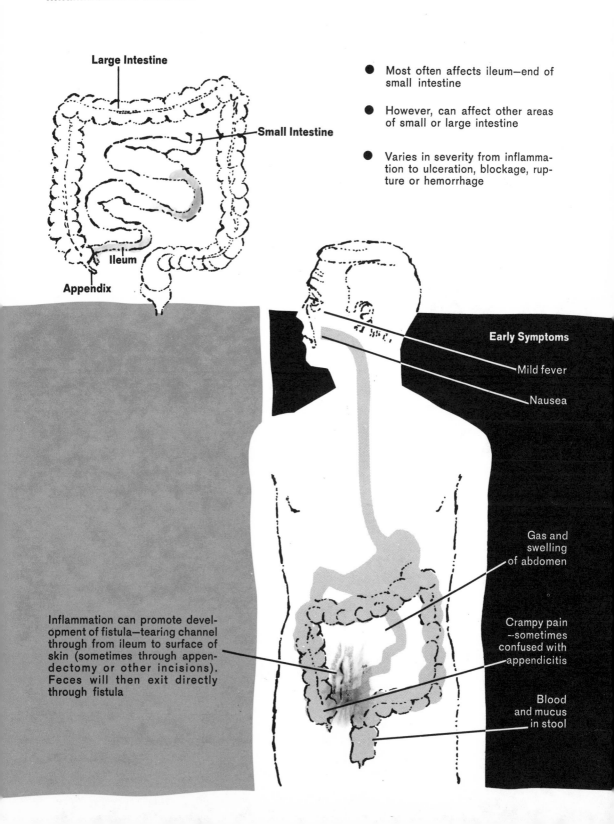

Large Intestine

Small Intestine

Ileum

Appendix

- Most often affects ileum—end of small intestine

- However, can affect other areas of small or large intestine

- Varies in severity from inflammation to ulceration, blockage, rupture or hemorrhage

Early Symptoms

Mild fever

Nausea

Gas and swelling of abdomen

Crampy pain —sometimes confused with appendicitis

Blood and mucus in stool

Inflammation can promote development of fistula—tearing channel through from ileum to surface of skin (sometimes through appendectomy or other incisions). Feces will then exit directly through fistula

the disease and its causes   This is an acute infectious disease of the skin usually caused by the streptococcus or staphylococcus bacteria. Impetigo is frequently seen in children. In young infants it may be extensive and very severe. The disease is highly contagious, and it is not unusual for several members of one family to be infected.

symptoms   Impetigo usually begins as a small blister which rapidly enlarges, ruptures, and discharges a cloudy material. These lesions form a crust the color of honey. Scratching them usually spreads the infection to other parts of the body. The eruptions form a characteristic picture readily identified by the doctor.

complications   As a rule there are no serious complications. However, impetigo has been related to nephritis in young infants.

prevention (or lessening of impact)   Because of the contagious nature of impetigo, strict hygienic measures must be used. Children should be isolated from others in school and at home.

The disease responds rapidly to antibiotic ointments which will be prescribed by the doctor.

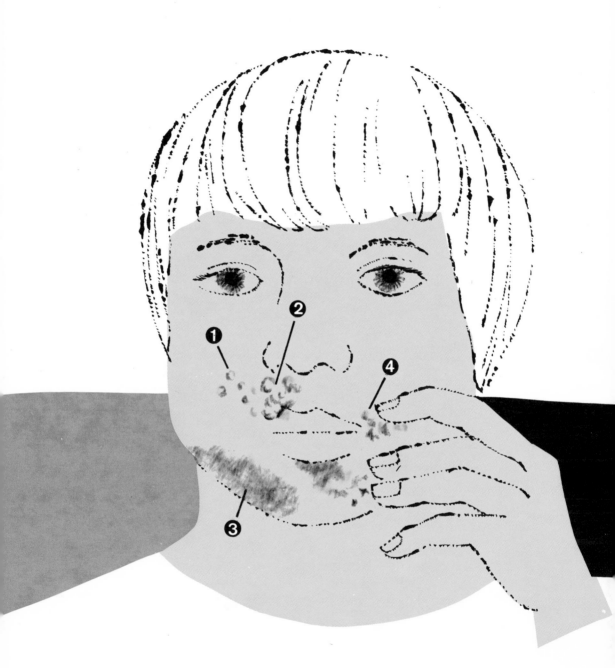

1. Small blisters on skin are first signs

2. Blisters enlarge rapidly, break, discharge cloudy pus

3. Skin becomes covered with pus filled eruptions, covered by crusty yellow scabs

4. Scratching spreads infection. Also contagious—spreading from child to child

the disease and its causes   Intestinal obstruction is a severe problem because it prevents the normal passage of food through the digestive tract. It may be caused by a variety of physical factors which mechanically obstruct the intestinal tract. These include tumors, foreign bodies, gallstones, parasites (such as worms), hernias, adhesions from operations, twisting of the intestine, etc.

There are also a number of possible non-mechanical causes of intestinal obstruction. These are called ileus by the medical profession and refer to chemical, bacterial, and circulatory problems which can prevent the normal passage of food through the intestines.

symptoms   The victim of acute intestinal obstruction usually finds himself suffering from abdominal pain, swelling of the abdomen, vomiting and constipation. The vomiting is more severe if the obstruction is high in the intestinal tract. Obstruction low down in the tract more often produces constipation and swelling. A wide variety of other symptoms may occur depending upon the cause, degree and length of blockage.

In the normal digestive process, the intestines move ingested material in regular rhythmic waves from the stomach down to the rectum along a coiled 28-foot length. In this process (called *peristalsis*), nutritional elements are extracted, absorbed into the bloodstream, and then circulated to the rest of the body. Blockage prevents this process from functioning normally and may set up a reverse peristalsis where the food becomes backed up—and where vomiting will occur, with loss of nutrients and water. In addition, the food that is trapped above the blockage may decompose and cause inflammation and bacterial infection of the bowel wall. The poisonous toxins that result may bring about a perforation of the intestinal wall that can cause peritonitis (inflammation of the lining of the intestines and abdomen). This in turn may lead to shock, high fever and disorientation.

The doctor diagnoses the disease by examination of the abdomen, X rays and laboratory tests. Surgery is almost always necessary to remove the mechanical type of obstruction, but the ileus type is usually cleared up by drugs and other medical measures.

complications   If intestinal obstruction is not attended to quickly, it can lead to such severe complications as perforation and peritonitis, gangrene, severe poisoning, disturbance of the body chemistry and dehydration. If untreated, any one of these can be fatal.

prevention (or lessening of impact)   If diagnosed early, intestinal obstruction can usually be handled by a program of antibiotics to fight infection, and surgery or drugs to remove the obstruction. The doctor also frequently prescribes a lot of fluids for the patient, to replace fluid loss. And to help decompress the disturbed bowel, the doctor may pass a tube down from the mouth to the blockage point.

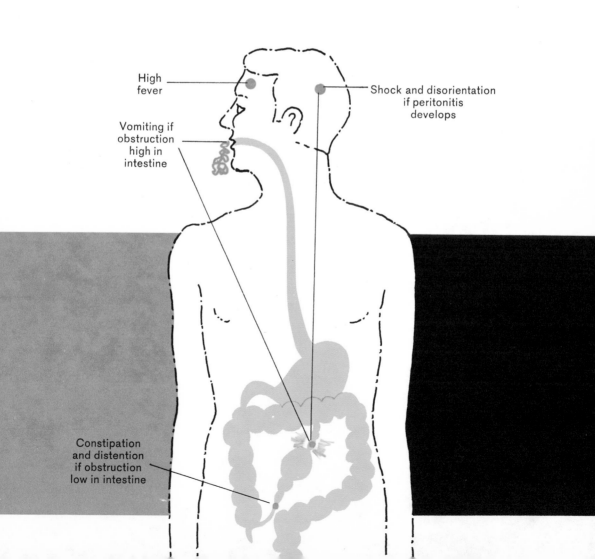

Blockage of movement of food through intestinal tract, with swelling and backup, from such causes as:

Mechanical Obstructions

Tumors

Gallstones

Worms and other parasites

Hernias

Adhesions

Twisting

Non-mechanical Obstructions (Ileus)

Chemical

Bacterial

Circulatory

High fever

Shock and disorientation if peritonitis develops

Vomiting if obstruction high in intestine

Constipation and distention if obstruction low in intestine

the disease and its causes   Iritis is a disease of the iris—the colored part of the eye. The function of the iris is to regulate the amount of light admitted to the interior of the eye. Infection and inflammation of the iris interfere with its ability to admit the correct amount of light—and thus cause vision problems.

Among the possible causes of iritis are infection from bacteria—particularly the Staphylococcus variety—and secondary infection from syphilis, gonorrhea, and TB. Diabetes may also cause iritis—and so may an injury to the eye.

symptoms   As the illustration shows, the iris becomes smaller and less distinct in color. Blue eyes turn green and darker eyes turn muddy in color. The pupil—the small black circle in the center of the iris—contracts in size and becomes sluggish in action.

Since the pupil is the opening through which the eye admits light, this sluggishness in bright light means that too much light will be admitted, causing discomfort. The eye is constantly tearing. The vision is blurred. There is pain—usually worse at night. It radiates from the eye to the forehead and to the temples.

complications   Since all parts of the eye are in intimate contact with each other, with fluid circulating between them, infections can easily spread. Involvement of the cornea, leading to serious long-term vision problems, is a possible complication. Glaucoma is another one. And blindness is, of course, the most serious potential hazard.

prevention (or lessening of impact)   Prompt treatment of all eye infections, and other underlying illnesses, is essential in preventing iritis. Once the disease is present, it requires careful treatment by an eye doctor. When the infection has been healed, surgical operations of various kinds may be necessary to bring the iris back to normal shape, and to aid in vision.

Iritis

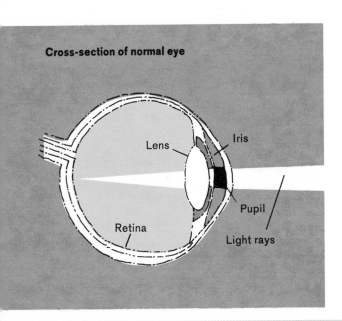

Cross-section of normal eye

Lens

Iris

Pupil

Retina

Light rays

Iris regulates amount of light admitted to interior of eye. Light rays from objects pass through pupil and lens of eye and transmit picture to retina. Iris allows size of pupil to expand in dim light to let maximum in . . . contracts size of pupil in bright light to prevent glare.

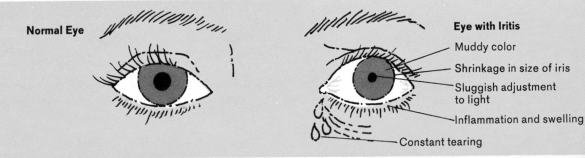

Normal Eye

Eye with Iritis

Muddy color

Shrinkage in size of iris

Sluggish adjustment to light

Inflammation and swelling

Constant tearing

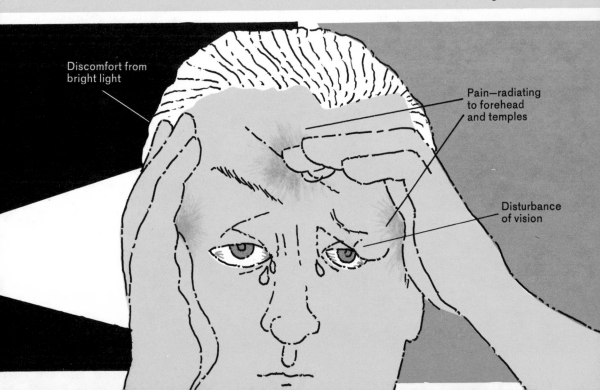

Discomfort from bright light

Pain—radiating to forehead and temples

Disturbance of vision

the disease and its causes Stones in the urinary tract are common and are found in both men and women, though rarely before the age of 20. There are different types of stones, each made up of assorted combinations of chemicals ordinarily excreted by the kidneys. It is not known exactly what causes these stones to form, but there are many theories. Some authorities think that patients have an inherited tendency toward the formation of stones, while others believe they simply might be the result of common family habits of diet, water intake, and mode of living.

When urine is concentrated it can predispose toward the formation of stones. Patients who do not take enough liquids may promote this condition. Another widely held theory is that stones may result from an abnormal change occurring in the colloid material which is present in the urine—the colloid material normally prevents the chemicals there from grouping together to form stones.

Other possible causes include the effect of vitamin D. When taken in quantity it can cause a heavy concentration of calcium to be excreted in the urine. Certain diseases of the parathyroid gland can act in the same way to form stones.

Gout is a common cause of kidney stones. The high uric acid content of the blood that is secreted into the urine by a gout sufferer will sometimes form uric acid stones.

Prolonged, complete bed rest sets the scene for the formation of kidney stones. It is one of the reasons patients are advised to get up and walk soon after an operation.

symptoms As the Medi-Graph shows, symptoms of urinary stones depend upon their location. And their location and movement determine whether the pain is steady, dull, and aching or excruciatingly sharp.

In about half the cases there is blood in the urine that is visible to the naked eye or under a microscope. However, the absence of blood does not mean there are no stones.

complications Prolonged or repeated attacks can cause a kidney to become enlarged and eventually to stop functioning. This can result in blood pressure changes, uremia, or infection. Without adequate drainage, kidney infections are very severe and can result in loss of the kidney.

prevention (or lessening of impact) It is important to determine the cause of the stone formation, if possible. Gout patients must be put on a medical program that will keep the uric acid crystals from solidifying into stones. Urinary tract infections should be treated. Any urine flow obstruction with which the patient may have been born must be corrected. Fluid intake should be high to dilute the urine. Weight increase should be avoided. Suitable vitamins must be prescribed. The doctor may take steps to increase the colloid character of the urine.

If a stone forms and does not pass by itself, it must be removed through a cystoscope, if possible, or surgically.

Kidney and Urinary Tract Stones

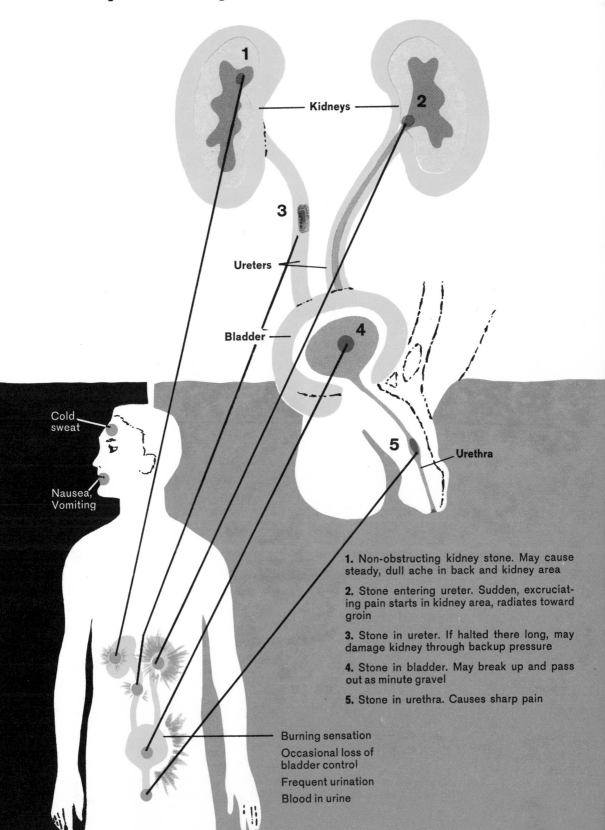

Kidneys

Ureters

Bladder

Cold sweat

Nausea, Vomiting

Urethra

1. Non-obstructing kidney stone. May cause steady, dull ache in back and kidney area

2. Stone entering ureter. Sudden, excruciating pain starts in kidney area, radiates toward groin

3. Stone in ureter. If halted there long, may damage kidney through backup pressure

4. Stone in bladder. May break up and pass out as minute gravel

5. Stone in urethra. Causes sharp pain

Burning sensation

Occasional loss of bladder control

Frequent urination

Blood in urine

the disease and its causes   Lead poisoning is becoming an ever increasing environmental problem—with increasing amounts of lead substances emitted in automobile exhausts, factory wastes, and industrial processes.

Among the specific ways lead poisoning is contracted is through prolonged working with paints with a lead base, inhalation of fumes of lead in burning batteries and solder, eating of food products contaminated with lead, drinking whiskey cooked in lead stills. or drinking water that has been stored in lead containers.

A particularly tragic problem is the eating of lead paint by children, particularly hungry ghetto children. The source here may be peeling wall or windowsill paint or lead-painted cribs, furniture or toys.

The bones store most of the lead. Prolonged exposure is required but since lead is poorly excreted by the body, exposure to heavy doses will sooner or later cause the accumulation of enough lead to trigger the illness.

symptoms   The prime symptom is colic—an agonizing abdominal pain. Not localized, it comes on suddenly and is often mistaken for a perforated ulcer. These colic attacks often recur and can be precipitated by overindulgence in alcoholic beverages.

In severe attacks of lead poisoning, neuritis (pain along the nerves) and paralysis often occur. The arms are most often involved and wrist drop is a common symptom. Anemia is also common—with the patient becoming quite pale in color.

Victims of lead poisoning also develop a "lead line"—a line of black along the edge of the gums at the tooth margin.

In children, a severe attack of lead poisoning can produce a form of encephalitis characterized by convulsions, delirium and coma. Mental retardation is a frequent result.

A doctor can diagnose lead poisoning by blood and urine tests. X rays of the liver may also reveal the presence of lead.

complications   Left unchecked, lead poisoning can damage the brain, with depression or even severe mental disturbances.

Severe cases of lead poisoning, particularly among children, can lead to death—especially if the disease has gone untreated so long that convulsions and coma have developed.

prevention (or lessening of impact)   Limiting lead paint to the exterior of buildings can help keep this hazard away from children. Watchful parents will also take care to check that there is no lead paint on interior walls, cribs and other furniture in the baby's room and on his toys. The fight to eliminate lead from the manufacture of gasoline will have to be waged to a successful conclusion. And care will have to be exercised in the handling of lead in paints and other industrial products and processes.

Early treatment of cases of lead poisoning can be effective. A doctor, when he has diagnosed the disease, can prescribe a drug which, given in repeated doses, can eliminate the lead from the body.

Lead Poisoning

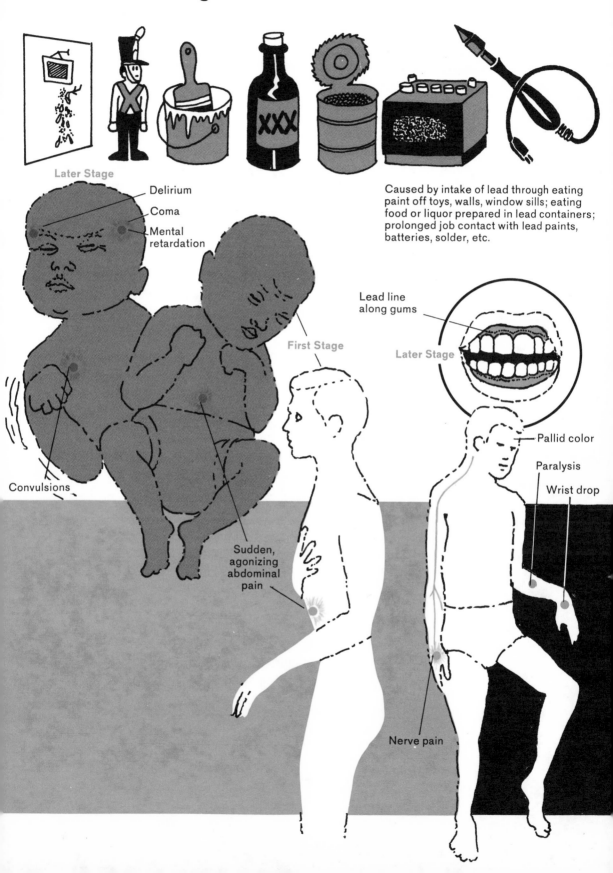

Later Stage

Delirium

Coma

Mental retardation

Caused by intake of lead through eating paint off toys, walls, window sills; eating food or liquor prepared in lead containers; prolonged job contact with lead paints, batteries, solder, etc.

Convulsions

First Stage

Sudden, agonizing abdominal pain

Lead line along gums

Later Stage

Pallid color

Paralysis

Wrist drop

Nerve pain

Leptospirosis
(Weil's Disease)

the disease and its causes   Leptospirosis is a blood infection caused by the spirochete-like organisms *leptospira*. (Spirochetes are corkscrew-shaped bacteria.) The leptospira get into the bloodstream and spread to various organs, with liver and kidney infection being most common.

Leptospirosis is a disease found primarily among animals such as rats, mice, cattle, hogs and dogs. Man is infected when water contaminated with urine of infected animals comes into contact with his skin. As a result, sewer workers, veterinarians, miners, farmers and soldiers are in the high risk group, particularly in countries with poor sanitation. Man may also be infected by the consumption of contaminated food or water.

The incubation period is 3–20 days.

symptoms   The disease comes on suddenly with high fever, marked aches and pains, headache, nausea and vomiting, chills and muscle pain. In most cases, the illness ends in 7–10 days.

The course of the illness is more severe in a type of leptospirosis called WEIL'S DISEASE, caused by the specific leptospira, *Icterohemorrhagiae*. Victims of Weil's disease may show signs of hemorrhaging in a number of places. Blood may appear in the stool, sputum, lining of the eyes, and under the skin. Nose bleeds may be a problem. Jaundice (yellowing of the skin and eyes) occurs at the end of the first week. The liver becomes enlarged and tender. Kidney failure may also occur in severe cases.

The doctor diagnoses leptospirosis by blood tests, including finding of the organism in the blood.

complications   Severe cases can develop meningitis, pneumonia and eye infections. Also, cases of kidney failure may result in death.

prevention (or lessening of impact)   Proper hygiene and sanitary measures, including safeguarding the freshness of the water supply and disposal of water contaminated with urine, can prevent leptospirosis. In treating a victim, the doctor concentrates on helping the kidneys to function and replacing blood loss. Specific antibiotics have been developed which are effective in treatment of the disease.

Leptospirosis
(Weil's Disease)

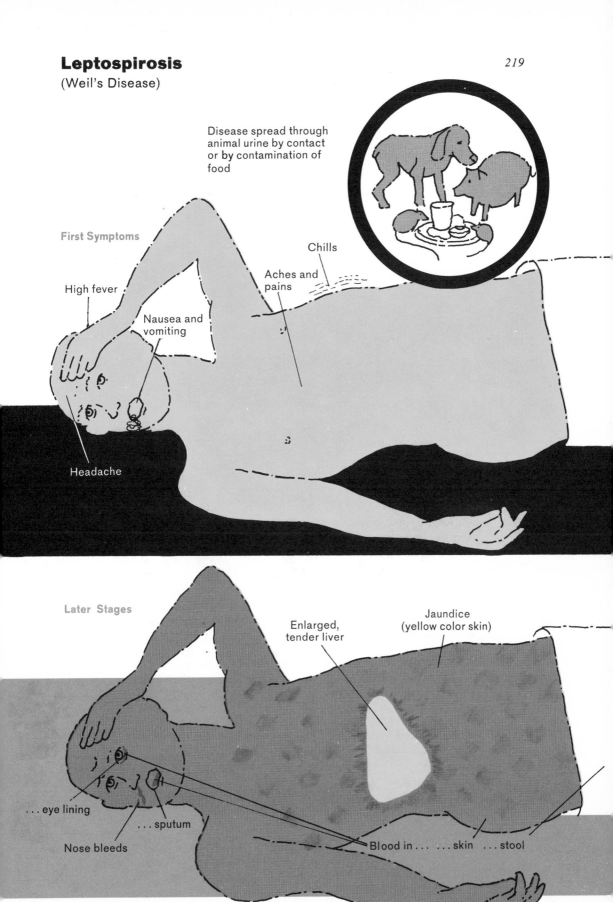

Disease spread through animal urine by contact or by contamination of food

First Symptoms

High fever

Nausea and vomiting

Chills

Aches and pains

Headache

Later Stages

Enlarged, tender liver

Jaundice (yellow color skin)

...eye lining

...sputum

Nose bleeds

Blood in... ...skin ...stool

Leukemia

(Cancer of blood involving abnormal increase of white blood cells)

the disease and its causes   There are many different types of leukemia, but all are a malignant disease of the white blood cells of the body. The cause of all types is still uncertain. Each type is determined by the specific blood cell involved and the length of time the illness lasts. Leukemia exists in both an acute and chronic form: it is detected when the blood is examined.

When the cell group known as the lymphocytes is affected, the disease is called lymphocytic leukemia. When the monocytes are involved, it is known as monocytic leukemia. And when the polymorphonuclear cells are involved, it is called myeloid leukemia.

The myeloid form attacks a younger age group than the lymphocytic. These two types are the ones seen most commonly, but almost all of what is noted here applies to leukemia in general.

Leukemia is more common in males than in females. The outcome of the disease depends upon the type, and whether it is in the acute or chronic form.

symptoms   In *acute* cases, as noted in the Medi-Graph, the onset is usually quite rapid and resembles an acute infectious disease. The earliest symptoms may be high fever, diffuse aches and pains, and severe weakness. Painful ulcerations of the mouth are not uncommon. There may be bone pain.

The course is unusually rapid, progressive, and downhill. There are hemorrhages of the mucous membranes of the mouth and into the skin. In the *chronic* case the disease develops stealthily and is discovered often during the course of a routine medical examination. The patient loses weight, appetite, and strength. He has night sweats and feels weak.

In the lymphatic form there is almost always swelling of the lymph glands. Sometimes the patient complains of pain in the abdomen in the area where the spleen lies. This is because that organ enlarges as the disease progresses. There is evidence of hemorrhaging—the patient bleeds from the mouth and develops blood spots under the skin. Weakness becomes more severe and the patient develops anemia.

complications   Because of the diminished resistance of the patient, he is subject to complications from secondary infections. Another serious problem is hemorrhage, frequently into the intestinal tract. Or it may involve any organ system.

prevention (or lessening of impact)   There is no way to prevent the onset of leukemia. There are many courses of treatment available which can prolong the life of the patient and even permit him to carry on his normal activity. Care must be taken to avoid secondary infection. There is no known cure, but with new research the outlook for patients with this illness continues to improve.

Leukemia

(Cancer of blood involving abnormal increase of white blood cells)

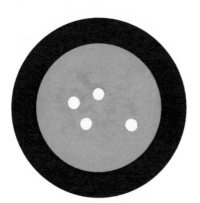

Normal Person
7,500 white blood cells
per cu.mm. of blood

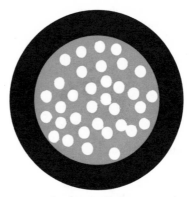

Leukemia Patient
100,000-1,000,000 white blood cells
per cu.mm. of blood

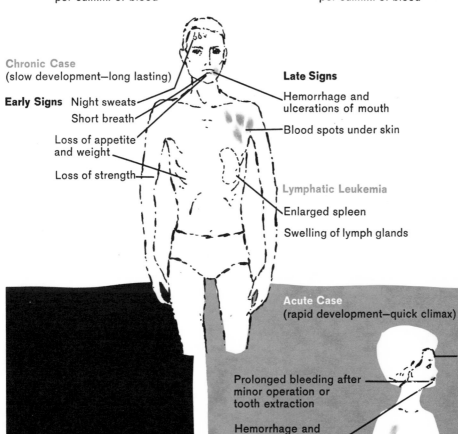

Chronic Case
(slow development—long lasting)

Early Signs Night sweats
Short breath
Loss of appetite
and weight
Loss of strength

Late Signs
Hemorrhage and
ulcerations of mouth
Blood spots under skin

Lymphatic Leukemia
Enlarged spleen
Swelling of lymph glands

Acute Case
(rapid development—quick climax)

High fever
Prolonged bleeding after
minor operation or
tooth extraction
Hemorrhage and
ulcerations of mouth
Bone pain
Blood spots under skin

the disease and its causes Leukoplakia is a chronic, painless disease which can affect any mucous membrane, as for example, the mouth and tongue or the vagina. Seen most often in the former area, it is an inflammation that develops slowly over many years from constant irritation, such as is caused by poor teeth or poor dentures, smoking in general, and pipe smoking in particular. Exposure to certain chemicals, including lead, is also thought to be a factor. The disease occurs almost exclusively in men after middle age.

symptoms This disease generally begins so slowly and is so painless that it is not detected until the patient has a routine examination. When the tongue is involved, it becomes dry and hot, and lags in speech. Membranes of the cheeks and gums become pearly white or grayish and, instead of remaining smooth, often become rough, with raised lesions that are thick, irregular, firm, and almost wartlike. Pipe smokers frequently develop a whitish spot on the lower lip which becomes thicker and less pliable as time passes.

complications The danger lies in the possibility that cancer can develop. This may be suspected when the areas involved become ulcerated or cracked.

prevention (or lessening of impact) The sources of mechanical, chemical, or heat irritation must be removed. All smoking must be stopped. Mouth washes will be suggested to cleanse the mouth and prevent secondary infections. The physician will have a biopsy made of any suspicious lesions and will arrange for surgery if there is any further indication of malignancy.

Leukoplakia

Affects mainly middle aged and older men

Caused by pipesmoking, poor teeth
or dentures, chemicals
or other irritants

White or gray lesions—
painless at first

Sometimes ulcerate or crack
and degenerate into cancer

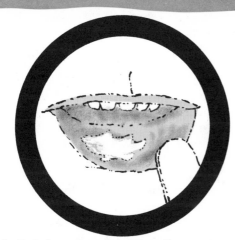

A. Early form—smooth patch on lip

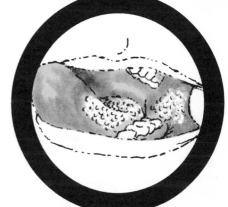

B. Moderately advanced form—raised
patches on tongue and cheek

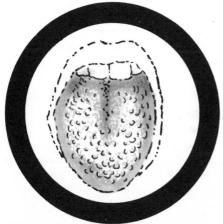

C. Advanced form—raised patches on tongue

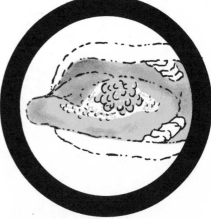

D. Degeneration into cancer

the disease and its causes SCABIES   Scabies is an infection of the skin caused by a parasite called the mange mite. The mite burrows into the skin of any part of the body, but most particularly between the fingers, in the elbow creases, groin, breast, and the small of the back. The slightly raised burrows are up to an inch in length and can be seen easily as dark gray lines beneath the skin.

Scabies spreads by contact with infected persons, their clothing, or bed linen contaminated with the adult female mange mite.

LICE   There are three types of human lice, each a separate species: the head louse, usually found at the back of the neck or scattered through the scalp; the body or clothes louse; and the crab, which lives on the hair in the pubic area.

These small, wingless parasites can play a sinister role in the spread of diseases such as typhus fever and relapsing fever. They also produce a particularly irritating form of skin disease.

Lice are found in any population group where personal hygiene is poor or where bathing or change of clothing is infrequent—such as in jails or among groups of soldiers under war conditions—or in cold climates. On rare occasions domestic animals may be the source of the infection.

symptoms SCABIES   There is severe itching which is worse at night. The rash appears as a number of small areas of redness with watery blisters. Scratching irritates the affected area, and it can become infected.

LICE   Human lice feed on the blood of the infected person. Head lice, usually found in children, produce a red lesion and severe itching which is aggravated by scratching. The eggs of the head lice are called nits and can be seen with the naked eye at the base of the hair shaft to which they become glued. They also become attached to clothing fibers, especially wool. At body temperature these nits hatch, go through a life cycle, and reach adulthood in 30 days.

complications SCABIES   There are no serious complications, nor is the mange mite involved in the spread of any specific diseases.

LICE   There can be secondary infection. The more serious complications, however, occur when infected lice transmit the diseases previously mentioned.

prevention (or lessening of impact) SCABIES   Since this disease is common under conditions of mass living where hygiene is neglected, known cases should be treated promptly. Infected clothing and linens must be sterilized. Medicines are available to eliminate the mites and cure the disorder.

LICE   Infected persons must be isolated and deloused—a process in which the adult lice as well as the eggs are killed. Each type of louse needs specific treatment. For head lice there is medication; sometimes the hair must be removed. When crabs are present, sexual intercourse should be avoided to prevent spread of the infestation. Contaminated clothing should be sterilized, and contact with other people limited.

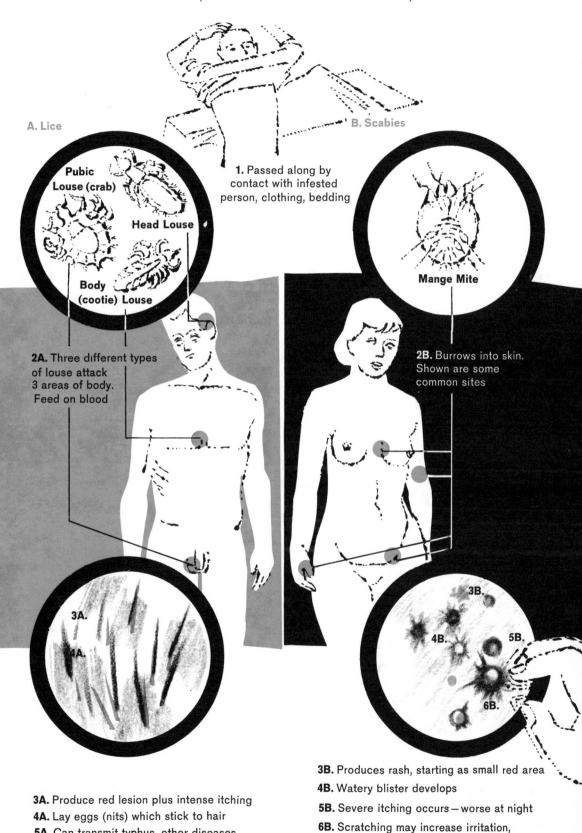

A. Lice

B. Scabies

Pubic Louse (crab)

Head Louse

Body (cootie) Louse

Mange Mite

1. Passed along by contact with infested person, clothing, bedding

2A. Three different types of louse attack 3 areas of body. Feed on blood

2B. Burrows into skin. Shown are some common sites

3A.

4A.

3B.

4B.

5B.

6B.

3A. Produce red lesion plus intense itching
4A. Lay eggs (nits) which stick to hair
5A. Can transmit typhus, other diseases

3B. Produces rash, starting as small red area
4B. Watery blister develops
5B. Severe itching occurs—worse at night
6B. Scratching may increase irritation, cause pus to develop

the disease and its causes Lung abscess is caused by an obstruction within the bronchial tree, which is the network of bronchial tubes and smaller branches, as illustrated in the Medi-Graph. Infection sets in around the obstruction and breaks down lung tissue, after which the abscess forms. The causes of lung abscess are varied and are the result of specific pneumonias, as a result of cancer of the bronchus, or any other cause of bronchial obstruction. The swallowing or inhalation of vomitus or a foreign body is another frequent cause of lung abscess.

The abscess may develop in as short a time as 5 days—or take 6 weeks or longer, depending upon the cause and the bacteria involved in the infection. It is seen most often in alcoholics, patients weakened by illness, or in epileptics—because these patients may not have the normal cough reflex or be conscious of the need to clear obstructions from their bronchial tree.

symptoms The onset is rapid, usually with chills and very high fever. Pain is severe and localized in the area of the chest over the infected part of the lung. There is shortness of breath and a bluish color change in the face. Cough is severe and produces a foul-smelling, thick sputum of variable color, sometimes mixed with blood. The patient is acutely ill and requires immediate medical attention.

complications The complications depend on the primary cause of the obstruction and the extent of infection throughout the body. In some instances, infected matter carried into other parts of the body can set up secondary abscesses. Abscess of the brain occurs in this manner.

prevention (or lessening of impact) People involved in extensive dental work should take care not to breathe in any foreign particles. If there is the slightest suspicion that this has happened, they should be carefully observed for some time thereafter. Epileptics, following a seizure, and patients in coma from any cause, should be watched for signs of respiratory infection. Once the disease is established, medical or surgical steps must be taken promptly. Since the lung may be left useless by the destructive changes of an abscess, infections should never be neglected.

Lung Abscess

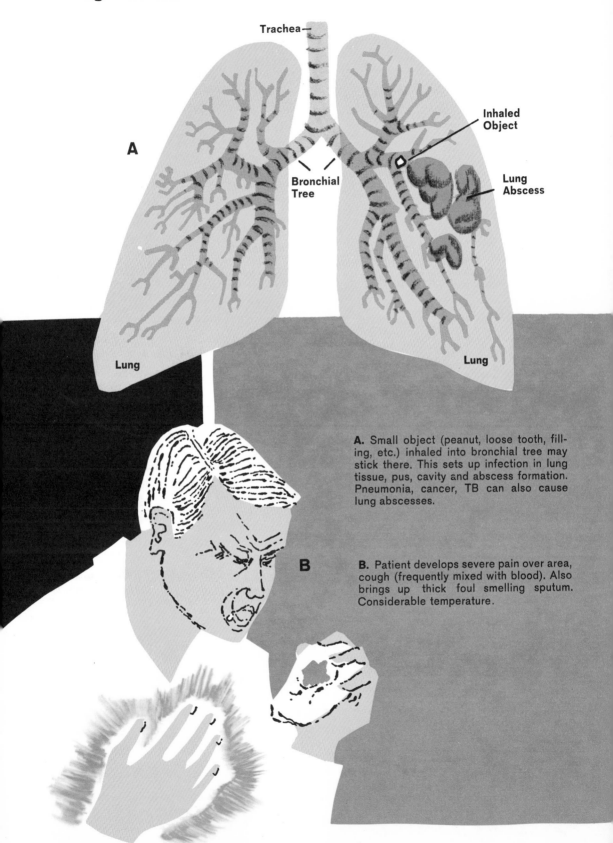

Trachea—

A

Bronchial
Tree

Inhaled
Object

Lung
Abscess

Lung

Lung

B

A. Small object (peanut, loose tooth, filling, etc.) inhaled into bronchial tree may stick there. This sets up infection in lung tissue, pus, cavity and abscess formation. Pneumonia, cancer, TB can also cause lung abscesses.

B. Patient develops severe pain over area, cough (frequently mixed with blood). Also brings up thick foul smelling sputum. Considerable temperature.

the disease and its causes   This is a chronic disease which, in its limited or discoid form, attacks the skin of the face, the mucous membrane of the mouth or lips, the hands, forearms, etc. As long as it remains in the discoid form, it is no serious threat to life. However, a skin rash frequently heralds the onset of other potentially dangerous symptoms. The disease can become generalized or disseminated. Then, in addition to attacking the skin it attacks other parts of the body such as the pleura (the membrane that lines the lungs), the pericardium (the membranous sac which surrounds the heart), the peritoneum (the membrane that lines the abdominal walls), and the joints.

The disease attacks primarily women, and appears in the age group 15 to 40. The cause is not known, but the illness often follows infection, injury, or exposure to sunlight.

Lupus erythematosus is hard to distinguish from a condition brought on by the use of certain medicines prescribed to control high blood pressure.

symptoms   In the limited form described in the upper half of the Medi-Graph, there is generally no pain or itching. Flare-ups are often related to exposure to sunlight or to the use of cosmetics or other skin irritants.

In the severe, generalized form, symptoms depend upon the organ system involved. Early symptoms may include low-grade fever, painful, inflamed joints, pleuritic pain, weight loss, and shortness of breath. The skin eruption mentioned above and described in the Medi-Graph may appear early and precede by many years the development of other more serious symptoms.

The blood system may be involved. Very often X rays show the presence of fluid in the pericardial sac or pleural space.

As the disease progresses, arthritic pain becomes more severe and there is swelling and pain in different joints, all resembling rheumatoid arthritis.

High blood pressure can develop with swelling of the lymph glands, particularly those in the neck.

complications   Once organ systems are involved, complications can include high blood pressure with heart damage, severe kidney disease, and central nervous system disorders causing epilepsy, neuritis, and stroke. There can also be severe anemia.

prevention (or lessening of impact)   A patient with the discoid form should avoid exposure to sunlight and should follow the program of medication prescribed by the doctor.

In the disseminated or generalized form, the organ system involved must be treated to lessen the severity of the disease and curb its destructive effects. While there is no known way of preventing lupus erythematosus, good control may be obtained by specific medications which will be outlined by the physician.

Lupus Erythematosus

Type 1: Limited form — attacks skin

Reddish-purple butterfly pattern

May also occur elsewhere:
on mucous membrane
of mouth or lips,
on hands and forearms,
etc.

Usually no itching or pain

Tends to recur

Sometimes covered by shiny gray scales

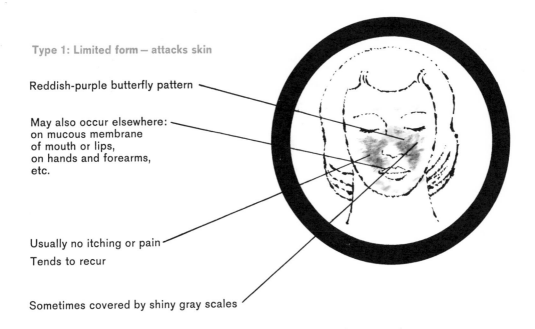

Type 2: Severe form — attacks other sections of body

Early symptoms:

Joint pains   Weakness and weight loss   Swelling of lymph glands   Smaller rash — may
look like hives

Fever

May go on to strong attack on . . .

. . . Central
Nervous System
epilepsy
neuritis
stroke

. . . Heart
pericarditis
myocarditis
high blood pressure

. . . Lungs
pleurisy

. . . Kidneys
nephritis and nephrosis

. . . Joints
arthritic tenderness and swelling

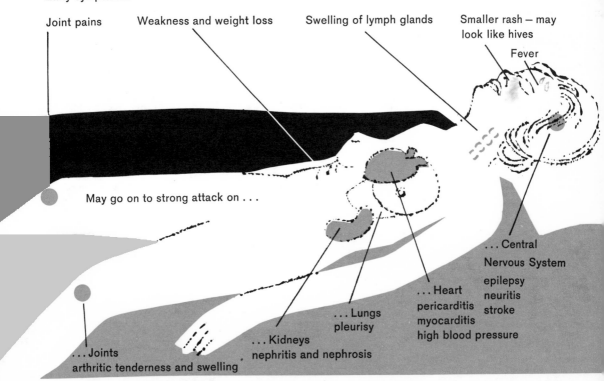

the disease and its causes Malaria is a disease which occurs in a pattern of attacks that alternate chills with fever. There are 4 main types of malaria that affect man. While their patterns differ somewhat, they will be discussed together here.

Malaria exists in all areas where the mosquito is a problem. While the disease is caused by a parasitic protozoa *(plasmodium)*, it is transmitted to man by the bite of the *Anopheles* mosquito. Well over 100 million malaria cases occur each year.

The incubation period from the bite of an infected mosquito to the outbreak of the disease depends on which one of the 4 types is contracted. It can vary from 10 days in the common type to 6 weeks in the less common variety.

symptoms Each type of malaria has its own characteristic course but in all 4 types of malaria, the patient suffers chills, fever, headache, muscle ache, anemia and an enlarged spleen. In the cold stage of the cycle, the victim suffers chills with chattering teeth, uncontrollable shaking, and a cold, blueish skin. This gives way to a period of high fever—up to 106°. The attack ends after 8–10 hours with a drenching sweat, and the temperature drops to normal. The cycle occurs with some regularity—each attack usually milder than the preceding one.

A doctor makes the diagnosis of malaria by finding the parasite in the blood.

complications Blackwater fever is a most serious problem resulting from one form of malaria. This name comes from the fact that the blood breaks down (for reasons unknown), causing the urine to become black in color. Kidney failure or anemia may be the result.

If the malaria affects the brain *(cerebral malaria)*, convulsions, delirium and death are common.

Rupture of the spleen is also a possible complication.

prevention (or lessening of impact) Elimination of the *Anopheles* mosquito and its breeding areas is the most important element in preventing the disease.

If you are in a tropical region where you are exposed to malaria, you should take preventive medication as directed, screen your bed at night, keep the air moving with a fan, and wear suitable protective clothing. Insecticides and repellents are also useful.

Some of the drugs that are used to prevent the disease can also be used to lessen its impact. Quinine and atabrine are familiar to World War II veterans of the South Pacific. However, newer products requiring smaller suppressive doses are now in use.

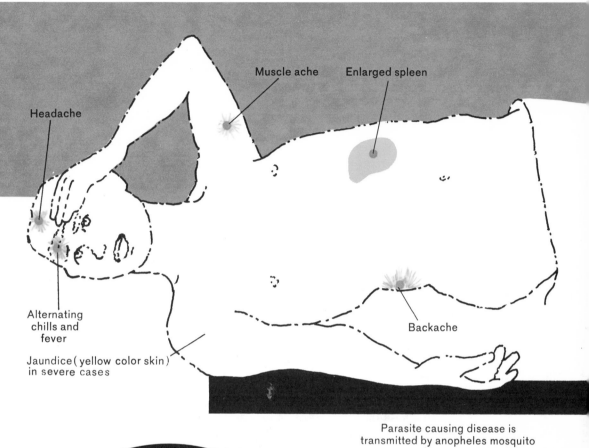

Headache

Muscle ache

Enlarged spleen

Alternating chills and fever

Jaundice (yellow color skin) in severe cases

Backache

Parasite causing disease is transmitted by anopheles mosquito

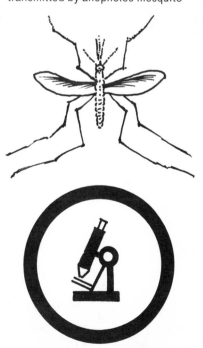

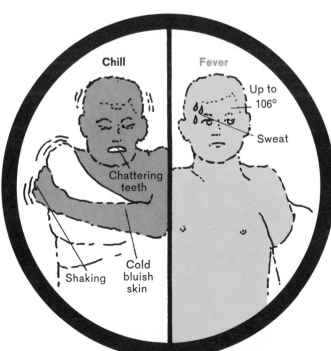

Chill

Fever

Up to 106°

Sweat

Chattering teeth

Shaking

Cold bluish skin

Cycle of attacks. Each one usually milder

Diagnosed by finding parasite in blood sample

the disease and its cause   This is a disease of the mastoid bone—the spongy part of the skull just behind the ear. Mastoiditis almost always occurs as a secondary consequence of infections of the middle ear. These infections may have been caused by diphtheria, scarlet fever, measles, or even a cold.

A couple of decades ago, mastoiditis was a dreaded disease, but with the advent of the antibiotics it is becoming a rarity.

symptoms   The outstanding symptom is pain over the mastoid bone during an ear infection. This pain is very severe and is aggravated by pressure on the bone. Pain also radiates from the mastoid area to the eyes and teeth.

The mastoiditis sufferer usually has a fever. Depending on the nature of the bacteria that have caused the infection, it may be quite high. If the infection progresses further, the accumulation of pus may cause perforation of the eardrum. At this point, there is considerable swelling and pain in the mastoid area with the ear being pushed down and forward.

complications   The mastoiditis sufferer's hearing may be impaired, depending upon the amount of middle ear involvement and the extent of destruction of bone and nerve tissues.

The most serious possibility is the spread of the infection to the brain, causing the development of brain abscesses and meningitis—leading to death.

prevention (or lessening of impact)   Prompt treatment of all middle ear infections with appropriate antibiotics should prevent the development of mastoid infections. Mastoiditis can also be prevented if upper respiratory infections are treated before they reach the middle ear.

Even if the disease does develop, systemic antibiotics and sedatives are usually effective in combating it. Occasionally, surgery may be necessary to prevent loss of hearing and other complications.

Mastoiditis

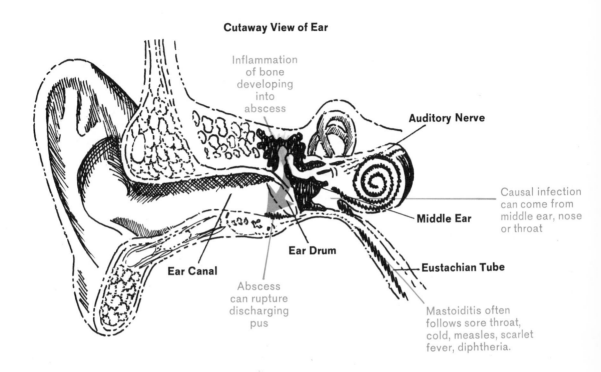

Cutaway View of Ear

Inflammation of bone developing into abscess

Auditory Nerve

Causal infection can come from middle ear, nose or throat

Middle Ear

Ear Drum

Ear Canal

Eustachian Tube

Abscess can rupture discharging pus

Mastoiditis often follows sore throat, cold, measles, scarlet fever, diphtheria.

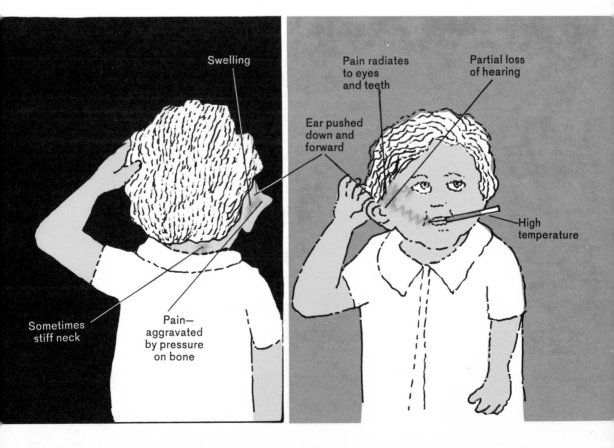

Swelling

Pain radiates to eyes and teeth

Partial loss of hearing

Ear pushed down and forward

High temperature

Sometimes stiff neck

Pain— aggravated by pressure on bone

the disease and its causes   Measles is a highly contagious disease of childhood, although an occasional case crops up among adults. An uncomplicated case of measles is no problem for a healthy older child to handle—though it may be dangerous for young children under the age of 3 or 4, or adults (particularly pregnant women).

Measles is a virus disease, like a cold, and spreads the same way—by direct contact with an infected individual or with discharges from his nose and throat. There may be an incubation period of anywhere from one to two weeks after exposure to an infected child before the child who has been exposed begins to develop obvious symptoms.

symptoms   Measles starts with the symptoms of a bad cold: fever, a hard cough, and red, watery eyes. However, these cold symptoms do not respond to antibiotics or other drugs. The fever usually goes higher each day until the fourth day—when a rash appears behind the child's ears. During the next 3 to 4 days, this rash spreads over the face and neck and down the rest of the body. Individual blotches reach their strongest intensity within 24 hours after they appear, and then begin to fade. All traces of the rash disappear by about the fifth day after it first appeared behind the ears.

The fever stays high for the first day or two after the rash appears. A day or two after the cold symptoms begin—and a day or two before the rash appears—Koplik spots appear inside the mouth, next to the lower rear teeth. These are tiny white specks within red patches, usually so small that they are hard to recognize.

complications   If the child is not given proper bed rest and care, complications such as ear infections, pneumonia, bronchitis and encephalitis can develop. It is a good idea to keep anyone with cold symptoms away from a child with measles—since the cold germs can help bring on these complications. If the high fever continues more than 3 days after the rash begins, or if the fever goes down and then back up again, this may be a sign that complications are developing.

prevention (or lessening of impact)   Measles vaccine is now in use. It is very effective and may eventually eliminate the disease among children or susceptible adults. For those people not immunized, an injection of gamma globulin serum can provide immunity against measles for 2 to 6 weeks. Therefore, many doctors use this serum for pregnant women, young children under the age of 3 or 4, or older children in poor health who are exposed to measles.

Many doctors also feel it is unnecessary to prevent older children from getting measles, feeling they should catch it and get it over with. Gamma globulin is administered in a dose which will hold the illness to a mild case. For most people, one attack of measles confers a lifelong immunity against developing the disease again.

Measles (Rubeola)

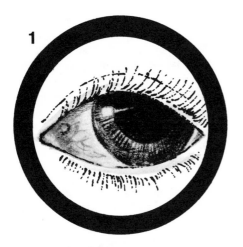

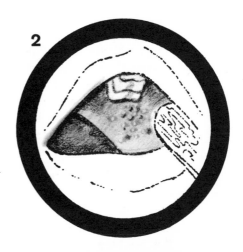

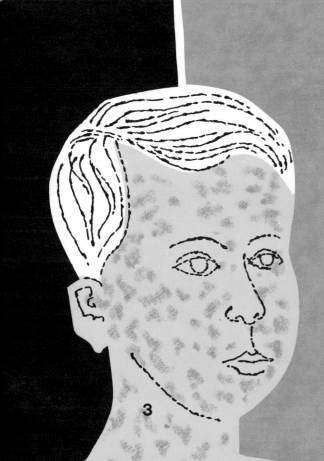

1. Inflammation of Eye

On second day of fever, eyes become bleary, swollen, and congested. Pimples frequently appear in corner.

2. Appearance of Koplik Spots

On third day of fever, Koplik Spots may appear. These are tiny red patches with whitish specks which appear on inside of cheeks and other areas of mucous lining of mouth.

3. Rash

On fourth day of fever, blotchy rash may appear behind ears. It spreads to face and down trunk of body. Rash begins to disappear four or five days after its first appearance—fading first where it appeared first.

Ménière's Disease (and Labyrinthitis)

Chronic Disease   Acute Disease

the diseases and their causes   Ménière's disease is a chronic disorder of the inner ear, or balance center. The acute form of the illness is called labyrinthitis. Among the causes of this disease are middle ear infections, meningitis, toxic reaction to drugs like streptomycin and aspirin, injuries that cause the blood to hemorrhage into the inner ear, and disorders of the blood vessels of the inner ear. Emotional tensions precipitate the disease in some cases.

Ménière's disease appears most commonly among people in their 40's— but no age group is spared.

symptoms   Ménière's disease usually is associated with mild deafness, and a head noise called tinnitus. This is a high-pitched buzzing or ringing noise— generally heard in one ear only.

Attacks of severe dizziness, which are aggravated when the person changes position, are a major sign of Ménière's disease. This is usually accompanied by nausea and vomiting. The dizziness—a strong feeling of swaying or rocking—starts without notice and may last from a few minutes to several hours.

In labyrinthitis, deafness or ringing or buzzing in the ear rarely occur. Nystagmus (uncontrolled movements of the eye) is a frequent sign noted in acute labyrinthitis. This can be so severe that the patient has to remain immobile, because any motion may intensify the problem.

Attacks of labyrinthitis vary in intensity and duration, lasting from days to weeks. In milder cases they resemble seasickness.

complications   While the interference with normal life can be severe, most patients can function, although their movements must be slow and careful when the attack breaks out. Of course, activities like driving or working at heights cannot be undertaken.

Permanent deafness is a potentially serious problem with the progression of Ménière's disease.

prevention (or lessening of impact)   Mild cases are treated by the doctor with anti-seasickness types of medication like Dramamine.

Low salt diets and diuretics have also been helpful in some cases. Where extreme emotional tension seems to precipitate the attack, psychotherapy may be the solution.

In some severely persistent cases, an operation to cut the eighth cranial nerve, which supplies branches to the ear, may be the last resort.

Ménière's Disease (and Labyrinthitis)

Chronic Disease   Acute Disease

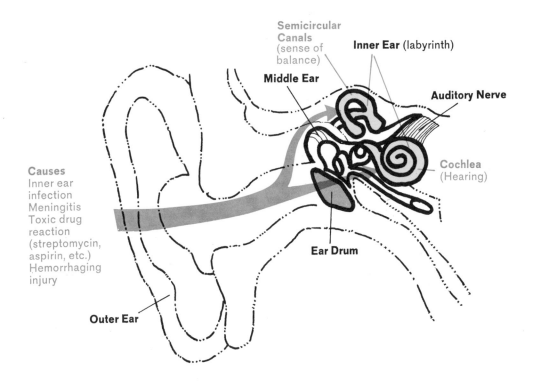

Causes
Inner ear
infection
Meningitis
Toxic drug
reaction
(streptomycin,
aspirin, etc.)
Hemorrhaging
injury

Some Common Symptoms

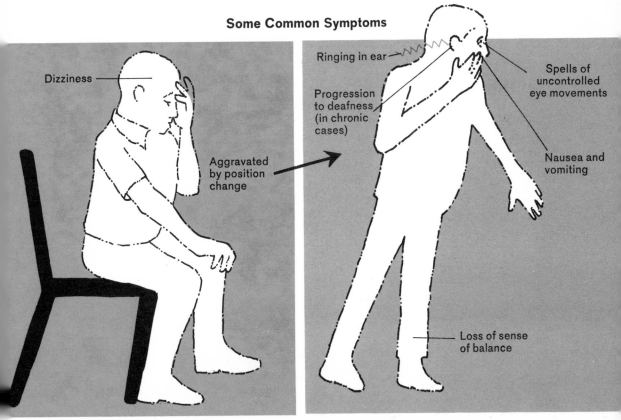

the disease and its causes Meningitis refers to any infectious disease attacking the meninges, which are the membranes covering the brain and spinal cord. In the form most commonly seen, the inflammation is caused by the meningococcus and pneumococcus bacteria. These germs are found in the upper respiratory tract of 2% to 5% of normal individuals who may act as carriers; or, under certain circumstances, they may develop the illness as the bacteria spread from the nose and throat to the brain, usually via the bloodstream. The disease is also spread by an infected person through nose and throat secretions. Meningitis may also develop as a secondary infection following acute infections of the sinus cavities or middle ear. The incubation period of this form of the disease is about one week. It occurs most often in the winter months, and generally more in males than in females. Children, young adults, and older persons are most susceptible.

symptoms Much depends on the resistance of the patient and the virulence and type of bacteria. In a severe case, symptoms may start with sudden chills, fever, violent headache, and vomiting. Coma may follow rapidly. Blood spots may appear on the skin. The patient goes into shock and death may occur within a period of several hours.
Fortunately, most cases are not so catastrophic. These begin with the signs of an upper respiratory infection, chills, fever, and headache. There is nausea. In young children there may occasionally be diarrhea. A blotchy red rash may or may not appear. There is wide fluctuation in temperature. The patient complains of muscle aches, severe headache, and there is marked stiffness of the neck. The more quickly the diagnosis is established, the shorter the course of the illness and the fever.

complications Hydrocephalus, a deformity in which the head is enlarged, is a common complication in infants. At all ages visual and hearing disturbances can occur due to nerve damage. Occasionally the heart is involved. Chronic headaches are a frequent complication.

prevention (or lessening of impact) Use of antibiotic drugs for carriers and persons exposed to meningitis is a most effective preventive step and should never be neglected. Infections of the nose, upper lip, ear, and sinus should be treated promptly to prevent spread to the brain.

Meningitis

Inflammation of membrane covering
brain and spinal cord.

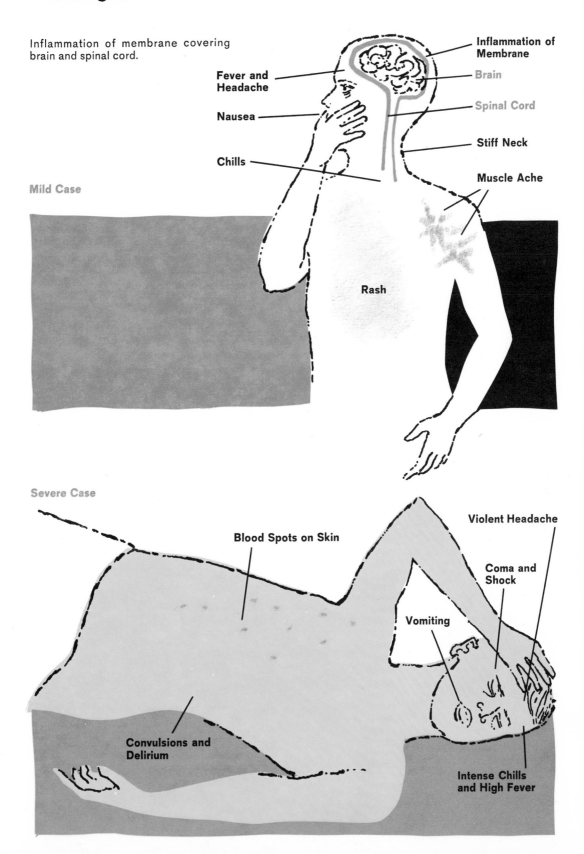

Inflammation of Membrane

Brain

Fever and Headache

Spinal Cord

Nausea

Stiff Neck

Chills

Muscle Ache

Mild Case

Rash

Severe Case

Blood Spots on Skin

Violent Headache

Coma and Shock

Vomiting

Convulsions and Delirium

Intense Chills and High Fever

Menopause
(Change of life)

the disease and its causes   MENOPAUSE (commonly known as the *Change of Life*) is a term describing the characteristic physical changes which take place in most women between the ages of 45–55—though in some cases these changes take place earlier or later. Menopause takes place because the woman's ovaries stop producing adequate amounts of the female hormone estrogen.

In some women, the menopause occurs quickly and creates only minor problems. With others, however, this change of life can last 3 or 4 years, with many physical and emotional problems.

Contrary to some folklore, most women do not lose sexual desire after reaching the menopause.

symptoms   The most common physical symptom is the "hot flush"—a feeling of warmth which suddenly rolls over the body, neck and face. There is also the "hot flash"—a sudden surge of heat over the entire body, accompanied by a drenching sweat.

Menopause typically begins with a change in the woman's menstrual pattern. Her periods become irregular in their timing and in the amount and duration of menstrual flow. Finally, her periods cease completely. Other sex characteristics show changes. The breasts and uterus tend to shrink, pubic and armpit hair diminish, while facial hair increases.

On the emotional side, nervousness, feelings of weakness and irritability are frequent. Some women are easily excited while others sink into a depression. However, these symptoms do not affect everyone. Many women go through menopause with only mild symptoms that cause little physical or psychological discomfort.

complications   Several problems may crop up in menopausal women that can be considered complications. Once menstruation has ceased, a renewal of vaginal bleeding requires immediate investigation to rule out the possibility of tumor development. Some women experience marked emotional depression and may need psychological therapy.

Circulatory problems such as hypertension and the beginning of arteriosclerosis may also be linked to menopause. And the bones tend to decalcify and soften *(osteoporosis)*.

prevention (or lessening of impact)   The female sex hormone estrogen, now produced artificially by drug manufacturers, can make up for much that is lost when a woman's ovaries stop producing sex hormones at the menopause. So in the case of severe, prolonged menopausal symptoms, a doctor may feel that the sufferer should receive the benefits of hormonal therapy.

At present a large group of doctors also feel that all women of menopausal age should be placed on estrogen therapy. Women with a history of breast tumors or fibroid tumors of the uterus probably should not use this hormone. In any case, it requires strict supervision by your doctor.

Menopause

(Change of life)

Usually occurs between ages 45-55 because ovaries stop producing adequate amounts of estrogen (female sex hormones)

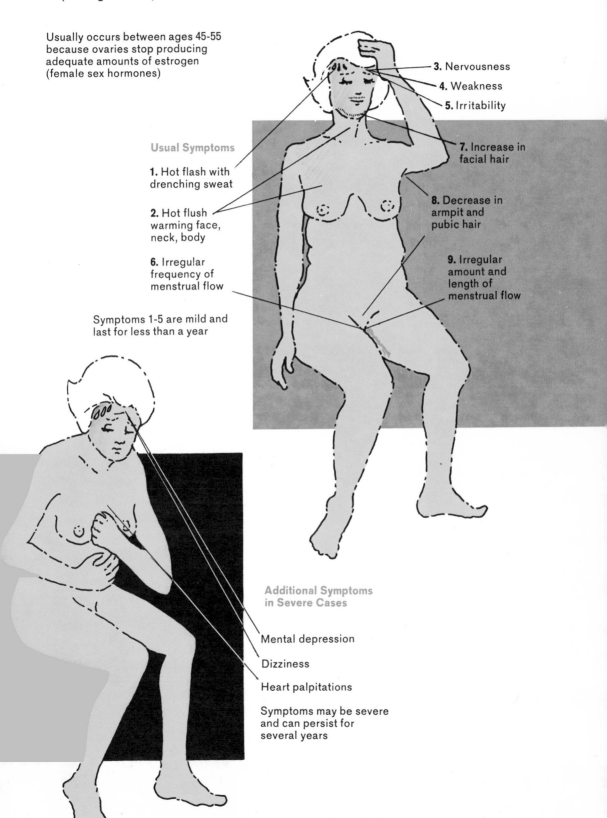

Usual Symptoms

1. Hot flash with drenching sweat

2. Hot flush warming face, neck, body

6. Irregular frequency of menstrual flow

Symptoms 1-5 are mild and last for less than a year

3. Nervousness

4. Weakness

5. Irritability

7. Increase in facial hair

8. Decrease in armpit and pubic hair

9. Irregular amount and length of menstrual flow

Additional Symptoms in Severe Cases

Mental depression

Dizziness

Heart palpitations

Symptoms may be severe and can persist for several years

the disease and its causes   Mercury poisoning is becoming an increasing threat, with the growth of water pollution problems. Contamination by industrial dumping of mercury wastes has in some cases affected drinking water. More frequently, fish have picked up these mercury wastes in streams, lakes and oceans—to such an extent that government sources are now warning against the eating of a number of types of fish.

In addition, mercury compounds have been used as fungicides sprayed on wheat and other grains. This has affected man directly, through eating bread made from mercury-contaminated grain—or indirectly through eating the meat of pigs, ducks and game birds which have fed on the mercury-infected grain. Young infants are particularly susceptible to mercury ingested with food.

Mercury poisoning also occurs among workers who breathe in mercury vapors in laboratories, instrument factories, and gold and silver refineries.

symptoms   Where the body is continually accumulating small amounts of mercury, the symptoms of mercury poisoning may be mild at first but build up with increasing severity. The symptoms can include weakness, fatigue, loss of interest, numbness, tingling of the hands and feet or the area about the mouth. The victim may then begin to suffer visual and hearing problems, and personality changes (including fits of rage and depression). Coordination may be affected, with clumsiness of speech, difficulty in writing, staggering gait and spastic limbs.

In cases of mercury poisoning from the sudden intake of large amounts of mercury, the symptoms are acute. These include severe pain in the mouth and throat, nausea, vomiting, bloody diarrhea, kidney involvement and anemia.

complications   In both the slow accumulative poisoning and the sudden intake of large amounts, the victim—if untreated—can go on to paralysis and eventually coma and death.

prevention (or lessening of impact)   Medicines containing mercury (such as the antiseptic *bichloride of mercury*) must be kept out of the reach of young children—as must other substances with a large mercury content.

The more subtle poisoning arising from contamination of foods requires strict enforcement and spread of public health regulation. The contamination of our rivers and lakes by mercury compounds, with their effect on fish life and ultimately on human beings, can only be controlled by effective laws and policing. This means strict controls on industrial dumping and on the use of mercury compounds as fungicides and pesticides.

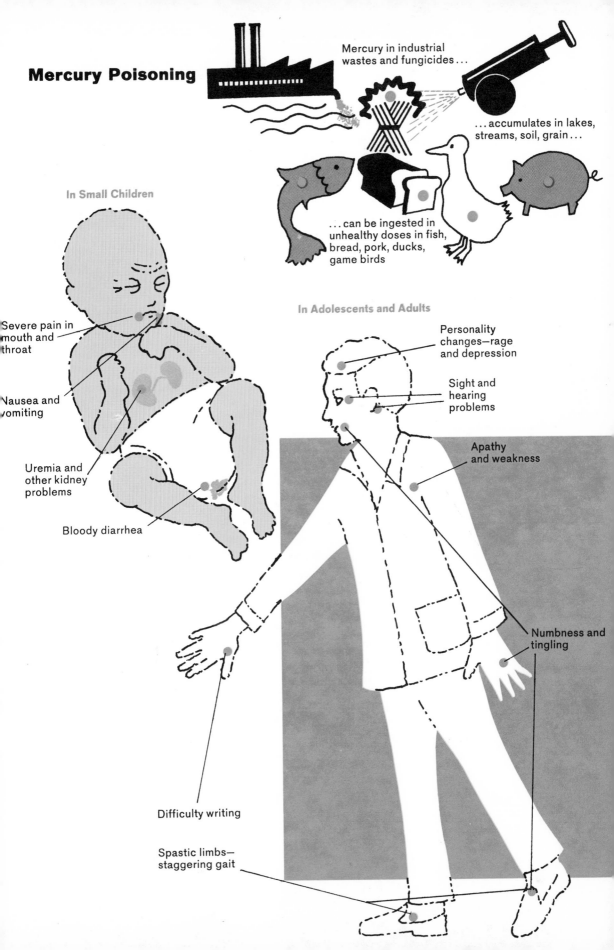

Mercury Poisoning

Mercury in industrial wastes and fungicides...

...accumulates in lakes, streams, soil, grain...

...can be ingested in unhealthy doses in fish, bread, pork, ducks, game birds

In Small Children

Severe pain in mouth and throat

Nausea and vomiting

Uremia and other kidney problems

Bloody diarrhea

In Adolescents and Adults

Personality changes—rage and depression

Sight and hearing problems

Apathy and weakness

Numbness and tingling

Difficulty writing

Spastic limbs— staggering gait

the disease and its causes   Migraine is a specific type of headache which occurs, in most cases, when the larger arteries of the scalp stretch and the arteries within the brain widen or dilate. The cause is not known. Emotional disturbances seem to play a part, but there is not much evidence to confirm this as a specific cause. Most patients have a strong family history of migraine headache. It usually begins in childhood or adolescence and tends to become less severe as the patient gets older. Migraine is seen considerably more often in females than in males, and interestingly enough, occurs less often during pregnancy. Usually it disappears during the fifties or sixties.

The attack occurs at irregular intervals and almost always is localized in one part of the head, though not always the same part in each attack. Occasionally it involves the entire head.

symptoms   The headache develops in a rather typical and somewhat dramatic sequence of events. The patient is often aware of a headache coming on when she gets up in the morning. She may be slightly confused and complain of some visual disturbance, or speak of a visual aura in which she sees bright spots or different visual patterns. Occasionally there is a momentary loss of sight. The headache follows, beginning as a dull, boring, throbbing pain and eventually affecting the whole side of the head. The patient becomes pale and weak, and benefits from lying down in a darkened room. If there is severe pain, nausea and vomiting can occur. At its height, the pain of the headache may be almost unbearable. Mental confusion, depression, and extreme irritability are common. The patient may be pale and cold, and sweat profusely. Gradually the attack subsides, often after she falls into a deep sleep. When she awakes, she is better, although she may feel groggy for as long as 24 hours.

complications   There are no serious complications from migraine headache.

prevention (or lessening of impact)   Patients who know that certain actions precipitate a migraine headache would obviously do well to avoid such actions. Those with strong emotional problems may benefit from psychotherapy. Medicines are available and are moderately effective if taken early in the attack. Once the headache develops the patient rarely can swallow any medicine without vomiting, and it may have to be given by injection.

There is no specific cure for migraine headache. The best one can hope for is that the severity of the attack be reduced by prompt recognition of early symptoms, and the use of medication before the headache develops.

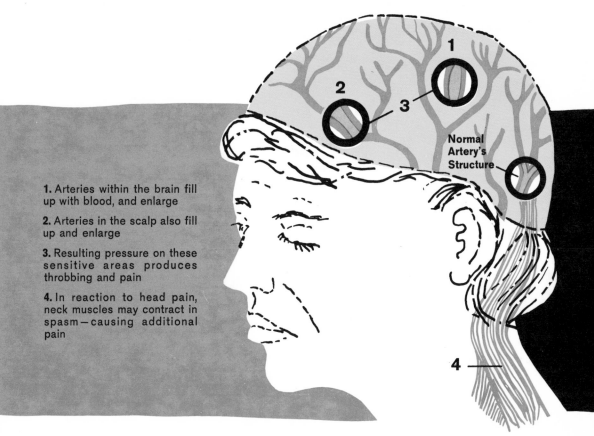

1. Arteries within the brain fill up with blood, and enlarge

2. Arteries in the scalp also fill up and enlarge

3. Resulting pressure on these sensitive areas produces throbbing and pain

4. In reaction to head pain, neck muscles may contract in spasm—causing additional pain

Normal Artery's Structure

Progress of a Migraine Headache

Early Stage

Full Blast

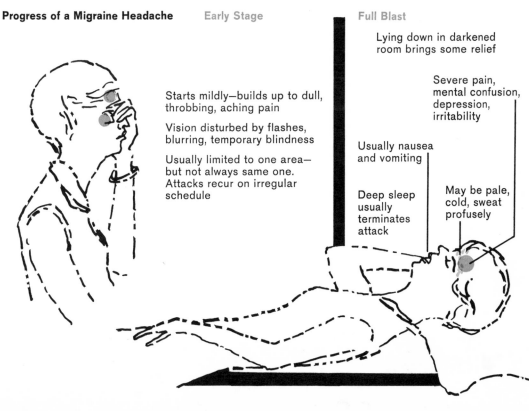

Lying down in darkened room brings some relief

Severe pain, mental confusion, depression, irritability

Starts mildly—builds up to dull, throbbing, aching pain

Vision disturbed by flashes, blurring, temporary blindness

Usually limited to one area— but not always same one. Attacks recur on irregular schedule

Usually nausea and vomiting

Deep sleep usually terminates attack

May be pale, cold, sweat profusely

the disease and its causes   This is a mildly contagious disease caused by a virus not yet identified, which causes a swelling of the lymph glands and changes in the white blood cells. It may be transferred during kissing, tests reveal, and possibly by other forms of direct contact not yet defined. The disease occurs in children and young adults. The incubation period is about 2 weeks, and the illness itself lasts from 2 to 6 weeks.

symptoms   Mononucleosis begins quite suddenly with weakness, headache, and a sore throat that resembles tonsillitis. Temperatures vary from 100° to 103°. Within a few days, the lymph glands become enlarged and tender. Lymph glands at the front and back of the neck, armpit, and groin are the ones involved. The swellings vary in size from small, or pea size, to walnut size. In the majority of cases, the liver and spleen also become enlarged and tender. There may be intestinal symptoms such as nausea, vomiting, and pain, and in cases where the liver is involved, jaundice may occur. Weakness of the extremities follows the course of the illness. A generalized rash resembling German measles may appear during the early stages of the disease, and frequently there is a mild cough. Specific blood tests are used to establish the diagnosis and follow the disease.

complications   Complications include hepatitis, encephalitis, severe nosebleeds, or rectal bleeding. Convulsions may occur. A rare but serious complication is rupture of the spleen.

prevention (or lessening of impact)   There is no known method of preventing infectious mononucleosis. It is advisable to rest well and limit activities during the recuperative stage in order to shorten the length of the illness. Since it is not certain exactly how contagious this disease is or the variety of ways in which it may be transferred, it is advisable to avoid contact with people known to have it. Complications can be anticipated and dealt with by the family doctor as they develop. Mononucleosis itself is predictable and recovery is generally uncomplicated and complete. It often occurs in epidemic outbreaks, especially among teenagers in the same school or social group.

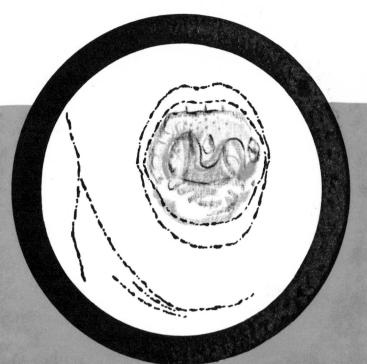

First Stage

Weakness, headache, sore throat. Yellow, white or gray patches appear on tonsils or other throat area.

Second Stage

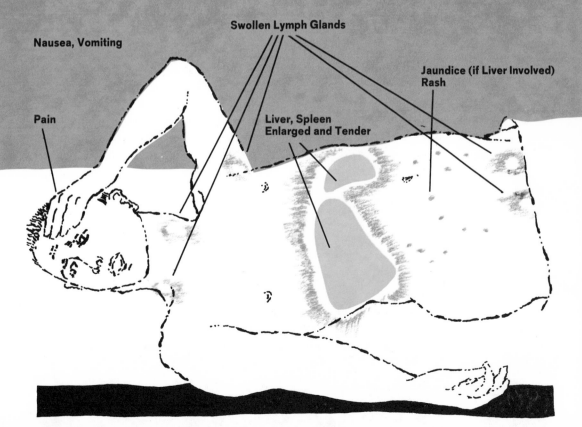

Nausea, Vomiting

Pain

Swollen Lymph Glands

Liver, Spleen Enlarged and Tender

Jaundice (if Liver Involved) Rash

the disease and its causes   This is a disease of the central nervous system, affecting principally the white matter of the brain and spinal cord, and causing progressive deterioration. The cause is not known, but many theories are advanced. These include infections, abnormal enzymes, chemical toxicity, non-specific illnesses in which there is high fever, injuries, pregnancy, and psychological trauma. While there is no agreement on the direct cause, there seems to be little doubt that relapses are occasionally precipitated by some of the conditions just mentioned.

The course of the illness varies considerably because so large an area of the central nervous system is involved. Symptoms depend upon the area involved and the degree of nerve tissue destruction.

Multiple sclerosis usually develops between the ages of 20 and 40. Both sexes are affected equally. The disease is quite common throughout the world, particularly in northern European countries. It is seen least often in Africa and Asia.

symptoms   It is difficult to give a clear, exact description of the symptoms of multiple sclerosis. Both the course of the illness and the symptoms vary. The more common disturbances are described in the Medi-Graph, but it must be emphasized that the order in which these symptoms occur is different in each case.

The symptoms cover a broad range of conditions, but all of them are rarely seen in one patient. A characteristic of the disease is that it recurs frequently, with long periods of time between relapses. During those periods the patient functions normally. Some patients with multiple sclerosis become depressed, but many characteristically present a false picture of cheerfulness.

complications   At the onset of this illness—which can run from 15 to 30 years after it begins—it is very difficult to foresee the future of a given case. Such complications as occur do so in the later stages of the disease and are related to the growing disability of the patient and the effects of constant bed rest. These include infections, bed sores, bladder and kidney infection, and kidney stones. However, very few patients become so disabled that they are bedridden. Thus, complications are not usually a problem.

prevention (or lessening of impact)   There is no known method of preventing, curing, or counteracting the long-term deterioration of a multiple sclerosis patient. But it is important to avoid frequent relapses. Maintenance of good health can contribute to this. Unusual fatigue, infection, and injuries should be avoided where possible. Although there is no great evidence that pregnancy increases the severity of the disease, it probably does precipitate relapses and is best avoided. Exercise, massage, physiotherapy, and rehabilitation are all of tremendous importance to the patient. He should be encouraged and helped by trained, professional therapists to pursue his activities and interests to the best of his ability.

Multiple Sclerosis

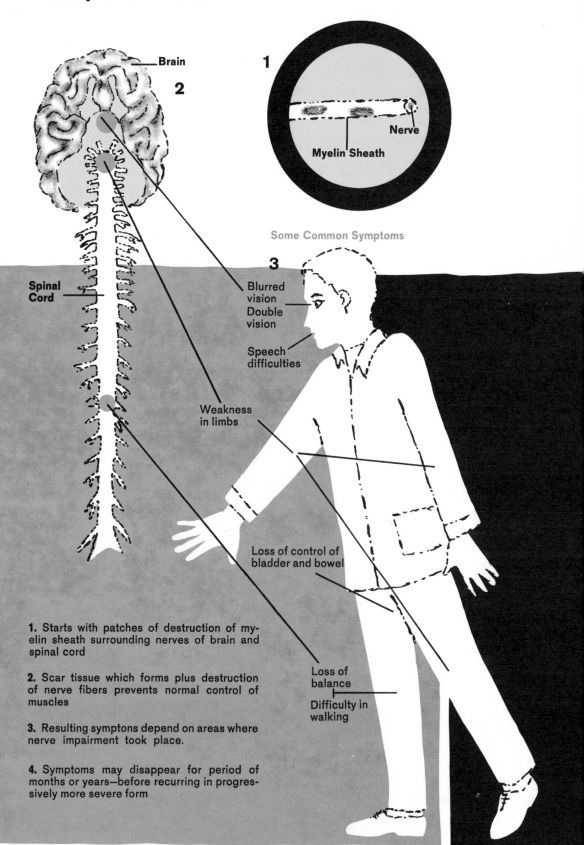

Brain

2

1

Nerve

Myelin Sheath

Some Common Symptoms

3

Spinal Cord

Blurred vision
Double vision

Speech difficulties

Weakness in limbs

Loss of control of bladder and bowel

Loss of balance

Difficulty in walking

1. Starts with patches of destruction of myelin sheath surrounding nerves of brain and spinal cord

2. Scar tissue which forms plus destruction of nerve fibers prevents normal control of muscles

3. Resulting symptons depend on areas where nerve impairment took place.

4. Symptoms may disappear for period of months or years—before recurring in progressively more severe form

the disease and its causes Mumps is a disease of the salivary glands caused by a virus. It is spread by direct contact with someone who has mumps, or with the secretions—such as saliva or nasal discharge—of that person. Although most people are susceptible to this disease, it is most common in children 5 to 15. Generally a case of mumps gives lifelong immunity, but it is not a rare thing to get mumps a second time. The incubation period is 12 to 21 days, and it is contagious from the time the cheek lining becomes red and swollen, and the glands begin to swell, until the swelling disappears. Newborn infants generally have immunity for the first eight months of life.

symptoms The early symptoms may be very mild, with low-grade fever, some general aches and pains, and stiffness where the ear and jaw meet, or in front of the ear. The gland in front of the ear swells—one side usually two or three days before the other. Sometimes the glands under the jaw become swollen. It hurts to open the mouth wide, and the area is sensitive to touch. Since the salivary fluids become scanty during the disease, sharp-tasting foods such as lemon irritate the mouth and glands and cause pain. Mumps usually lasts 10 days.

complications Boys past the age of puberty and male adults may develop infection of the testicles. When this occurs, it starts in the second week of the disease, beginning with pain and swelling of the testicles. Temperature goes up and the patient feels sick all over. Unless both testicles are involved there is little danger of sterility, but the disease can result in the destruction of the testicle involved.

Either sex is subject to the complication of an infection of the pancreas. This begins about the 7th day and is marked by pain in the abdomen and digestive disturbances which may last about a week.

Still another complication can develop toward the end of the first week. This is encephalitis, in which the lining of the brain is involved. There is severe headache, stiff neck, and a high fever. There may even be delirium. However, death from this form of encephalitis is rare, and most patients recover completely.

prevention (or lessening of impact) A mumps vaccine is available which can eventually eliminate this illness. Therefore, it is suggested that all children be vaccinated with it. There is also a skin test for those who don't know whether they have had mumps and want to check on their immunity. The care of a patient with mumps is simple, but the complications can be serious and require specific treatment.

Mumps

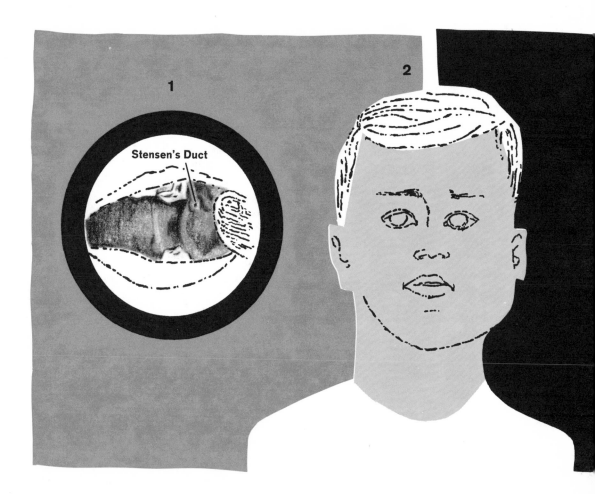

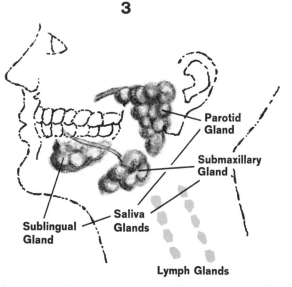

1. Swelling in Mouth

On first day, opening in cheek lining at level of second molar tooth (Stensen's duct) becomes red, swollen and nippled in appearance.

2. Swelling of Glands

On second day, parotid gland (one of saliva glands, under ear lobe) swells up. Hard swelling enlarges to cover jawbone at angle near ears. Other saliva glands may become swollen. Swelling usually spreads to other side of face after day or two.

3. Telling Mumps from Swollen Glands

Mumps affect saliva glands — parotid, submaxillary and sublingual. Ordinary case of swollen glands refers to swelling of lymph glands in neck — usually after sore throat.

the disease and its cause   This is a disease of the nervous system that affects the muscles of the eyes, face, larynx, pharynx, respiration and swallowing—making them exceedingly weak and easily fatigued.

The disease affects both sexes—but women twice as often as men. It can strike at all ages—although the peak for women is in the late 20's and early 30's, while for men it is in later periods of life. Its cause is unknown.

When the disease strikes, it usually takes several weeks for the first attack to develop clearly. It then becomes gradually more severe for a long period of time. The course of the disease is marked by frequent periods of apparent improvement, followed by relapses.

In 10%–20% of the cases, there is an associated tumor of the thymus gland.

symptoms   The outbreak of the disease is usually preceded by an emotional upset or an infection. In 90% of the cases the first symptom is drooping of one or both eyelids. Eye muscle weakness also causes double vision, while face muscle weakness creates a relatively immobile, expressionless look. In cases where laryngeal and pharyngeal muscle weakness develops, the patient has difficulty swallowing—and may choke while drinking fluids. The voice takes on a nasal quality.

In advanced cases, a person with myasthenia gravis may be so weak that she cannot hold anything in her hands, keep her eyes open, or even feed herself.

Atrophy of muscle groups takes place when the patient has suffered from the disease over a long period of time. However, after 10 years, if the damage has not been too great, the severity of attacks levels off and the course of the disease is usually more benign.

complications   Attacks of myasthenia gravis are aggravated by infections, fatigue, alcohol, and certain drugs (particularly those of the quinine family). Death may be caused by respiratory failure (suffocation) due to paralysis of the chest muscles.

prevention (or lessening of impact)   Fortunately, if diagnosis is made early, there are drugs available which can dramatically control the symptoms of the disease in mild cases.

In more severe cases, drugs may be of little avail. Prevention of infection and the use of a respirator to help breathing are among the measures that must be taken.

Myasthenia Gravis

Neuromuscular disease that
can weaken action of
voluntary muscles of

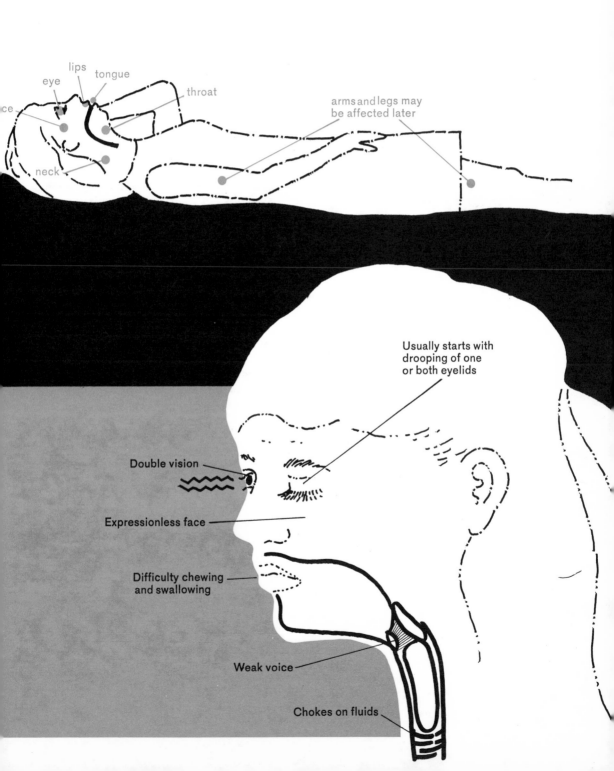

eye
lips
tongue
throat
ce
neck
arms and legs may
be affected later

Usually starts with
drooping of one
or both eyelids

Double vision

Expressionless face

Difficulty chewing
and swallowing

Weak voice

Chokes on fluids

the disease and its causes   This disease is a generalized inflammation of blood vessels which affects primarily the tiny blood filters of the kidney called glomeruli. It occurs most frequently in childhood, often follows an upper respiratory infection, and is a common complication of scarlet fever. Nephritis generally begins from 1 to 6 weeks after a preceding infection has cleared up, and seems to result from a hypersensitivity reaction to that infection, particularly when it is caused by streptococci of a specific group. It also has been shown to follow or be associated with infections such as endocarditis, pneumonia, and gastroenteritis. Prolonged cold, exhaustion, and lowered resistance may be factors. The disease is more common in males, without regard to race or climate.

symptoms   Acute nephritis begins quite slowly. The patient does not feel particularly ill. The eyelids or face may swell and there may be headache, slight fever, moderate weakness, tenderness over the back in the area of the kidneys, or some generalized, vague abdominal pain. On examination the doctor finds specific changes in the urine analysis. The urine may decrease in amount and become smoky or reddish in color. There is cause for concern when the urine output stops completely or diminishes to a very low level.

Blood pressure can be high. And when, in more severe cases, blood pressure is very high, there may be headache, drowsiness, and vomiting. Muscular twitchings may occur, and occasionally there are convulsions and coma. Anemia, a condition in which the blood is lacking either in quantity or quality, is another possible symptom.

The majority of acute nephritis patients recover within 6 to 8 weeks, but a small group succumbs to uremia or congestive heart failure.

complications   The most serious complications are uremia, high blood pressure, and coma, as well as the development of a chronic form of nephritis. This last may crop up years after the disease appears to have been controlled.

prevention (or lessening of impact)   Patients exposed to or showing evidence of streptococcus infection or scarlet fever should be treated with appropriate antibiotics and made to follow the program prescribed by the doctor. Urine is usually checked two or three times a week, a special diet is provided, and bed rest is ordered. Particular care is taken to prevent reinfection.

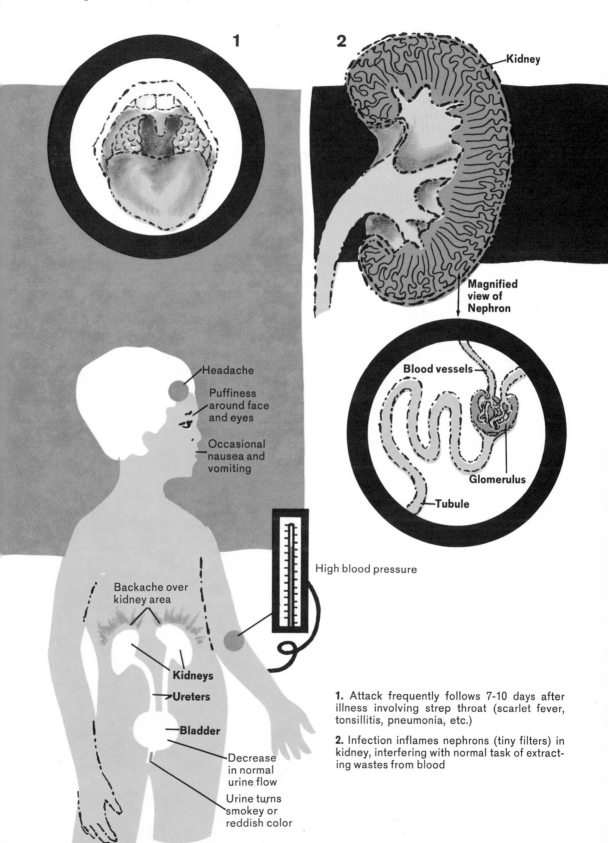

1

2

Kidney

Magnified view of Nephron

Blood vessels

Glomerulus

Tubule

Headache

Puffiness around face and eyes

Occasional nausea and vomiting

High blood pressure

Backache over kidney area

Kidneys

Ureters

Bladder

Decrease in normal urine flow

Urine turns smokey or reddish color

1. Attack frequently follows 7-10 days after illness involving strep throat (scarlet fever, tonsillitis, pneumonia, etc.)

2. Infection inflames nephrons (tiny filters) in kidney, interfering with normal task of extracting wastes from blood

the disease and its causes   Neuritis is an inflammatory or degenerative disease of the nerves which reduces their ability to function.   One nerve or many nerves can be involved.

Multiple neuritis involves many nerves and can be caused by a large number of things among which are the following: poisons, including arsenic, lead and mercury, methyl alcohol and benzine derivatives; dietary deficiencies caused by chronic alcoholism, lack of vitamins, diabetes, and occasionally pregnancy; infections of the central nervous system; infections such as diphtheria and infectious mononucleosis; and blood vessel disorders such as arteriosclerosis.

Single nerve involvement can result from infections such as herpes zoster (shingles); injury to the nerve such as stretching, tearing, or compressing it; tumors of the nerve root; and unknown causes such as those resulting in so-called Bell's palsy.

symptoms   The Medi-Graph lists symptoms common to most forms of neuritis although the areas involved may differ and the causes vary.

Interestingly enough, certain chemicals or diseases affect specific, peripheral nerves. Lead poison, for example, often results in the so-called wrist drop, while arsenic may lead to the development of the foot drop. Both wrist and foot drop may be seen as a result of alcoholism. Vitamin deficiencies usually involve the lower extremities first and then spread to involve other areas of the body. Sciatica (nerve pain spreading down the leg from the buttocks) is usually caused by a herniated intervertebral (slipped) disc.

complications   Complications depend upon the cause of the neuritis.   In the case of poisons, paralysis and its attendant problems are inevitable and death can result unless the cause of neuritis is treated promptly and corrective measures are provided.

prevention (or lessening of impact)   Any person with a specific illness capable of causing neuritis should be alert for the symptoms shown in the Medi-Graph. The danger of using chemicals or drugs indiscriminately, without suitable precautions and supervision, must be emphasized. Insecticides should be clearly labeled to indicate what offensive material they contain and what precautions should be taken in using them.

Problems caused by lack of vitamins and other deficiency states should be treated early, before they lead to irreversible changes and muscle paralysis. Effective medications and vitamins are available for these deficiency states.

When the underlying cause of the neuritis is mechanical, such as pressure on a nerve, the treatment will be directed toward correcting that condition. Nerves heal slowly and treatment, to be effective, should be begun at the earliest possible moment.

Neuritis

Inflammation of nerves caused by . . .

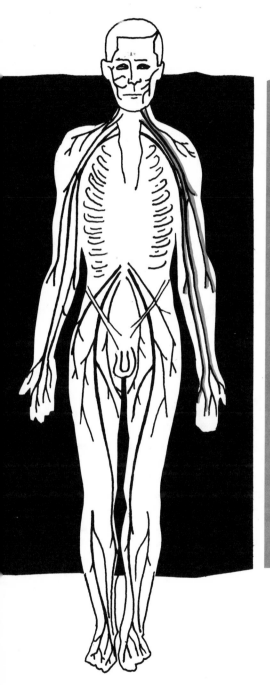

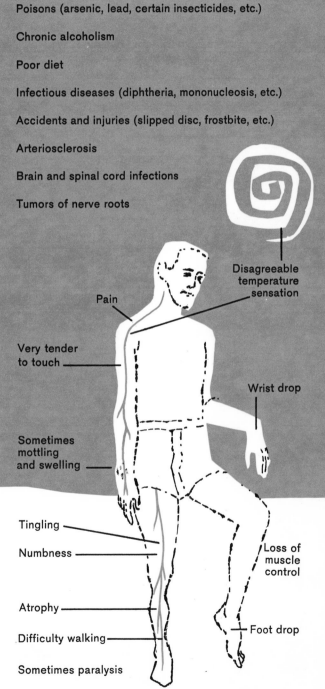

Poisons (arsenic, lead, certain insecticides, etc.)

Chronic alcoholism

Poor diet

Infectious diseases (diphtheria, mononucleosis, etc.)

Accidents and injuries (slipped disc, frostbite, etc.)

Arteriosclerosis

Brain and spinal cord infections

Tumors of nerve roots

Disagreeable temperature sensation

Pain

Very tender to touch

Wrist drop

Sometimes mottling and swelling

Tingling

Numbness

Loss of muscle control

Atrophy

Difficulty walking

Foot drop

Sometimes paralysis

the disease and its causes   There are many other names for this condition: irritable heart, soldier's heart, effort syndrome, nervous heart, and cardiac neurosis. All reflect the fact that the disease is psychosomatic in origin. This term means that there is no physical basis for the symptoms the patient displays—or that the symptoms are out of all proportion to the patient's physical problems.

In many cases of neurocirculatory asthenia there appears to be an inherited constitutional weakness in this direction. However, the specific cause of the disease appears to be anxiety and strain. Frequently it appears as a complication of some organic heart disease or other serious illness. It is found most often in young adults, more often in females than in males. Tobacco, coffee, and alcohol seem to aggravate the condition.

symptoms   The symptoms are real enough. There is unusual weakness, palpitations of the heart, shortness of breath with very little exertion. The patient complains of a constant dull ache in the chest, about the region of the heart. Occasionally there is a sharp chest pain. Breathing is rapid and there are frequent deep sighs. The patient shows the classic signs of anxiety—dizziness, faintness, sweating, tremors of the hands, and unusual nervousness. As the Medi-Graph shows, there are ways to distinguish these from organic heart systems.

complications   Since there is no real disorder to account for this condition other than anxiety, the only complication likely to occur is increased anxiety and emotional involvement.

prevention (or lessening of impact)   Removal of the patient from stressful situations can help. Psychotherapy is often helpful.

If the patient can learn to live a placid life, free of those pressures which create anxiety in him, the condition is likely to be improved. In such an atmosphere there need be no limitation on his activities.

Patients who have had some history of heart disease and are fearful and anxious for the future are among those who develop neurocirculatory asthenia. Help for them consists of treatment for their condition and reassurance that they are not necessarily in mortal danger.

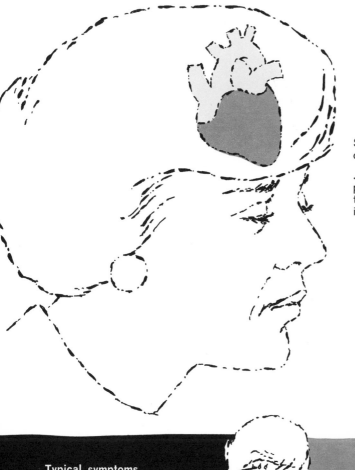

Symptoms of heart trouble that have no organic basis . . .

. . . Or if the patient has an organic heart problem and worries about it, the symptoms are out of all proportion to her physical problem

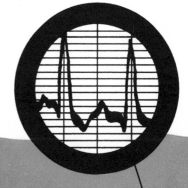

Typical symptoms

Sweating

Dizziness and faintness

Frequent deep sighing

Breathlessness

Sharp chest pain
or deep ache

Palpitations

Tremors

**Reason they don't indicate
organic problems**

Pain in lower left chest, where patient thinks pain should be, but rarely site of true problems

Physical activity doesn't produce electrocardiograph changes

Physical activity doesn't increase symptoms — frequently relieves them

Feeling of weakness

Numbing of extremities

the disease and its cause   This is a disease which involves infection and inflammation of the testicles. Its characteristics are pain, swelling, and a feeling of heaviness in these organs.

Orchitis most commonly occurs as a complication of mumps among men in the 15–25-year-old age group. Orchitis may break out in up to 25% of these mumps cases. However, it may also occur secondarily to a number of other diseases, such as gonorrhea, chicken pox, bruncellosis and bacterial prostate infection.

symptoms   When it follows mumps, orchitis usually appears about 7–10 days after the typical facial swelling of mumps—though it may occur in mumps cases where there is no facial swelling. Orchitis usually involves only one testicle which can become enormous in size and very painful. Fever, chills, and a feeling of weakness are other symptoms.

The symptoms of orchitis usually subside in 3–10 days.

complications   Atrophy of the testicle and sterility are the main complications. Atrophy of one testicle occurs in about 50% of the cases. Sterility is not common—occurring only in the infrequent cases where both testicles are involved. Another infrequent complication is the development of blood clots that travel to the lungs (pulmonary emboli).

prevention (or lessening of impact)   Prompt treatment of prostatic infection and gonorrhea can prevent orchitis in the infrequent cases where these infections are the primary threat.

A mumps vaccine is available which can prevent that disease. But once mumps is present, there is no way of preventing orchitis from developing in 25% of the cases.

Orchitis

Inflammation of testicles caused by infection resulting from mumps, VD, TB, chicken pox, prostate infection, etc.

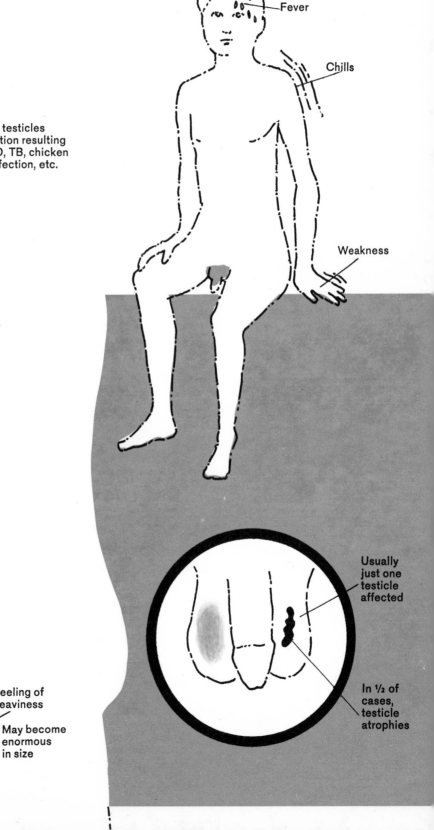

Fever

Chills

Weakness

Swelling of testicle

Pain

Feeling of heaviness

May become enormous in size

Usually just one testicle affected

In ½ of cases, testicle atrophies

the disease and its causes   This is a chronic disease involving the joints, and one which is likely to affect most people if they live long enough. It is sometimes referred to as a degenerative joint disease, because as one grows older there is degeneration of the joint cartilage and some overgrowth of bone. People who are overweight are affected, particularly in the weight-bearing joints such as the knees and hips. Osteoarthritis also affects the vertebrae of the back and the joints of the fingers. Unlike other forms of arthritis which can result from infection and inflammation, this disease is primarily the result of aging, and wear and tear. It is, however, often associated with repeated joint injury.
Both men and women are affected. It occurs in women about the time of the menopause and seems to affect their hand joints much more often than the hand joints of men.

symptoms   The condition develops slowly, with few obvious symptoms. Mainly there are joint aches and pains, and stiffness. These appear to be related to exercise of the particular joint involved. Medication generally gives relief. The stiffness is pronounced after the patient has been at rest, and tends to disappear when he is active. As the illness progresses, the osteoarthritic patient develops the characteristics shown on the Medi-Graph—knobby fingers, some grating of the joints on motion, and the formation of bony spurs, which are small projections off the bones.

complications   There are no serious complications. Sometimes there is pain, and because of this the activities of the patient become limited. In severe cases joint changes may interfere with normal activity. The joints are deformed and the back is stiff. Usually this does not affect the patient's general health or curtail his normal life span.

prevention (or lessening of impact)   Patients who are overweight must take steps to lose weight in order to lessen the strain on the joints. Those who are overactive are advised to get extra rest. Mild exercise and physiotherapy tend to lessen the severity of the disease and keep the joints mobile. Poor habits of diet should be improved. Any known infection should be treated and eliminated even though there is no positive relationship between infection and osteoarthritis.
When the lower spine is involved, patients can use bed boards and corsets to make themselves more comfortable. There are no specific medicines for this disease, and simple remedies are usually suggested.

Osteoarthritis

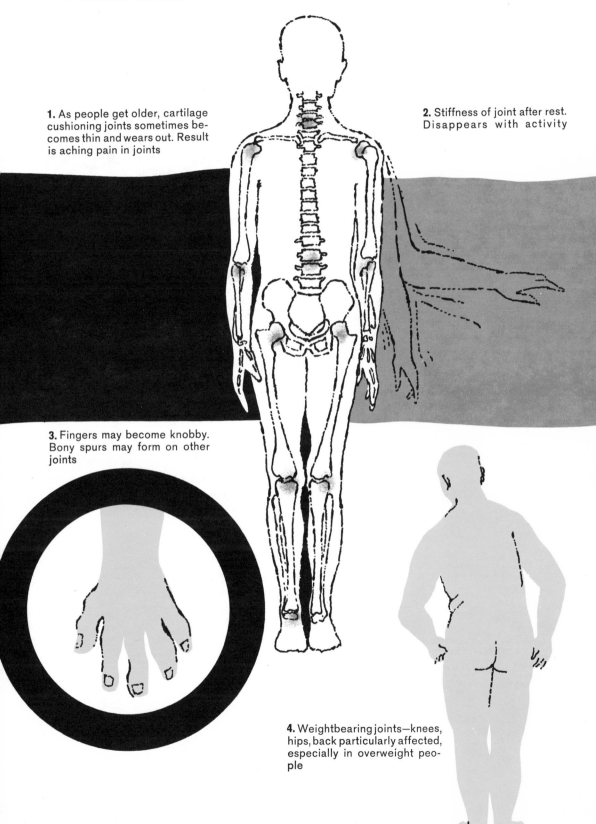

1. As people get older, cartilage cushioning joints sometimes becomes thin and wears out. Result is aching pain in joints

2. Stiffness of joint after rest. Disappears with activity

3. Fingers may become knobby. Bony spurs may form on other joints

4. Weightbearing joints—knees, hips, back particularly affected, especially in overweight people

the disease and its causes   This is an infection of the bone, often related to blood poisoning. Three types of osteomyelitis are generally recognized. The first, acute osteomyelitis, is most common in childhood. Its cause can be an abscess or any bodily infection carried by the blood. TB, pneumonia, and typhoid fever are among the diseases whose germs can get into the bloodstream and cause osteomyelitis by attacking the bones.

The second type, secondary osteomyelitis, is due to a specific problem at the bone site. Among these are compound fractures of the bone from accident or injury, dental infection, and penetrating wounds.

Chronic osteomyelitis is the third type. It describes persistent, resistant cases of osteomyelitis which originate as acute or secondary cases and gain a deep hold because they aren't treated promptly.

symptoms   An osteomyelitis victim has certain generalized symptoms, such as fever, chills, and feelings of weakness. More specific is pain, usually over the bone area where the disease has attacked. The overlying skin tissue becomes red, swollen, hot, and very tender to the touch. It looks as if an abscess had developed.

A symptom of secondary osteomyelitis is the appearance of a draining, non-healing wound near a bone area. For example, a draining dental infection that does not heal may be due to the development of osteomyelitis of the jaw. An X ray examination enables the doctor to make a prompt diagnosis. Chronic cases are easier to recognize, since the wound is open and draining small bits of bone.

complications   These can arise especially when the disease is not diagnosed promptly. One danger is multiple osteomyelitis—the spread of the infection to several bones at once. Severe destruction of the bone and prolonged disability also result. Amputation may become necessary if the diagnosis is delayed—or if the infection does not respond to treatment.

prevention (or lessening of impact)   Prompt treatment of all primary infections with appropriate antibiotics today usually prevents the development of osteomyelitis. In the case of compound fractures, corrective surgery and careful follow-up care can also stop development of the disease.

However, if osteomyelitis does develop, quick identification of the cause is needed. Treatment with adequate surgical drainage and antibiotics should suffice to prevent a serious problem.

Osteomyelitis (Infection of Bone)

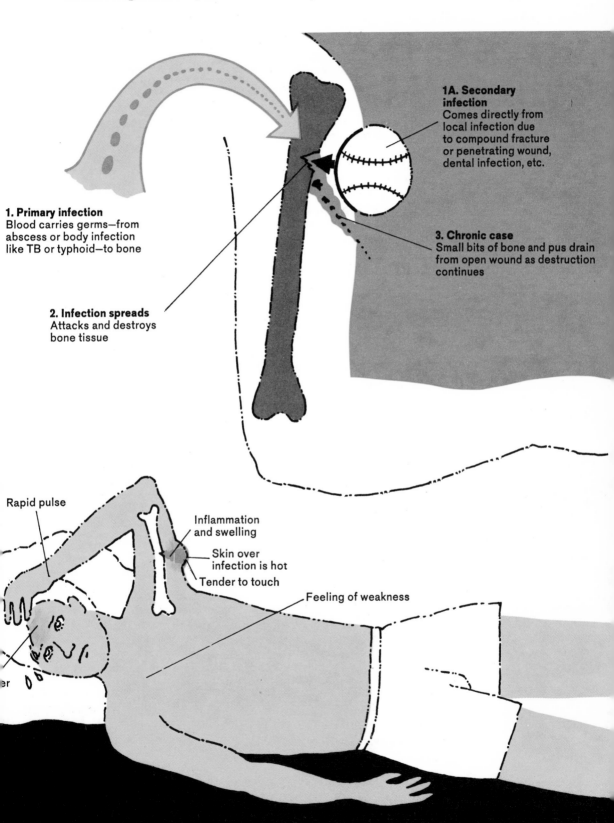

1A. Secondary infection
Comes directly from local infection due to compound fracture or penetrating wound, dental infection, etc.

1. Primary infection
Blood carries germs—from abscess or body infection like TB or typhoid—to bone

3. Chronic case
Small bits of bone and pus drain from open wound as destruction continues

2. Infection spreads
Attacks and destroys bone tissue

Rapid pulse

Inflammation and swelling

Skin over infection is hot

Tender to touch

Feeling of weakness

the disease and its causes   Ovarian infections are usually the result of infections elsewhere in the body. Organisms such as the gonococcus, the strepto-coccus, and the tubercle bacillus enter the genital area in the course of illnesses such as gonorrhea, scarlet fever, strep throat, and tuberculosis. The infection may spread from an adjacent organ, such as the Fallopian tube or uterus, or it may be carried through the blood from distant sites. Sometimes a sizable abscess develops in the ovary, as shown in the Medi-Graph.

symptoms   In an acute ovarian infection there is some abdominal pain and swell-ing, nausea, and vomiting. The patient may have a temperature of 101° to 103°. The neighboring bowel and bladder are frequently irritated by the infection, resulting in frequent urination and sometimes diarrhea. The involved side is tender to touch and, on examination, shows signs of spasm. When the right side is involved and the white blood cell count is high, it is easy to mistake the illness for appendicitis.

The patient shows the usual signs of an abscess in the body as the ovarian infection progresses: severe pain, high fever, and an increase in nausea and vomiting. Sometimes the abscessed mass can be felt ex-ternally and the patient reports it to be very tender to the touch.

Frequently, at this point, the illness quiets of its own accord and the patient appears to recover completely. But the condition tends to be-come chronic, with intermittent flare-ups of pain and discomfort often associated with the menstrual cycle.

Occasionally the abscess in the ovary can rupture into the rectum, bladder, or vagina.

When the infection is caused by the tubercle bacillus, the symptoms are similar but the disease tends to be more chronic, worsening along with the worsening condition of the tubercular patient. There is loss of weight and general disability. Often fluid forms in the abdomen. Alto-gether, the patient becomes generally weakened.

complications   When both ovaries are involved, the tissue destruction results eventually in sterility.

When an ovarian abscess ruptures into neighboring areas, there can be further infection throughout the body.

When the cause is gonorrhea, arthritis is a common complication.

In its chronic state this disease can be distressing to a patient who is repeatedly disabled, frequently without warning.

prevention (or lessening of impact)   When gonorrhea or tuberculosis is identi-fied as the cause of the acute infection, immediate therapy is required. Antibiotics may be effective if treatment is begun early. If unresponsive to antibiotics, the infection may be treated surgically, particularly where only one ovary is involved, for by avoiding the spread of the infection to the healthy ovary, sterility may be avoided.

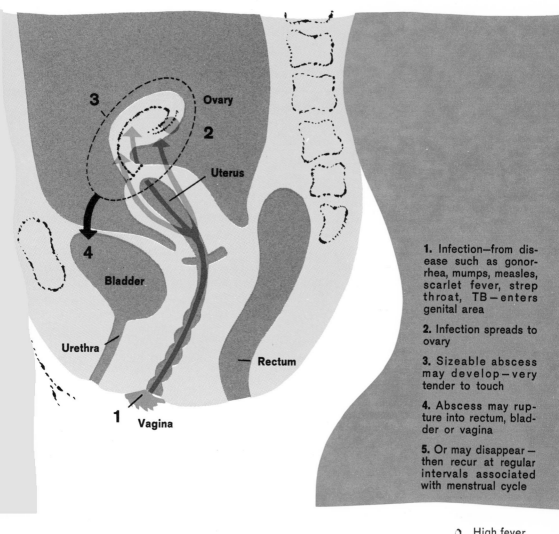

1. Infection—from disease such as gonorrhea, mumps, measles, scarlet fever, strep throat, TB—enters genital area

2. Infection spreads to ovary

3. Sizeable abscess may develop—very tender to touch

4. Abscess may rupture into rectum, bladder or vagina

5. Or may disappear—then recur at regular intervals associated with menstrual cycle

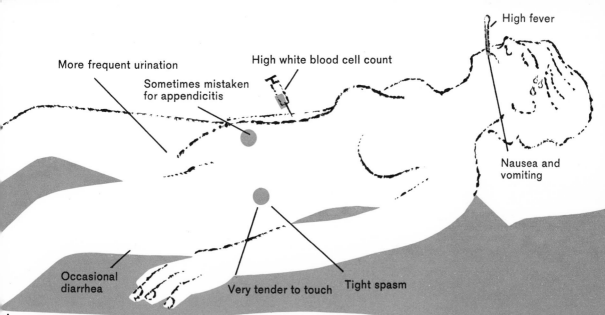

the disease and its causes   The pancreas is a gland involved in the digestive process. The disease known as pancreatitis occurs when this gland is attacked by excess enzymes liberated into it, for reasons that are not known. It occurs in middle age, slightly more often in females, and most frequently in patients with alcoholism, peptic ulcer, and gallstones. Direct injury and pregnancy are also causes.

The disease can be mild or severe, depending upon the degree and type of involvement of the pancreas. Often a patient is subject to the illness after he has eaten a heavy meal.

symptoms   Pancreatitis begins very suddenly, with severe upper abdominal pain radiating into the back and lower chest. Frequently there is nausea and vomiting. The patient is very anxious and restless, and in severe cases, shock-like. In this latter state, he is cold, sweaty, and extremely weak. His face, lips, and fingernails have a bluish color. Such severe or hemorrhagic cases can be fatal 50% of the time. Most mild cases recover in a short time.

There may be jaundice (liver involvement with yellowing of the skin and eyeballs) in both the mild and severe forms of pancreatitis. Temperature and pulse do not change as a rule, but there is bloating of the abdomen and constipation.

Recurrence of pain, nausea, or vomiting may indicate further injury to the pancreas or the development of complications.

complications   With a severe case of pancreatitis, there can speedily be such drastic complications as shock and death. In a milder case, complications include abscess of the pancreas, cyst formation, internal hemorrhage, and fistula formation. A frequent complication is the development of a chronic form of pancreatitis with recurrent bouts of pain and other symptoms.

prevention (or lessening of impact)   There is no specific way this disease can be prevented. Patients with gallstones or peptic ulcers should have corrective treatment without delay because of the frequent association of these conditions with pancreatitis.

Pancreatitis (Acute)

Mild Case

1. Anxiety and restlessness

2. Nausea, bloating and vomiting

3. Severe abdominal pain radiating to back and chest

Severe Case

1. Shock symptoms, cold, sweaty, weak

2. Face, lips, fingernails turn blue

3. Excruciating pain and spasm or rigidity of abdomen

4. Hemorrhaging and deterioration of pancreas

Duodenum

Colon

Stomach

Kidney

Pancreas

Advanced Hemorrhagic Pancreatitis

Complete destruction of pancreas can occur—halting its production of digestive juices and insulin. If patient recovers, he may be left with digestive difficulties and diabetes.

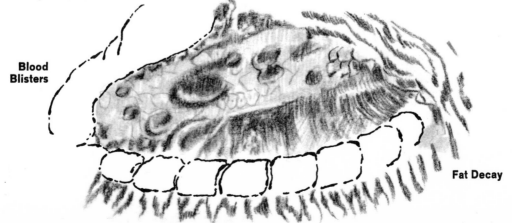

Blood Blisters

Fat Decay

the disease and its causes Very little is known about the cause of this disease, but it is believed to be the result of degenerative changes in certain areas of the brain occurring in old age. Head injuries have been mentioned as a cause, but evidence doesn't support this. A condition resembling Parkinson's disease follows encephalitis and sometimes syphilitic infection of the central nervous system. It occurs more often in men than women, and mostly in their fifties and sixties.

symptoms The onset is very slow, and often years may pass before either the patient or his family observes that he is becoming disabled. Although he is otherwise in good health, he shows slowly increasing body rigidity, associated with tremors of the head and limbs. There may be various tics, twitches, muscle spasms, and other involuntary movements. Salivation increases and drooling is common. The patient's face takes on a blank expression. He becomes slower in his movements. His arms no longer swing when he walks, and indeed, walking becomes difficult. Even his voice tends to lose its natural inflections and becomes weak and monotonous.

Usually one side of the face and body is involved, followed in a year or so by the other side.

Some patients have greater muscle rigidity, others have more tremor. Although the patient may have difficulty talking in the later stages of the disease, his mental sharpness is not affected. In severe cases, the patient may become completely immobile and unable to care for himself.

complications Parkinson's disease is a slowly progressive one. Although no recoveries are recorded, death rarely occurs from this illness and the life span of the patient is not usually shortened.

In those patients confined to bed, pneumonia, bladder infections, kidney stones, and bed sores all are likely to develop. These undermine the general health of the individual and open the way to secondary infections that cause death.

prevention (or lessening of impact) The useful life of a patient can be prolonged with good nursing care and rehabilitation techniques. He should be encouraged to perform whatever skills he has as long as he is able. Moderate exercise and physiotherapy are helpful. Drugs are available to control the tremor and the excess salivation. The benefits of these, however, are limited.

Current research holds out hope for an eventual substantive cure. Encouraging results have been obtained with the new drug levodihydroxyphenylalanine (L-DOPA). Experimental brain surgery has opened another promising avenue toward control of this disease.

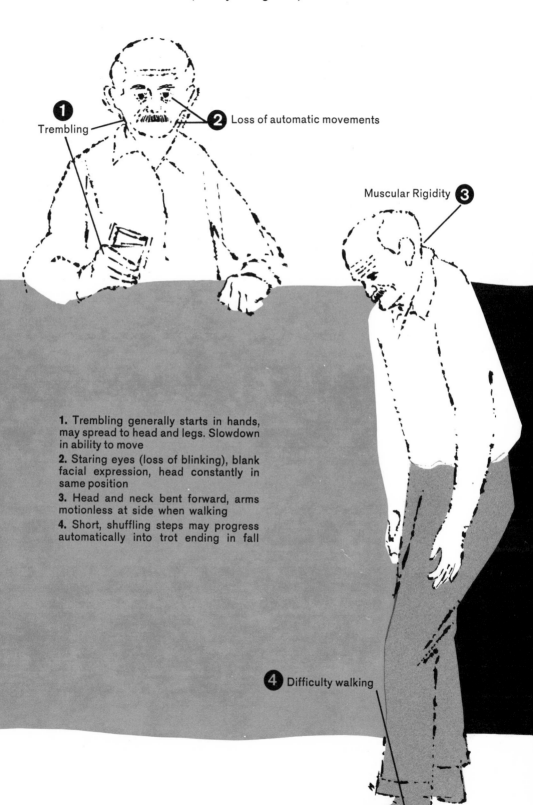

1. Trembling

2. Loss of automatic movements

3. Muscular Rigidity

4. Difficulty walking

1. Trembling generally starts in hands, may spread to head and legs. Slowdown in ability to move

2. Staring eyes (loss of blinking), blank facial expression, head constantly in same position

3. Head and neck bent forward, arms motionless at side when walking

4. Short, shuffling steps may progress automatically into trot ending in fall

the disease and its causes Pellagra is a dietary deficiency disease in which the vitamin substance nicotinic acid, in particular, is lacking. Nicotinic acid is found in high quantities in lean meats, liver, tomatoes, spinach, peas, turnip and mustard greens.

Pellagra is extremely common, especially in areas where poverty and ignorance force people to live on unbalanced diets. Even people of means can get pellagra if they live on a diet rich in carbohydrates and fat, but low in proteins, minerals, and vitamins.

Some people get this disease because they have an organic illness which makes it difficult for them to consume or make use of nicotinic acid compounds.

Alcoholics are frequent victims of pellagra because they eat poorly. And food faddists who tend to eliminate some of the foods with anti-pellagra nicotinic acid sometimes get this disease.

symptoms There is usually what is known as the 3 D's of pellagra—*diarrhea, dementia,* and *dermatitis.*

The patient complains of a scalded sensation in the mouth. The edges of the tongue become irritated, red, and ulcerated. Skin lesions are common on all the extremities. They begin as reddened areas which peel and form large blisters. These eventually clear up at the center, but when they heal, some areas of the skin take on a parchment-like appearance.

There is usually weakness and loss of weight, frequently associated with diarrhea. There may be fever, muscle weakness, prostration, irritability, memory loss, and headache.

Dementia may take the form of mental depression and psychosis, as the result of pellagra.

complications Complications are seen most often in children who are undernourished. They appear underdeveloped and obviously in ill health. Unless the diagnosis is made and corrective measures are taken, they will develop poorly, both physically and mentally.

prevention (or lessening of impact) A diet containing foods with sufficient nicotinic acid will prevent pellagra. Vitamin preparations containing this chemical can be bought, but it is better to plan a diet that includes the necessary foods.

Pellagra

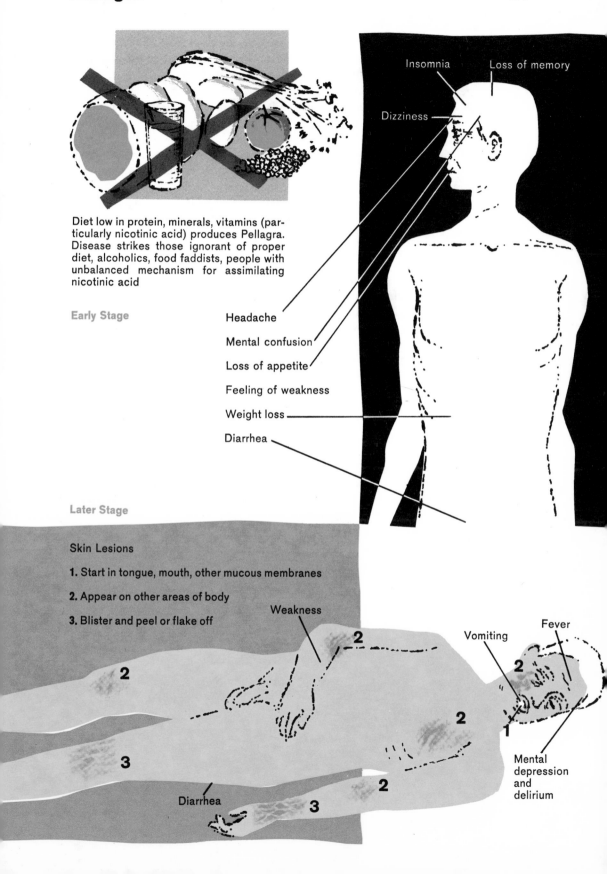

Diet low in protein, minerals, vitamins (particularly nicotinic acid) produces Pellagra. Disease strikes those ignorant of proper diet, alcoholics, food faddists, people with unbalanced mechanism for assimilating nicotinic acid

Early Stage

Insomnia

Loss of memory

Dizziness

Headache

Mental confusion

Loss of appetite

Feeling of weakness

Weight loss

Diarrhea

Later Stage

Skin Lesions

1. Start in tongue, mouth, other mucous membranes

2. Appear on other areas of body

3. Blister and peel or flake off

Weakness

Vomiting

Fever

Diarrhea

Mental depression and delirium

the disease and its causes   Acute pericarditis is an inflammation of the pericardium—the outer lining of the heart. The nature and severity of the primary infection will determine the course of the pericarditis, which is generally the result of an infection elsewhere in the body. However, it also can be directly associated with heart disease or with uremia, cancer, injury, and air or foreign bodies in the pericardial sac that surrounds the heart.

In this discussion, we are dealing with benign (viral) pericarditis—the most common type. The acute form is frequently preceded by a respiratory infection.

The disease is found in all ages but more usually in younger adults. While the course of this illness can be stormy, it is usually over in a few days to two weeks.

symptoms   The symptoms are noted on the accompanying Medi-Graph. There is sometimes an irregular heart rhythm. The pain is often related to pleurisy which frequently accompanies pericarditis. Sometimes it will feel like the form of heart attack known as acute coronary occlusion. The pain can be continuous, or come and go, and it can be quite sharp. Often a patient gets relief by sitting up.

complications   Blood, fluid, or pus can collect in the pericardium in a quantity sufficient to press upon the heart and interfere with its normal activity. This complication is not frequent, but it can be serious when it occurs. More frequent complications are involvement of the heart muscle and lung membrane.

prevention (or lessening of impact)   There is no known method of preventing this disease. A patient with pericarditis must be watched carefully for signs of complications and promptly treated if and when they develop, to avoid more serious problems.

Bed rest and antibiotics may be sufficient if the initial infection responds to treatment. When fluid collects, techniques are available to reduce the pressure on the heart. Surgery is sometimes indicated and can be quite helpful.

Pericarditis

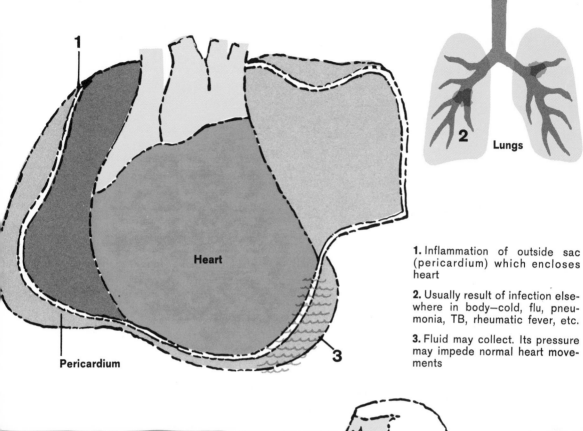

Heart

Pericardium

Lungs

2

1. Inflammation of outside sac (pericardium) which encloses heart

2. Usually result of infection elsewhere in body—cold, flu, pneumonia, TB, rheumatic fever, etc.

3. Fluid may collect. Its pressure may impede normal heart movements

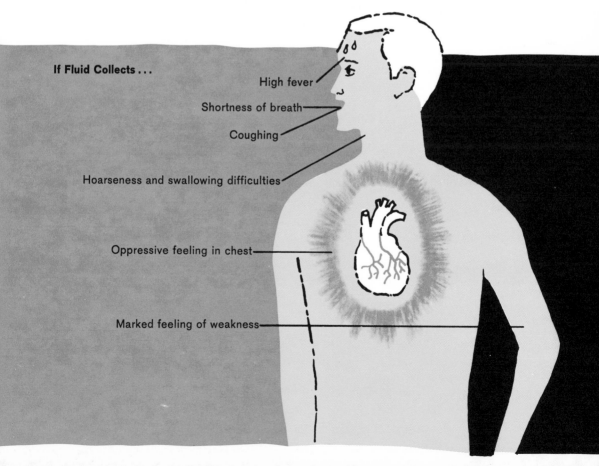

If Fluid Collects . . .

High fever

Shortness of breath

Coughing

Hoarseness and swallowing difficulties

Oppressive feeling in chest

Marked feeling of weakness

Pernicious Anemia
(Lack of red blood cells)

the disease and its causes This is a blood disease in which the body does not produce red blood cells in sufficient quantity and quality to sustain a normal, active life. The disease occurs because of the inability of the victim to absorb adequate amounts of vitamin B_{12}—which stimulates production of healthy red blood cells. The stomach of a normal person produces a substance called *intrinsic factor* which—together with hydrochloric acid—is responsible for this B_{12} absorption. Pernicious anemia sufferers do not produce either intrinsic factor or hydrochloric acid. As a result, they do not produce a normal supply of red blood cells.

Most cases of pernicious anemia develop in people in their 40's and 50's. The disease strikes both sexes equally, and occurs most frequently among fair-haired, blue-eyed people who tend to premature graying of the hair.

symptoms The disease comes on gradually with an increasing feeling of fatigue and weakness, shortness of breath and headache. A sore, beefy red tongue is a common symptom. The skin frequently acquires a pale coloration.

Digestive problems may occur, such as loss of appetite and diarrhea. Heart and circulation problems may occur, such as chest pain, rapid pulse, palpitations. Mental symptoms may occur, such as drowsiness, memory loss and depression.

If the disease is allowed to progress, the spinal cord is affected, with weakness and numbness of the limbs—eventually leading to a loss of their control.

The doctor's examination may reveal an enlarged liver and spleen. He can make a positive diagnosis of the disease by blood tests and the absence of hydrochloric acid in the stomach's secretions.

complications When the disease is untreated or treatment delayed, the most serious effects are on the nervous system. The victim loses the ability to control his body movements, including bowel and bladder control.

In his weakened condition, the pernicious anemia sufferer is also susceptible to secondary infections. And it has also been noted that cancer of the stomach is 3 times more common in patients with pernicious anemia.

prevention (or lessening of impact) No treatment is yet known that will restore the intrinsic factor and hydrochloric acid to the gastric juice of the stomach. However, in 1926 it was discovered that adding large amounts of liver to the diet would control pernicious anemia.

More recently, it has been found that large doses of vitamin B_{12} have the ability to powerfully stimulate the formation of red blood cells. Once the diagnosis has been made and the doctor has started the program of B_{12} injections, the patient's pallor, anemia, and other symptoms clear up in a quick and dramatic fashion. However, the treatment is not a cure. Therefore, the patient must continue it under his doctor's direction to maintain his health.

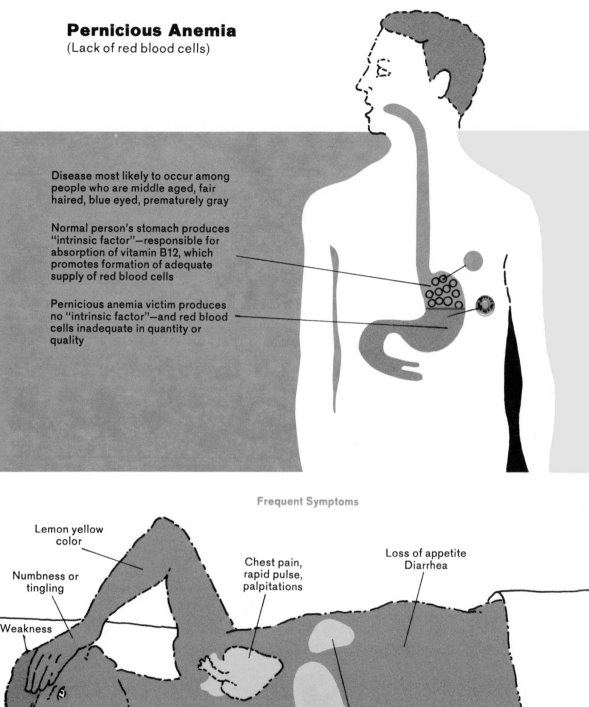

Pernicious Anemia
(Lack of red blood cells)

Disease most likely to occur among people who are middle aged, fair haired, blue eyed, prematurely gray

Normal person's stomach produces "intrinsic factor"—responsible for absorption of vitamin B12, which promotes formation of adequate supply of red blood cells

Pernicious anemia victim produces no "intrinsic factor"—and red blood cells inadequate in quantity or quality

Frequent Symptoms

Lemon yellow color

Numbness or tingling

Weakness

Chest pain, rapid pulse, palpitations

Loss of appetite
Diarrhea

Drowsiness, memory loss, depression

Shortness of breath

Beefy, smooth, sore tongue

Enlarged liver and spleen

Poor coordination of hands and feet

the disease and its causes   Phlebitis is a common inflammatory disease involving the veins of the body. Almost any vein may be affected, but the disease is most common in the lower extremities. It occurs most often after an operation, after pregnancy, and in association with other blood vessel disorders or serious illnesses.

The exact cause is unknown, but it seems that slowing of the blood flow, changes in the blood vessel wall, and changes in the clotting mechanism are all involved. Injury and infections elsewhere in the body also seem to play a part.

symptoms   There may be pain along the vein in the beginning, but not always. The affected vein feels like a long, hard cord and is tender to touch. The skin over it is red and hot. Walking may cause pain. Low-grade fever is usually present.

When the deep veins of the leg are involved, the disease is harder to identify. There is pain in one or both calves which gets worse if the foot is bent forcefully toward the knee. The leg may swell and feel warm on the affected side. The patient is quite uncomfortable if his calf is squeezed.

Phlebitis can travel by direct extension from the legs into the abdominal blood vessels.

complications   There are no great risks or problems in superficial (surface) phlebitis. When deep veins are involved there is usually clot formation (phlebothrombosis). The danger is that a piece of the clot may be carried to the lungs. When this happens the result is calamitous.

prevention (or lessening of impact)   Because phlebitis occurs so frequently after surgery, it has become the practice to get patients up and walking as soon as possible. Activity seems to improve circulation and prevent the development of phlebitis. Therefore, prolonged bed rest in any illness should be avoided where possible.

Once phlebitis is present, anticoagulant drugs are generally used in an attempt to keep the disease from extending further and to prevent the development of blood clots. Surgery is another effective means of limiting the spread and preventing an embolus from forming and traveling to a distant organ.

Phlebitis

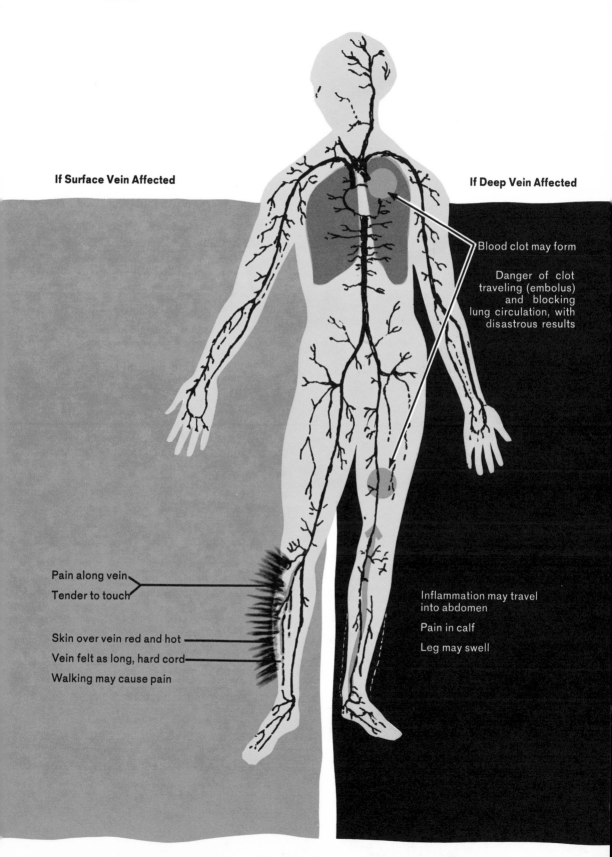

If Surface Vein Affected

If Deep Vein Affected

Blood clot may form

Danger of clot
traveling (embolus)
and blocking
lung circulation, with
disastrous results

Pain along vein
Tender to touch

Skin over vein red and hot

Vein felt as long, hard cord

Walking may cause pain

Inflammation may travel
into abdomen

Pain in calf

Leg may swell

the disease and its cause This is a birth defect in the skin over the base of the spine. It occurs because the skin fails to close completely over the midline of the spine. As a result, cysts are formed, the inside walls of which often contain hair follicles and sweat glands. The cyst cavities also often collect loose tufts of hair.

These pilonidal cysts frequently are present without the victim's knowledge until, because of injury or infection, they become painful.

symptoms The victim becomes aware of a pilonidal cyst because of pain, swelling, and a redness over the area at the base of the spine. An abscess develops which may burrow under the skin to either side of the spine, forming a sinus (tunnel). When opened, this discharges large amounts of pus, blood, and often tufts of hair. The pilonidal cyst may open spontaneously, or it may have to be opened surgically to relieve the victim's discomfort. New cyst infections develop periodically, along with new sinus formations.

complications In some cases, the cyst can become as large as an egg—presenting a serious impediment to working and everyday living.

As with any other infection, the poisons from the pilonidal cyst may spread to other parts of the body or cause blood poisoning. In rare instances, the underlying bone (the sacrum) can become infected—causing the disease osteomyelitis.

prevention (or lessening of impact) Infected pilonidal cysts should be opened and drained surgically if they do not soon open spontaneously or with the aid of measures like sitz baths. Strict cleanliness and use of antibiotics in the area may prevent further flare-ups.

In cases of chronic infection and disability, surgery to remove all sinus tracts in the area is usually curative. It may be that considerable abnormal tissue must be removed, and sufficient time must be spent in the hospital to allow complete healing.

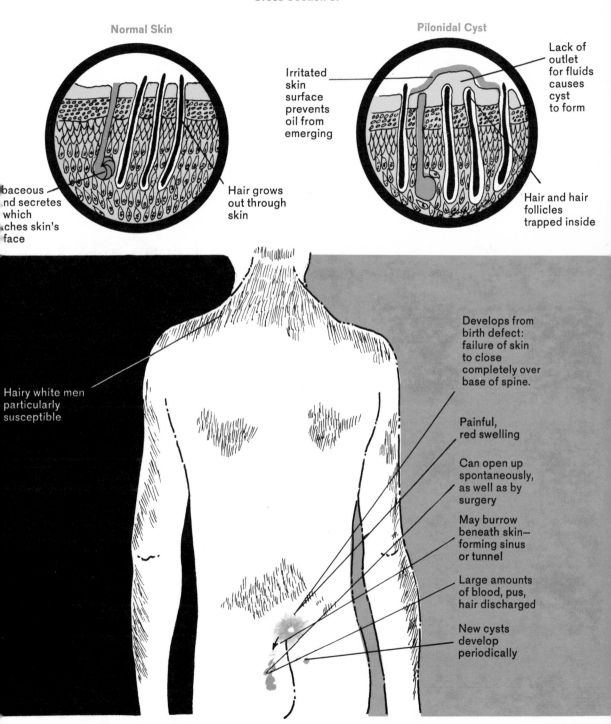

Cross Section of

Normal Skin

Pilonidal Cyst

Irritated skin surface prevents oil from emerging

Lack of outlet for fluids causes cyst to form

baceous nd secretes which ches skin's face

Hair grows out through skin

Hair and hair follicles trapped inside

Hairy white men particularly susceptible

Develops from birth defect: failure of skin to close completely over base of spine.

Painful, red swelling

Can open up spontaneously, as well as by surgery

May burrow beneath skin—forming sinus or tunnel

Large amounts of blood, pus, hair discharged

New cysts develop periodically

the disease and its causes   This is a small, round worm which infects the small and large intestines of humans. It is found most often in children, but frequently all the members of one family can be infected.

The eggs of the worm enter the body through contaminated food or water and pass into the small intestine where they develop into adult worms. Then the fertilized females wander to the anus and deposit a new crop of eggs there. Sometimes they even enter the vagina and Fallopian tubes.

symptoms   There is intense itching and irritation of the anus and the surrounding area. Since the adult female pinworms migrate and lay their eggs in the anal area at night, the symptoms are much more marked at that time.

complications   There are no serious complications. This is a mild but annoying illness. Occasionally there is secondary infection around the anus.

prevention (or lessening of impact)   Personal hygiene is the most important factor in controlling this disease. After bowel movements the anus should be carefully cleaned and the hands thoroughly washed. Infected children should have their nails clipped short and scrubbed before eating, because when they scratch the anal area, they embed the microscopic-sized eggs under the fingernails. Then, in eating, the pinworm eggs can come off the fingernails onto the food, starting the infection cycle again. Children should also be warned to keep their hands out of their mouths.

Stool examinations or rectal smears should be taken, as directed by the physician, to make certain no living worms remain after treatment. Pinworm infestation responds well to drug therapy, but reinfections are frequent unless the entire family is treated.

Pinworm

Causes itching of anus—particularly at bedtime

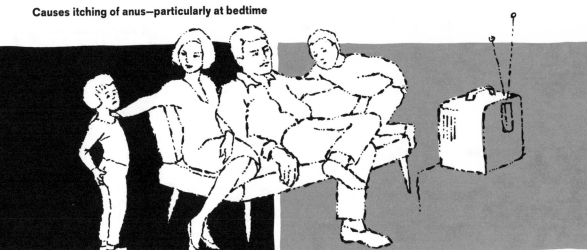

Pinworm generally spreads throughout family, starting with children

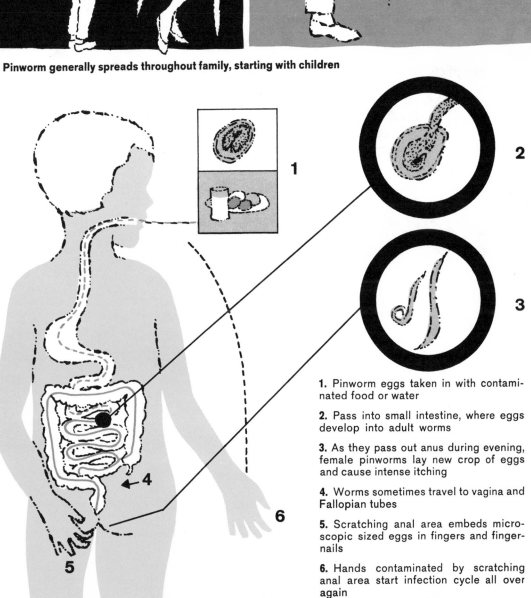

1. Pinworm eggs taken in with contaminated food or water

2. Pass into small intestine, where eggs develop into adult worms

3. As they pass out anus during evening, female pinworms lay new crop of eggs and cause intense itching

4. Worms sometimes travel to vagina and Fallopian tubes

5. Scratching anal area embeds microscopic sized eggs in fingers and fingernails

6. Hands contaminated by scratching anal area start infection cycle all over again

the disease and its causes This is an acute disease of the skin which is said to be self-limiting because it runs a definite course and then clears up. On rare occasions in children it spreads to the extremities and face, but in adults it is usually limited to the shoulders, trunk, and pelvic areas. The cause is unknown. It is not contagious, nor is it a serious disease. A single attack gives immunity. It is important primarily because it is often confused with certain contagious diseases and more serious lesions.

symptoms It usually begins with the appearance of a herald patch—a large, salmon-colored area that breaks out on the body or neck. A generalized body rash breaks out 7 to 10 days later. In the rash pattern, the lesions have a characteristic appearance—bright red with yellowish scaling. They usually appear in lines that parallel the lines of the ribs and other skin cleavages. Patients with pityriasis rosea have no discomfort, and there is no itching.

complications There are no serious complications.

prevention (or lessening of impact) There is no known way to prevent this disease. Since it is self-limiting, it requires no treatment and actually responds to none. It is included here because it is so frequently a matter of concern, not because it is a serious illness.

Pityriasis Rosea

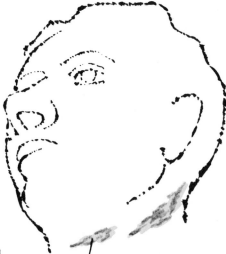

1. Herald Patch Appears First
Salmon-colored, with a scaly surface, large patch appears on body or neck

Herald Patch

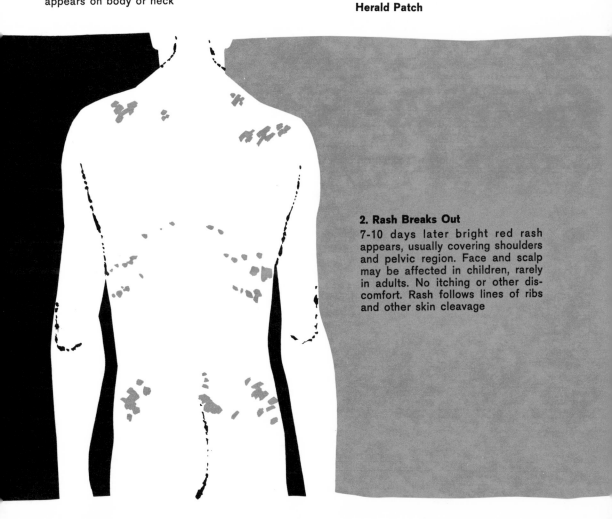

2. Rash Breaks Out
7-10 days later bright red rash appears, usually covering shoulders and pelvic region. Face and scalp may be affected in children, rarely in adults. No itching or other discomfort. Rash follows lines of ribs and other skin cleavage

3. Rash Lasts 6-10 Weeks
Rash gives off yellow flakes or scales. Single attack usually results in immunity from subsequent recurrence

the disease and its causes   Pleurisy is an inflammation of the delicate membrane
lining part of the chest cavity which houses the lungs. Pleurisy is almost
always the result of infection elsewhere in the body. This is particularly the case with lung infections such as pneumonia and tuberculosis.
Tumors, blood clots, and certain generalized diseases also can involve
the pleura.
When the inflammation is accompanied by an accumulation of fluid in
the pleural sac, it is known as pleural effusion, or wet pleurisy. In dry
pleurisy, pain is caused by the pleural membranes rubbing together—as
explained in the Medi-Graph.

symptoms   The onset is usually quite rapid, with severe pain in the chest. Coughing, deep breathing, and change of position aggravate the condition. The
pain may radiate to the abdomen, neck, shoulders, or back.
The type of symptoms that appear will be determined by the nature of
the primary infection. If there is pneumonia, cough and fever will be
present. If there is a blood clot to the lungs, the patient will spit blood.
Whatever the disease responsible for the pleurisy, the symptoms will
relate to that disease.

complications   Complications can be held to a minimum if the cause of the
pleurisy is identified promptly and treated forthwith. The usual complication is accumulation of fluid in the pleural sac. This may be clear,
bloody, or pussy, creating in the latter case a condition known as
empyema. When there is fluid, there is some collapse of lung tissue
which adds to the discomfort of the patient as well as to the seriousness
of the illness. But always the underlying infection determines how
serious the complications are likely to be.

prevention (or lessening of impact)   Prompt recognition of pleurisy and its cause
is important. When this is done, and proper medical care is given, the
patient can be made much more comfortable and complications avoided.

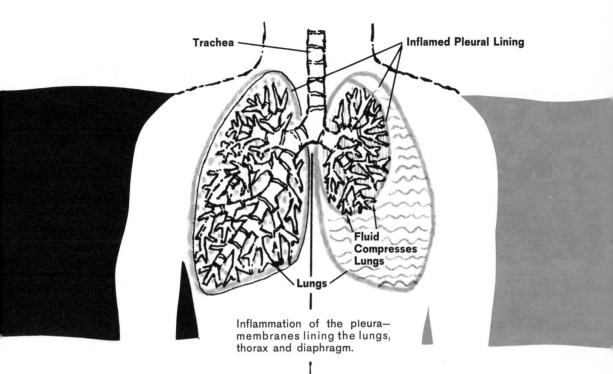

Trachea

Inflamed Pleural Lining

Fluid Compresses Lungs

Lungs

Inflammation of the pleura—membranes lining the lungs, thorax and diaphragm.

Dry Pleurisy
Painful inflammation of the pleura lining, aggravated by breathing, coughing, sneezing, or anything else causing inflamed layers of lining to rub together.

Wet Pleurisy
Inflammation plus accumulation of fluid, collapsing lung, making breathing difficult.

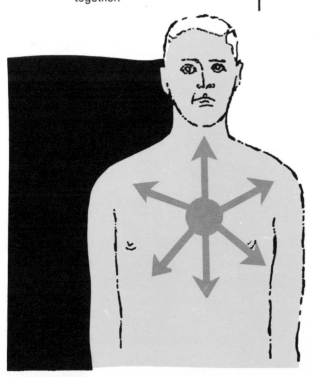

Most common symptom is severe pain in chest, particularly when breathing. Pain may radiate to abdomen, neck, shoulders or back. Pleurisy can be a complication in the wake of other diseases affecting lungs, such as pneumonia, TB, flu, etc.

the disease and its causes   Pneumonia is an acute infection of one or both lungs. At one time lobar pneumonia was the typical form seen. However, sulfa drugs and antibiotics have been so effective in dealing with it that this type is rarely seen today—although it still occurs. The exact diagnosis depends on the bacteria isolated, X ray evidence, and the visible symptoms.

The type of pneumonia most common now is virus, or atypical, pneumonia. Despite the name and the belief that a virus is involved, the precise cause is not known. It is this form of bronchopneumonia which is discussed here and described in the Medi-Graph.

symptoms   The onset is usually slow. There are minor upper respiratory symptoms, low-grade temperature, chills and headache. Appetite is poor. The throat may be dry or scratchy. Pain beneath the breastbone is common along with a cough when the patient breathes deeply. After a few days the dry cough becomes looser, with thick sputum that may be streaked with blood. Temperature can rise as high as 104° in the first few days, but the fever generally drops back to normal about the 5th to 7th day.

Convalescence from pneumonia is slow and it may take weeks for a patient to lose his cough and his feeling of weakness. Very often patients have virus pneumonia in a form so mild they do not know they have it. There is no temperature, a mild cough, and some feeling of weakness. The presence of the disease is made known in such cases only when routine chest X rays are taken and the lung infection is revealed.

Virus pneumonia is not seen often in a severe form, but it can and does attack chronically ill, debilitated patients.

complications   These are rare. Occasionally the membranes that surround the lungs fill with fluid. And infrequently, the brain and heart become involved.

prevention (or lessening of impact)   Since the precise cause of this disease is unknown, there is no known method of preventing it. Cold shots and vaccines are available and are helpful to some, but they are not proven preventives. It can only be suggested that one should avoid exposure to infected individuals, follow a sensible diet, and get sufficient rest.

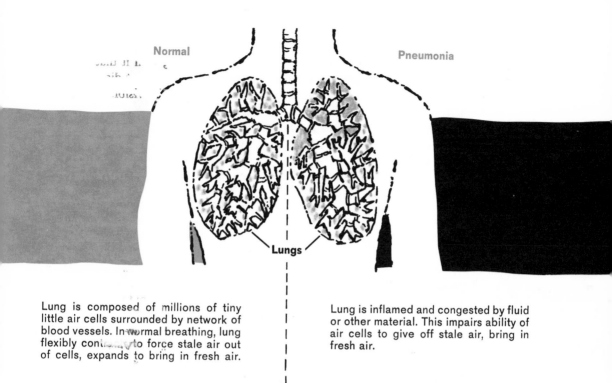

Normal

Pneumonia

Lungs

Lung is composed of millions of tiny little air cells surrounded by network of blood vessels. In normal breathing, lung flexibly contracts to force stale air out of cells, expands to bring in fresh air.

Lung is inflamed and congested by fluid or other material. This impairs ability of air cells to give off stale air, bring in fresh air.

Typical Symptoms of Virus Pneumonia

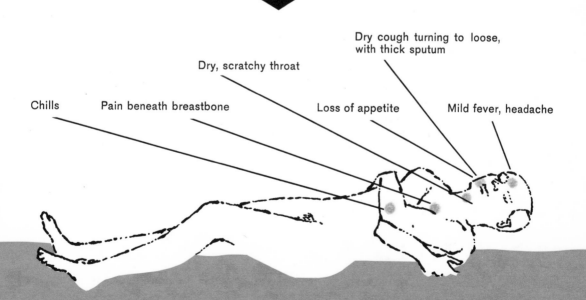

Dry cough turning to loose, with thick sputum

Dry, scratchy throat

Chills

Pain beneath breastbone

Loss of appetite

Mild fever, headache

the disease and its causes   Poliomyelitis, or infantile paralysis, is an acute virus infection of the central nervous system. It is spread in two ways: through the intestinal tract by means of food and water that have been contaminated by convalescent patients, healthy carriers, fleas, insects, pests, or animals; and through the secretions from the nose and throat of an infected person. The incubation period is 7 to 14 days, and the disease is usually over in 10 to14 days. One attack gives lifelong immunity but only to the specific type of polio involved. Infants have a high degree of natural immunity. However, the disease hits hardest at young children. Youngsters with recent tonsillectomies seem to be particularly susceptible during epidemics.

symptoms   The onset is usually sudden, with fever, headache, drowsiness, and irritability. The neck becomes stiff and the spine rigid. Muscles can be quite tender. By the third day the temperature may drop, only to rise again by the 5th day as muscle paralysis develops. While any group of muscles may be involved, usually it is those of the lower extremities or back.
Bulbar polio is a severe form in which the base of the brain is involved. In such a case, swallowing becomes difficult and speech and breathing are interfered with. It is often fatal.
A mild or "abortive" type of polio is also seen. All the early symptoms may be present, but no paralysis develops. Because the attack is so mild, diagnosis is difficult and often is never made.

complications   There are secondary complications, particularly pneumonia and kidney infection. Other problems arise in relation to the areas involved and the degree of nerve damage, and these depend upon the severity of the illness.

prevention (or lessening of impact)   Two effective vaccines are now available. One is the "killed" Salk vaccine which is given by injection. The other is the "live" Sabin vaccine taken by mouth. Anyone who starts on the Salk vaccine may continue with the Sabin provided each vaccine is taken exactly as recommended. In that way maximum protection is provided. Every infant should be routinely immunized. For that matter, unless otherwise advised by the physician, everyone should be protected by one or both of these vaccines.

After day or two of fever, headache and weakness, patient begins to develop such symptoms as:

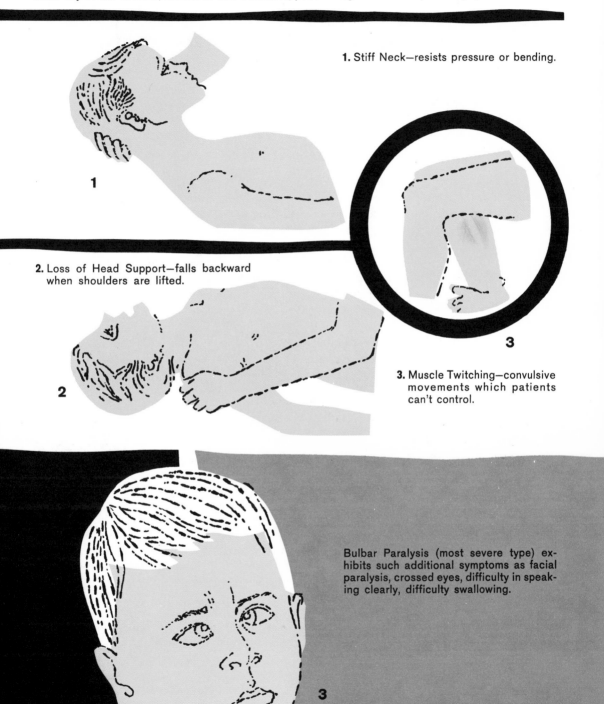

1. Stiff Neck—resists pressure or bending.

2. Loss of Head Support—falls backward when shoulders are lifted.

3. Muscle Twitching—convulsive movements which patients can't control.

Bulbar Paralysis (most severe type) exhibits such additional symptoms as facial paralysis, crossed eyes, difficulty in speaking clearly, difficulty swallowing.

the disease and its causes PROSTATIC ENLARGEMENT The prostate is a gland located at the base of the bladder. This gland sometimes enlarges and continues to enlarge as a man gets older. The cause of this enlargement is not known; it affects about 30% of all men, married and single, by the time they reach 50 years of age; and there is no known relationship to other infections or to individual sex habits.

CANCER Cancer of the prostate accounts for 1 out of every 10 deaths from cancer in men. As with most malignant diseases, the cause is not known.

symptoms PROSTATIC ENLARGEMENT The symptoms of prostate enlargement are shown in the accompanying Medi-Graph. The patient urinates more frequently and feels the urge to urinate several times during the night. As the disease progresses and the prostate enlarges, the bladder becomes thin, weak, and less efficient. There is difficulty starting the stream of urine. Waste products are retained in the blood, leading to generalized weakness. In the final stage, the patient cannot pass urine at all.

CANCER Cancer of the prostate can be undetected until it has spread to involve other organ systems or bones, because very often there are no symptoms and no discomfort to the patient. Sometimes there may be mild discomfort on urination, or blood in the urine—as shown in the Medi-Graph. If there is pain, it is felt in the area just below the rectum. Sometimes the cancer is discovered when a prostate condition is treated surgically and routine biopsy reveals its presence. Bone pain in the lower back, or lung involvement which is discovered in a routine chest X ray, may be the first indication that the disease is already beyond control.

complications PROSTATIC ENLARGEMENT Complications in prostatic enlargement develop when obstruction, due to enlargement, prevents the free passage of urine and stagnant urine collects. There is back pressure and infection involving the ureter, urinary tract, and the kidneys. At a late stage of the illness, the patient may be in great pain because the bladder is so overstretched. Uremia may be an end result of this condition.

CANCER Complications in cancer of the prostate develop when the cancer is not diagnosed early and it spreads beyond the prostate, out of control.

prevention (or lessening of impact) PROSTATIC ENLARGEMENT Since there is no known method of preventing enlargement or cancer, men after 50 should have a physical check-up at regular six-month intervals, including a urine analysis and prostatic examination. Where enlargement is present, the doctor will advise treatment before urinary obstruction becomes a problem.

CANCER The prime hope in cancer of the prostate is early diagnosis.

Prostate Gland Enlargement

Cancer of the Prostate

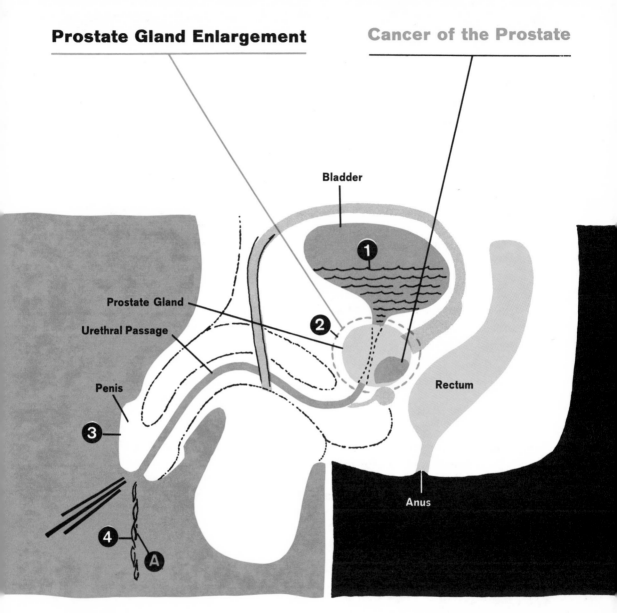

Bladder

Prostate Gland

Urethral Passage

Penis

Rectum

Anus

Enlargement

1. Difficulty clearing bladder of urine

2. Swelling of Prostate Gland constricts urethral passage through it

3. Difficulty starting urination

4. Lessening of force and quantity of urine

Cancer

Symptoms similar to Prostate Gland Enlargement plus

A. Occasional drops of blood in urine

B. Pain in pelvis and thigh bones as cancer spreads

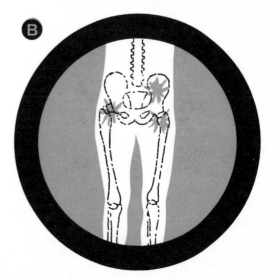

the disease and its causes   This is a chronic, recurrent skin eruption which
seems to run in families. The cause is unknown. Attacks are triggered
by emotional stress or shock; children often develop it after a strep
infection; sometimes it appears at the site of a skin injury. It is
neither infectious nor contagious, and there is little or no itching. Both
sexes, in all age groups, are subject to psoriasis—and it is more common in patients who drink a good deal of liquor.

symptoms   The disease begins without any warning and with no generalized symptoms. Small, flat, red patches appear which may or may not show a
tendency to peel. They spread by direct extension, and the surface
shows thin, silvery white scales. All of the infected area is covered with
these except for the narrow red rim. Itching, if present, is moderate.
In 75% of the cases the scalp, knees, elbows, and back are involved,
but it is not unusual to see psoriasis involving the nails. The disease may
be limited to one or two patches or cover the entire body.
If the surface scales are removed, a raw, red surface is exposed, with
minute bleeding points.

complications   There are no serious complications. Secondary infection can follow severe nail involvement, in which case the nail itself may have to be
removed.

prevention (or lessening of impact)   There is no known method of avoiding this
disease, and no known cure.
Good eating habits, the elimination of alcohol from the diet, vitamin
therapy, and the maintenance of good health can help limit the severity
of psoriasis flare-ups. Many medications to control the rash are available.

Psoriasis

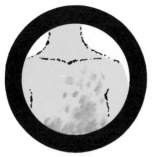

1. Starts as small red patches which enlarge and join together

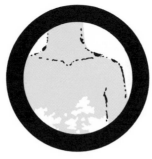

2. Patches usually become covered with silvery-white, scaly skin

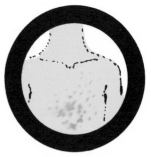

3. If scales fall off or are removed, red pinpoint area revealed underneath

Where Psoriasis Strikes

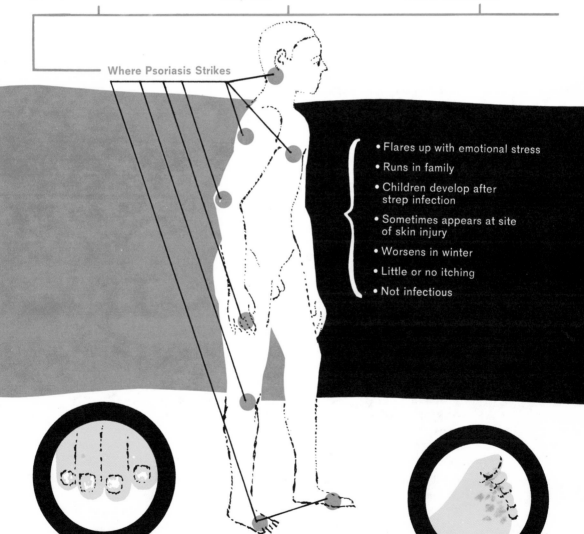

- Flares up with emotional stress
- Runs in family
- Children develop after strep infection
- Sometimes appears at site of skin injury
- Worsens in winter
- Little or no itching
- Not infectious

Nails become pitted or ridged with yellow spots — Soles of feet (and sometimes palms) may develop infection

Rabies Virus disease transmitted to man through saliva of rabid animals—particularly dogs and vampire bats

the disease and its cause This virus disease is transmitted to man through the saliva of an infected (rabid) animal. Dogs, bats, cats, skunks, foxes, squirrels, and raccoons are among the animals which transmit rabies— usually through bites but occasionally from scratches contaminated with their infected saliva.

The rabies virus affects the nervous system, eventually causing paralysis by damaging the spinal cord and brain. The disease is virtually always fatal to man, once its symptoms appear.

If the victim of a rabies bite is untreated, symptoms of the disease can appear anywhere from 10 days to a year later. The shorter incubation periods occur when bites have been inflicted close to the head or when there have been multiple bites.

symptoms The illustration shows the cycle of symptoms for a dog infected with rabies. In the case of a dog bite, it may be assumed that if the dog does not display rabies symptoms within 10 days, he does not have the disease. Human symptoms begin with a temperature that goes to 102°, headache, nausea, vomiting, and cough. The wound is usually painful and the pain radiates along the bitten arm or leg. Severe psychological disturbances take place, characterized by restlessness, depression, fear, rage, difficulty in speaking, and occasionally delirium.

Swallowing becomes difficult because of excruciatingly painful spasms of the throat muscles, so that the patient refuses to swallow anything, even water—hence the old name of hydrophobia for the disease. Speech becomes virtually impossible.

As the rabies virus presses its attack on the central nervous system, convulsions and blindness may occur. Paralysis of the breathing muscles, asphyxia, exhaustion, and general paralysis lead to death within 2–10 days.

complications This disease is invariably fatal unless antirabies vaccine is administered promptly following a bite from an infected animal.

prevention (or lessening of impact) Anyone thought to have been subjected to a bite or lacerations by a rabid animal needs immediate medical treatment with antirabies serum and vaccine. In cases of dog bite, the dog should be kept under observation for 10 days. If the dog does not exhibit symptoms of rabies during that period, the bite victim does not need vaccination. Since the vaccinations are given over a 14-day period, are painful, and cause some people to have severe reactions, the doctor must decide on the basis of the available evidence whether vaccination for dog bite is needed. If the dog escapes and cannot be observed, the bite victim should be vaccinated, especially if rabies has been previously reported in the area. All bites by bats and other wild animals necessitate vaccination.

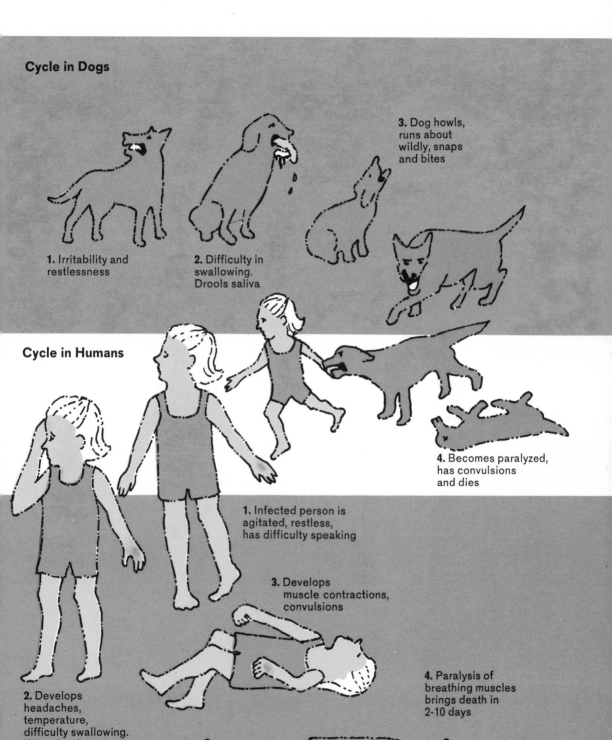

Cycle in Dogs

1. Irritability and restlessness

2. Difficulty in swallowing. Drools saliva

3. Dog howls, runs about wildly, snaps and bites

4. Becomes paralyzed, has convulsions and dies

Cycle in Humans

1. Infected person is agitated, restless, has difficulty speaking

2. Develops headaches, temperature, difficulty swallowing. Wound radiates pain

3. Develops muscle contractions, convulsions

4. Paralysis of breathing muscles brings death in 2-10 days

the disease and its causes This is a disease of the arteries of the hands and feet in which the fingers or toes become bloodless and white under certain conditions. Emotional upsets can bring about an attack. Cold weather, and even putting the hands in cold water, can also produce the change in color that is characteristic of Raynaud's disease. It occurs much more often in women than men, usually in the age group 20 to 40.

Occasionally Raynaud's disease occurs in association with other organic arterial diseases or with scleroderma (in which thickened, hard, rigid patches of skin develop), or cervical ribs (extra ribs in the neck which interfere with circulation), or with acute neck injuries.

symptoms When a patient with Raynaud's disease is exposed to cold, the fingers or toes may become bloodless and white. There is usually not much pain, but numbness is common. When warm again, the affected parts lose their white color and change from blue to red before turning normal. Between attacks, the fingers and toes appear normal. But when attacks are continuous or prolonged, small areas of gangrene can develop.

complications The only serious complication is gangrene, which is rare and most unusual. When it occurs, amputation may be necessary.

prevention (or lessening of impact) The patient with Raynaud's disease must take steps to prevent the development of gangrene and do what can be done to prevent attacks. She should keep her body and limbs warm. Any infection or associated illness should be treated. Emotional problems, which are thought to trigger attacks, should be handled professionally.

With proper care, Raynaud's disease rarely presents any serious problems.

Raynaud's Disease

Attacks precipitated by cold (low temperature) . . .

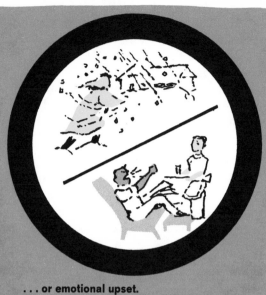

. . . or emotional upset.

When re-warmed, affected part goes through three stages of color:

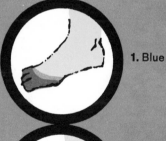

1. Blue

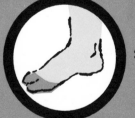

2. Red

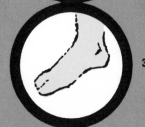

3. Normal skin color

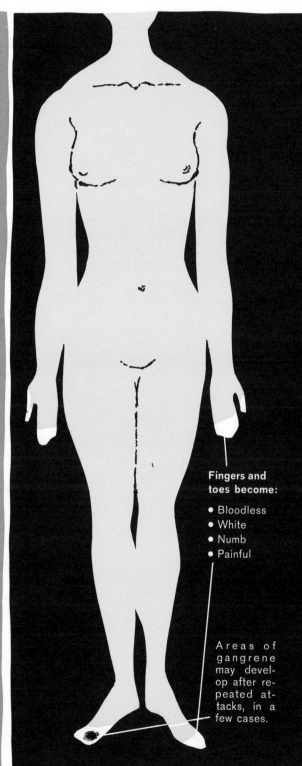

Fingers and toes become:

- Bloodless
- White
- Numb
- Painful

Areas of gangrene may develop after repeated attacks, in a few cases.

the disease and its causes   Rheumatic fever is a generalized infection caused by a bacterium or group of bacteria of the streptococcus family. It affects many different organ systems, including the central nervous system, the lungs, peritoneum, joints, and heart. The most likely point for the bacteria to enter the body is the throat, frequently the tonsils. The indication is that it is a sensitivity reaction in the patient which, under certain conditions, is responsible for the illness.

The disease occurs most often in young adolescents, equally divided between the sexes, and may involve several members of the family. It may also involve several families at a given time. Even epidemics have been reported. Crowded or unsanitary conditions seem to favor its occurrence.

symptoms   There is usually a sore throat for a week or two before the onset of such symptoms as sudden fever of 101° to 104°, accompanied by profuse sweats and pain in the joints. This pain usually involves the large joints, traveling from one to another. The joint becomes painful, red, hot, and swollen. As one improves and returns to normal, without damage, another becomes involved. There may be prolonged, unexplained fever without any other symptoms. Early in the illness there may be frequent unaccounted-for nosebleeds. St. Vitus' Dance frequently heralds the onset of rheumatic fever. In 1 out of 10 cases there is a rash on the arms, over the back, chest, abdomen, or armpits.

complications   Patients can recover completely from rheumatic fever. However, many suffer lifelong heart damage. Periodic flare-ups of this infection can increase the severity of the heart disease. Complications depend on the extent of damage. In very severe cases the damage can be overwhelming and the patient dies of heart failure. Rheumatic heart disease is discussed more fully under that heading.

prevention (or lessening of impact)   There is no effective preventive for rheumatic fever. One should avoid contact, if possible, with people ill with a streptococcus infection. At the sign of a sore throat proper drug care should be taken, particularly where there is a history of rheumatic fever. Early recognition and prompt treatment can cut down complications.

In the convalescent period, patients with heart involvement must take extra care and resume activities at a slow pace dictated by the family doctor. Since rheumatic fever frequently recurs, it is important to check with the doctor at regular intervals, and particularly during periods of other infections, or preceding elective surgery or extensive dental work.

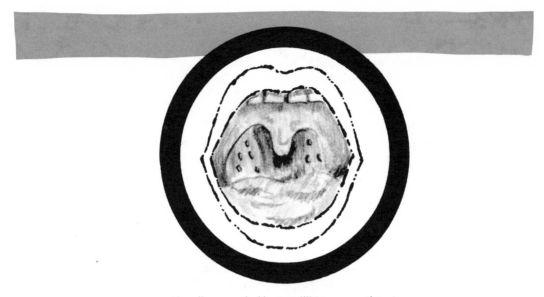

Usually preceded by tonsillitis or sore throat.

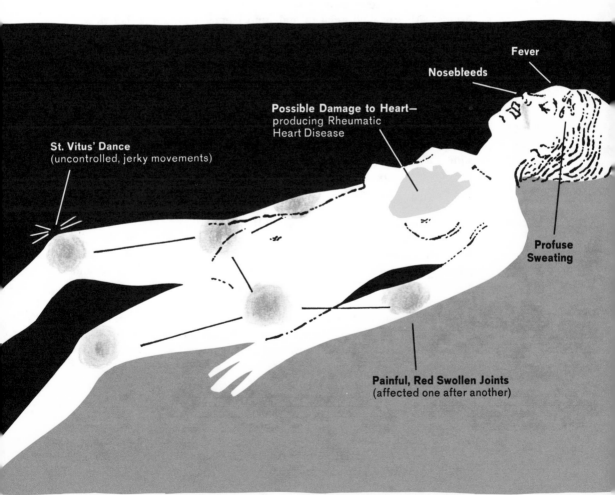

Fever

Nosebleeds

Possible Damage to Heart—
producing Rheumatic
Heart Disease

St. Vitus' Dance
(uncontrolled, jerky movements)

**Profuse
Sweating**

Painful, Red Swollen Joints
(affected one after another)

the disease and its causes   Rickets is a disease which results from a deficiency of vitamin D in the diet of infants (usually under the age of two). The only natural sources of this vitamin—which controls the deposition of calcium in the bones—are sunlight and certain foods such as eggs, sardines, tuna, herring, and salmon. Breast-fed infants get a fair amount of vitamin D from their mother's milk, but it needs to be supplemented with commercial preparations such as cod liver oil, or with milk to which vitamin D is added.

At present, in this country, the disease most often affects children who live under slum conditions where they are exposed to little sunlight.

symptoms   The onset of rickets is very slow, and very often the symptoms are so slight that the disease is overlooked. The infant is restless and seems to be uncomfortable without cause. There may be thickening over the ankle and wrist joints, painful areas on the body, sweating, low-grade fever, weakness, and poor growth. Pressure on the skull deforms it easily because it remains soft. Softening of the bones also causes deformities of the legs (bow legs) and pelvic and chest deformities. Fractures (broken bones) are common. The child is also more susceptible to respiratory infections, such as colds, grippe, pneumonia, etc.

Adults with so-called chicken and funnel breasts probably had rickets in infancy.

complications   The disease is rarely fatal in itself, but secondary infections are frequent and can result in death. Spasms of the larynx occur occasionally as well as convulsions. Tetany (a disease brought on by the influence of calcium in the blood) with convulsive spasms of the hands and feet, can be another complication.

In general, serious complications of rickets affect later life. A woman with a deformed pelvis can be severely handicapped during pregnancy. A patient with poor chest expansion due to rickets can be handicapped when he has a respiratory illness.

prevention (or lessening of impact)   The simplest way to prevent rickets is to take supplementary doses of a commercial product high in vitamin D. Fortified vitamin D milk should be used when there is a need. Exposure to sunlight can be of some help. A pregnant mother should make certain to include adequate amounts of calcium and vitamin D in her diet.

When the diagnosis is established and corrective measures are indicated, care must be taken to prevent deformity of the bones involved. A deformity which has already developed may have to be corrected orthopedically.

Rickets

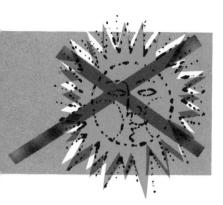

Develops in infants due to lack of Vitamin D

Sunlight prime source of Vitamin D, Mother's milk, egg yolk and cod liver oil can also supply infant's needs

Develops in Infants Between 3rd-18th Months

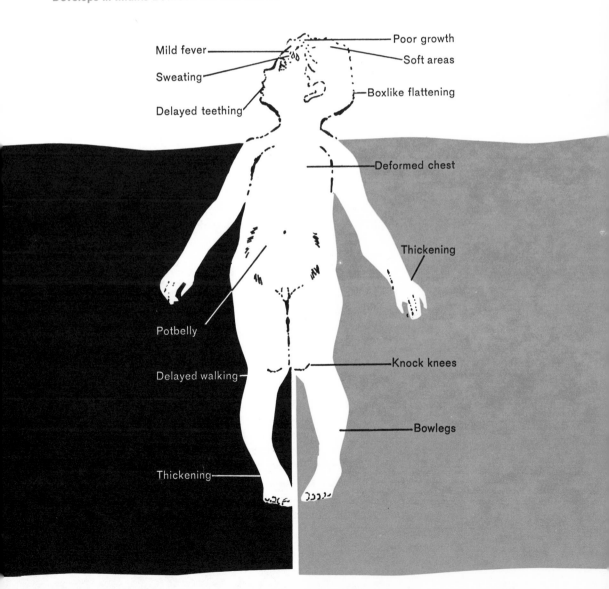

Mild fever

Sweating

Delayed teething

Poor growth

Soft areas

Boxlike flattening

Deformed chest

Thickening

Potbelly

Delayed walking

Knock knees

Bowlegs

Thickening

the disease and its causes This is one of the group of illnesses (others: *typhus, Q fever)* caused by a Rickettsia—a rod-shaped microorganism. The disease is transmitted to man by a tick which has been infected by Rickettsiae. The disease can be contracted either by the bite of an infected tick, by contamination of a skin wound through crushing a tick, or by tick feces getting into the wound.

Three types of ticks carry Rocky Mountain spotted fever in the U.S.: the wood tick in the Rocky Mountains and throughout the northwest, the dog tick in the east, and the Lone Star tick in Texas. Once these ticks pick up the Rickettsia, they remain infected for life—and also pass the disease on from generation to generation of ticks.

Since the ticks attach themselves to animals who roam wooded areas, the illness reaches its peak in man during the spring and summer seasons when the ticks are most active and man is most often exposed to them. The disease is found in most states in the U.S. but its highest toll is in the Rocky Mountain area.

The incubation period is from 3–12 days.

symptoms The disease breaks out suddenly with chills, headache, and aches and pains in the muscles and joints. The patient runs a fever and his temperature can reach 105°.

After 3 or 4 days, a characteristic rash breaks out. Composed of small red pimples, it first appears on the wrist, ankles, arms and soles of the feet. After a few days it spreads to the chest, abdomen, neck and face. In some places, the pimples come together and form black and blue areas because of bleeding under the skin. The fever continues during this phase.

If it is untreated, an attack of Rocky Mountain spotted fever may last 2 weeks—but this is shortened considerably with prompt attention from the doctor.

complications In severe cases, the lungs, liver and kidneys may be affected. Dehydration may cause particular kidney problems while pneumonia may infect the lungs. Heart failure is also a possibility in severe cases. These complications are particularly apt to occur in run-down youngsters and older people.

prevention (or lessening of impact) Persons living in areas where Rocky Mountain spotted fever is a problem should be vaccinated by their doctor, preferably in the spring. A series of 3 injections gives immunity to the disease for about a year—and, therefore, must be repeated annually.

People in tick-infested areas should also use insect repellents, wear protective clothing when in the woods and seek to eliminate the ticks by spraying. When ticks are found embedded in one's skin or on animals, they should be removed gently by tweezers after applying alcohol to them. Care should be taken to avoid crushing them.

In case the disease has been contracted, prompt diagnosis and treatment with antibiotics can bring the fever down within a few days and speed the patient's recovery.

Rocky Mountain Spotted Fever

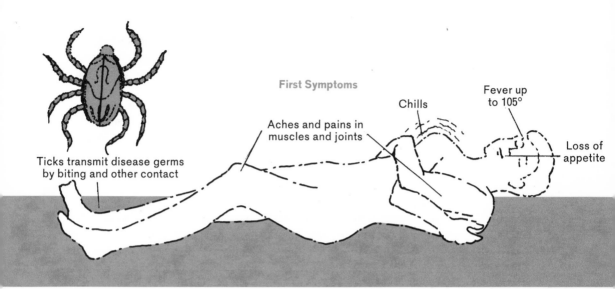

First Symptoms

Ticks transmit disease germs by biting and other contact

Aches and pains in muscles and joints

Chills

Fever up to 105°

Loss of appetite

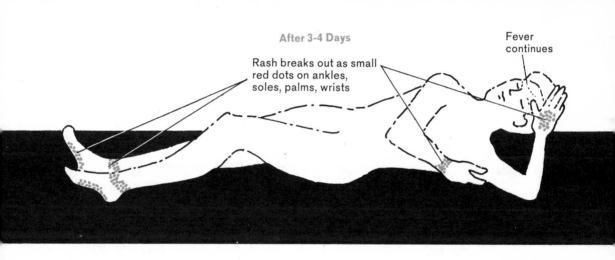

After 3-4 Days

Rash breaks out as small red dots on ankles, soles, palms, wrists

Fever continues

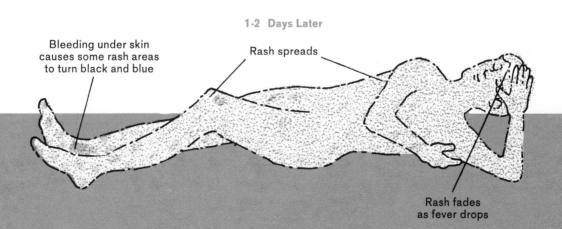

1-2 Days Later

Bleeding under skin causes some rash areas to turn black and blue

Rash spreads

Rash fades as fever drops

the disease and its causes   One of the most common parasitic diseases, this is
caused by the *Ascaris lumbricoides*—the giant intestinal roundworm.
It is called a parasite because it lives and feeds in man's digestive tract.
Man contracts the disease by taking in mature roundworm eggs from
soil polluted by infected humans or from contaminated food or drink.
Once ingested, the eggs go down the digestive tract to the small intestine
where they hatch and develop into the larvae stage. They then circle
around, migrating up—via the blood—to the lungs. From the lungs
they are coughed up into the mouth, swallowed again and return to the
intestine where they develop to full-size worms. Adult females are about
10–15 inches long; males are about half that size.

It takes the roundworm about 4 to 6 weeks to develop from the egg
form. The worm may then go on to live in the body for another 6
months. Females may produce as many as 200,000 eggs a day.

Both eggs and worms pass out through the digestive tract, primarily
through the anus—usually in the feces—though they may occasionally
emerge through the nose or mouth. In areas of poor sanitation, the feces
may then contaminate the soil or food and drink—and thus continue
the disease cycle.

symptoms   In the small intestine, the roundworms feed on man's partially digested
food. A heavy infestation may cause vague abdominal discomfort, loss
of appetite and occasionally diarrhea. When the larvae reach the lungs,
cough, blood spitting, and a form of pneumonia may develop.

The doctor diagnoses the disease by finding the characteristic roundworm
eggs in the patient's stool.

complications   A severe infestation in infants can cause death by pneumonia.
Occasionally roundworms migrate into the appendix and can cause acute
appendicitis. They may also produce intestinal obstruction.

prevention (or lessening of impact)   Prevention depends on proper personal hygiene and prohibiting the use of human feces as fertilizer. Prompt treatment of infected individuals also helps to prevent the spread of the
disease.

Treatment is relatively easy and effective, using a combination of
cathartics and drugs to clear out all the worms and eggs from the digestive system of the sufferer.

Roundworm (Ascariasis)

Signs of Disease

A. Loss of appetite and vague abdominal discomfort

B. Cough and blood spitting may occur during...

C. ...larval stage in lung

fertilized egg

worm hatching

Progress of Disease

1. Ingests fertilized eggs picked up from soil or food and drink contaminated by human feces

2. Eggs reach small intestine. Develop into larvae. Penetrate intestine wall

3. Migrate via blood to lungs

4. Larvae move up trachea to larynx, are swallowed again and re-enter digestive system

5. Develop into adult worms (10-15″ long) in small intestine

6. Severe infestation may cause intestinal obstruction, acute appendicitis, pneumonia

7. Worms pass out through anus, mouth or nose

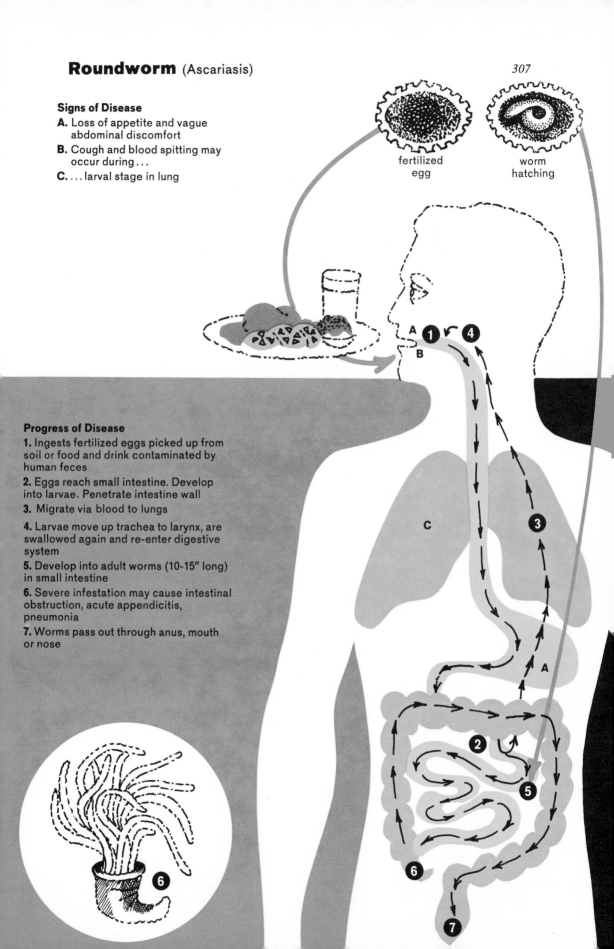

the disease and its causes Scarlet fever is a contagious disease caused by certain types of streptococcus bacteria. It is spread in many ways—by direct contact with infected patients, by healthy carriers, by contaminated food or milk, or by contaminated objects. The incubation period is 2 to 5 days. The disease occurs most often during the colder seasons and begins in the throat. Young children are affected most, but infants under a year are generally immune.

symptoms Scarlet fever develops rapidly, with a sore throat, temperature as high as 104°, and swollen neck glands. The back of the throat becomes covered with red spots, and the patient develops a pitted "strawberry" tongue which is really the minute swellings of the tongue glands. From 12 to 36 hours after the onset of scarlet fever, a red rash which is described as "blushing goose flesh" develops. Pressure of a finger on the skin leaves an easily visible white mark. When the rash fades about a week later, it is followed by a flaking of the skin on many parts of the body. Sometimes the teeth, fingernails, and hair are affected.

Attacks of scarlet fever may be very mild, presenting a slight quick rash and resembling simple tonsillitis; or they may be severe, with high fever, vomiting, and delirium. In severe cases there may even be bursting of small blood vessels under the skin. One attack of scarlet fever seems to assure almost certain immunity to future attacks.

complications The more serious complications affect the kidneys and the heart. Nephritis, which is a kidney ailment, may appear about the third week of the illness. One indication of nephritis is the patient's urine, which turns a reddish color.

The heart changes are related to and resemble rheumatic fever. Sometimes severe arthritis is seen with scarlet fever. Ear infections are common, as well as swollen glands with occasional abcess formations.

prevention (or lessening of impact) The severity and complications of scarlet fever can be reduced greatly by prompt and adequate treatment with penicillin. This drug is also used effectively in preventive care. A scarlet fever antitoxin is available, but often it is not recommended because so many people react severely to it. Many people are immune simply because they had the disease in a mild form at an earlier period and it was not recognized for what it was. The Dick test, which checks whether or not a person has immunity to scarlet fever, is often given by the doctor to those who may be exposed to the disease.

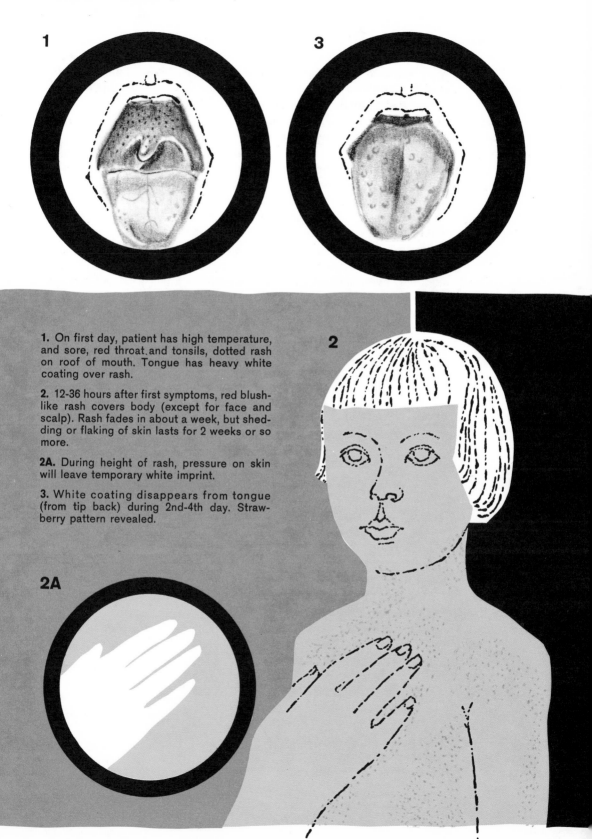

1. On first day, patient has high temperature, and sore, red throat and tonsils, dotted rash on roof of mouth. Tongue has heavy white coating over rash.

2. 12-36 hours after first symptoms, red blush-like rash covers body (except for face and scalp). Rash fades in about a week, but shedding or flaking of skin lasts for 2 weeks or so more.

2A. During height of rash, pressure on skin will leave temporary white imprint.

3. White coating disappears from tongue (from tip back) during 2nd-4th day. Strawberry pattern revealed.

the disease and its causes   This is a very important group of infections caused by a parasitic worm which gets into the human body mainly when people swim in contaminated waters. Schistosomiasis is very common throughout the Caribbean area and South America. Over the world, it is estimated that 50 million people suffer from its various forms.

There are 3 important forms but here we will discuss the type most prevalent in the western hemisphere—*Schistosoma mansoni.*

The life cycle of this disease starts with an infected human passing eggs of the parasite out in his feces which are—because of poor sanitation— discharged into fresh water streams, rivers, or lakes where people bathe. Here the eggs hatch into a form which infects snails as an intermediate host. Finally the schistosomes reenter the water to infect man by penetrating his skin while bathing.

The parasites then migrate through the body via the bloodstream, and develop into adult worms which live in the blood vessels of the victim's intestines, liver, and spleen. The adult worms attain a size of half an inch. The eggs of adult females are transported through the blood to the bladder and other organs of the body, with destructive results.

symptoms   While swimming in infected water, a person who has been invaded by the parasite may notice an itching or burning at the site of entry.

An allergic rash may break out at the site of infection. Usually the victim also suffers from headache, generalized aches and pains, and diarrhea. After maturation of the eggs into adult worms, the disease becomes more severe. The victim suffers from high fever, chills, and blood in the stool. Anemia may develop from the chronic blood loss. The liver and spleen become enlarged, and signs of pneumonia may develop. This stage may last up to 90 days.

Medical treatment brings gradual improvement, but most cases become reinfected because of the continuing unsanitary environment—and the symptoms become more severe with repetition.

The doctor makes a diagnosis by finding the characteristic eggs in the patient's stool or by rectal biopsy—taking a slice of rectal tissue and examining it under a microscope.

complications   Repeated infections in the intestine can cause ulcers and bleeding. In other instances, an individual who is constantly being reinfected finds his blood vessels becoming clogged by the eggs or the parasitic worms. This has a severely destructive effect on the organs involved. Cirrhosis of the liver may result. And in cases where this clogging affects the heart or lungs, death may occur from their failure.

prevention (or lessening of impact)   Effective prevention depends upon proper disposal of human feces and other waste products, and extermination of the intermediate snail host. Because of the increasing pollution of our streams and rivers, schistosomiasis could well become a threat in areas which have previously been free of it.

The doctor has at his disposal certain specific drugs which can eliminate this parasitic blood fluke from the body. However, to be effective the treatment must be given early. Once the patient develops advanced liver, lung, or heart trouble, his prospects are poor.

Schistosomiasis

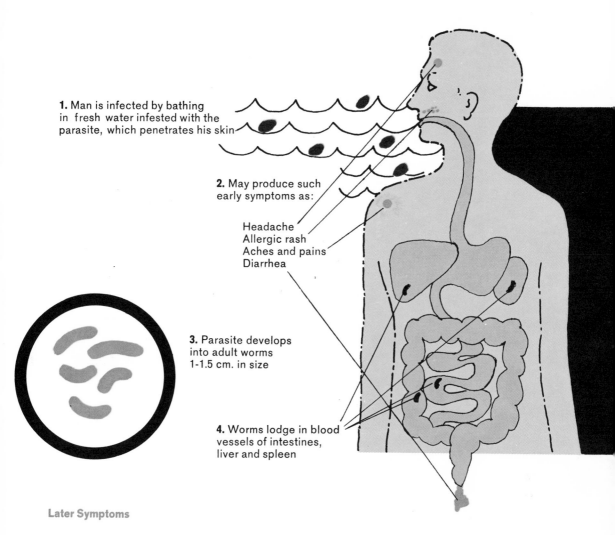

1. Man is infected by bathing in fresh water infested with the parasite, which penetrates his skin

2. May produce such early symptoms as:

Headache
Allergic rash
Aches and pains
Diarrhea

3. Parasite develops into adult worms 1-1.5 cm. in size

4. Worms lodge in blood vessels of intestines, liver and spleen

Later Symptoms

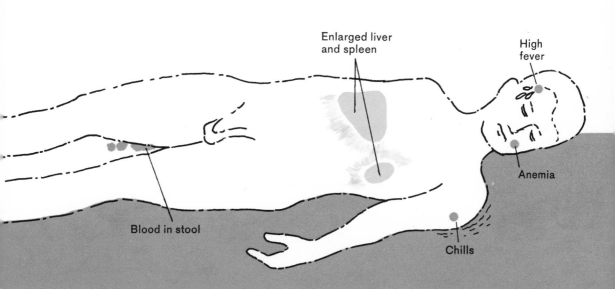

Enlarged liver and spleen

High fever

Anemia

Blood in stool

Chills

the disease and its causes   This is a chronic disease that affects the connective
tissue of the skin and other organs of the body. Both its cause and its
effective treatment are unknown at the present time.

It strikes people between the ages of 20–40 and attacks women more
often than men. Since this is a disease that affects almost all the organ
systems in the body, it is thought that a malfunction of certain blood
or immune mechanisms may play a part in its cause.

symptoms   There are many possible symptoms, depending on the site involved,
but the most common one is thickening of the skin. The tissue becomes
hard and rigid. This is often associated with symptoms of *Raynaud's
disease*. In this, the fingers and toes turn white or blue in cold weather
or under stress. In some cases the thickening and hardening of the skin
spreads to involve large areas of the arms and legs—and sometimes
even the entire body.

Calcium deposits may appear in the skin. Involvement of the esophagus
may lead to swallowing difficulty. A variety of gastrointestinal problems
may result from the disease.

Severe cases can lead to cardiac lesions and to high blood pressure with
accompanying kidney failure. Arthritis and general muscular weakness
may cut drastically into the patient's mobility. Fibrosis of the lungs is
another possible result.

Thus, the disease can strike widely throughout the body. It is frequently
diagnosed by a biopsy—taking a piece of tissue from the involved site
and examining it under the microscope.

complications   These depend upon the organ involved and the severity of the
involvement. Severe cases can lead to heart failure, anemia, pneumonia
and strokes. Any one of these may prove to be fatal.

prevention (or lessening of impact)   At the moment, prevention is impossible—
since the cause of scleroderma is unknown. For the most part, the course
of the disease is progressively more severe. However, there are cases of
spontaneous reversal and improvement, particularly among children.

Treatment with cortisone-type drugs is helpful in dealing with specific
problems and slowing the course of the illness. Physical therapy and
treatment of secondary bacterial infection can also help to ease the
patient's burden.

Scleroderma

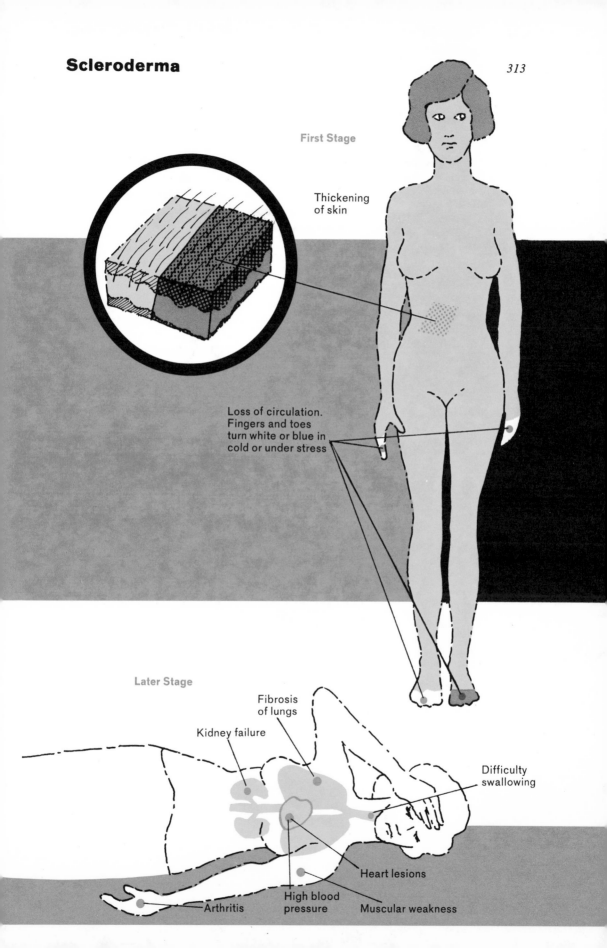

First Stage

Thickening
of skin

Loss of circulation.
Fingers and toes
turn white or blue in
cold or under stress

Later Stage

Fibrosis
of lungs

Kidney failure

Difficulty
swallowing

Heart lesions

Arthritis

High blood
pressure

Muscular weakness

the disease and its causes Scurvy is a dietary deficiency disease which results from a lack of vitamin C. It is becoming rare, particularly in adults, because a person must go without this vitamin for several months to develop the disease. However, it is not uncommon in infants who are fed a diet without enough citrus fruit or tomato juice.

Vitamin C is found in high amounts in orange and lemon juice, fresh fruits such as strawberries, cantaloupes, and bananas, and fresh vegetables such as cabbage and tomatoes.

symptoms The symptoms of infants with scurvy include loss of appetite, weakness, pallid skin, irritability, and lack of weight gain. When the baby teeth erupt, there is often bleeding of the gums. When the infant moves, there is pain in the legs caused by hemorrhage in the joints, and there are painful swellings about the joints. Blood spots appear on the skin. The patient has low-grade fever. There may be blood in his urine. Adults with scurvy lose weight, become weak, and develop pale skin. Their gums become tender and spongy, and eventually ulcerate. Large black and blue areas appear on the extremities, and there are frequently painful spots over the shinbones. There can be hemorrhage into the muscles of the calves, nosebleeds, and bloody vomiting. The teeth loosen and fall out.

Scurvy which involves the mouth must be distinguished from trench mouth or other local gum infections.

complications As a rule serious complications are rare. In advanced cases there can be hemorrhage and secondary infections. The loss of teeth is an important cosmetic problem.

prevention (or lessening of impact) Scurvy can be prevented by eating a balanced diet that includes adequate amounts of the foods mentioned as sources of vitamin C. Vitamin C in commercial form is easily available and should be taken by anyone who, for reasons of health, has to be on a rigid diet that eliminates foods high in this vitamin.

Scurvy

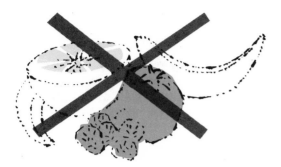

Lack of Vitamin C in diet causes Scurvy

Among best sources of Vitamin C are orange and lemon juice, tomatoes, cabbage, strawberries, cantaloups, bananas

Signs of Scurvy

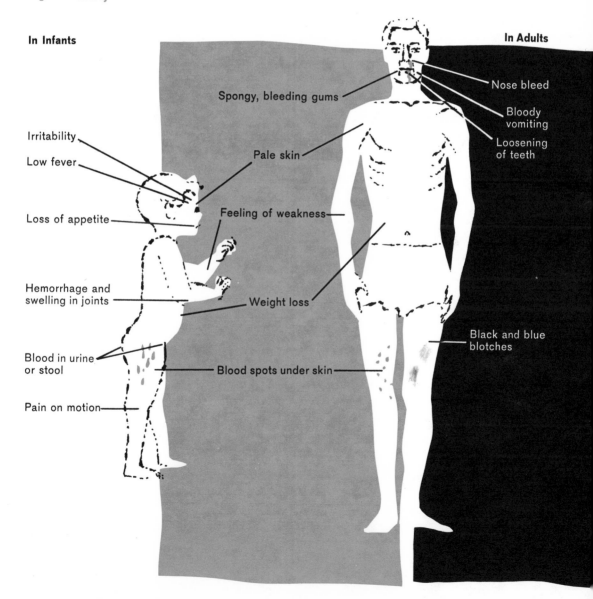

In Infants

In Adults

Spongy, bleeding gums

Nose bleed

Bloody vomiting

Loosening of teeth

Irritability

Low fever

Pale skin

Loss of appetite

Feeling of weakness

Hemorrhage and swelling in joints

Weight loss

Blood in urine or stool

Black and blue blotches

Blood spots under skin

Pain on motion

the disease and its causes This is a common type of skin disorder involving the scalp, eyebrows, cheeks, and the front of the chest. It occurs in adults and is common in both males and females. The cause is unknown, but several known factors play a part: It is frequently related to acne; it is thought to be involved with hormone action; it seems to be aggravated by foods such as chocolate, fatty or fried dishes, and seafood; it is not unusual to see it before or in association with the development of psoriasis.

symptoms There is a widespread eruption involving the entire skin of the scalp, and frequently breaking out behind the ears, too. The skin is red and covered with irregular patches on which there are greasy scales. These tend to flake and occasionally take on a yellowish color. The patches vary in size and shape, and are usually dry except for the area behind the ears, where oozing is common.

The eruption spreads slowly and may also be seen in the armpit, groin, and between the buttocks.

As a rule there is no itching and the patient is more disturbed by how this disease looks than how it feels.

complications There are no serious complications.

prevention (or lessening of impact) Seborrheic dermatitis tends to resist treatment and be chronic. However, there are specific medications a doctor will prescribe. Vitamins may be recommended. Good skin hygiene will certainly do much to prevent secondary infections and minimize unsightly appearance. The patient should most conscientiously omit from his diet any foods known to aggravate this disorder.

Seborrheic Dermatitis

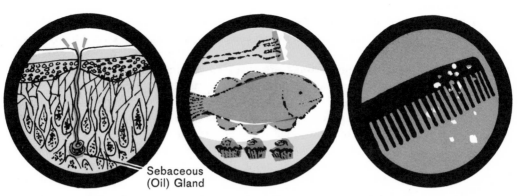

Sebaceous
(Oil) Gland

1. Caused by too much production of oil by glands of skin

2. Chocolate, seafood, fatty and fried foods may stimulate overproduction of oil

3. Milder forms range from dandruff to acne — but they are not necessarily preliminary to development of seborrheic dermatitis

Where Disease May Strike...

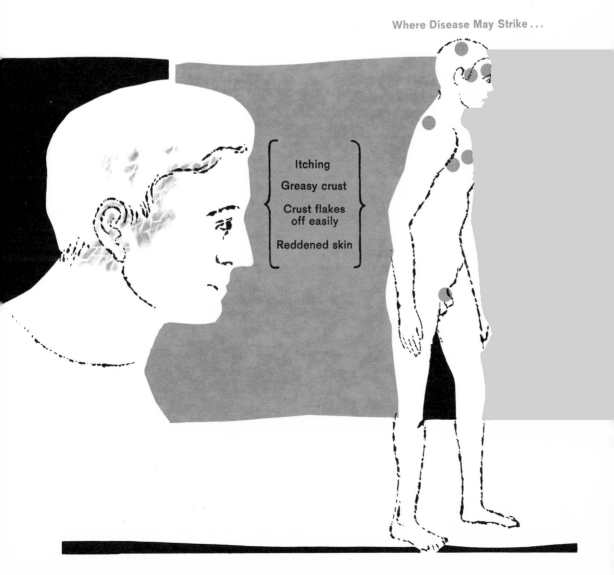

Itching

Greasy crust

Crust flakes off easily

Reddened skin

the disease and its causes   Shingles, also known as herpes zoster, is caused by a
virus which makes the nerve root become inflamed. Occasionally it is a
secondary result of certain diseases of the central nervous system in
which the nerve roots are involved. Tumor, syphilis, and other disorders are among the primary but infrequent causes.

There is also a relation between the virus of chickenpox and shingles,
and cases of chickenpox have been noted after someone has had contact
with a patient with shingles, and vice versa.

The red areas and water blisters that break out are similar to cold sores
except that they appear along the entire course of the nerve affected.
Every few days new crops appear. The disease is usually over in 4 to 6
weeks and, as a rule, involves only one side of the body. When the
blisters dry, they form shingle-like scabs which occasionally leave scars
when they heal.

symptoms   There can be skin sensitivity and aching pain along the course of the
nerve a few days before the redness appears. Sometimes there are fever,
chills, and weakness, but these disappear when the rash breaks out.
With the outbreak of blisters, there is uncomfortable, burning pain.
Even after the blisters are gone and the area is dry, the neuralgic nerve
pain may persist for some time.

If the eye nerve is involved, a severe form of herpes zoster can develop,
with such results as eye pain, tearing, sensitivity to light, and even the
formation of ulcers in the cornea.

complications   The only serious complication occurs when the eye is involved.
Without treatment and careful management, corneal ulceration and
blindness may result.

prevention (or lessening of impact)   There is no known method of preventing
shingles. The illness is mild in most cases, and presents few problems.
The doctor will examine the patient to see if there are any undetected
primary causes such as tumors or syphilis. And he will help the patient
guard against secondary infections by careful local care and good skin
hygiene. Such drugs as are available for treatment are used to try to
limit the spread of the infection and to make the patient as comfortable
as possible.

Shingles (Herpes Zoster)

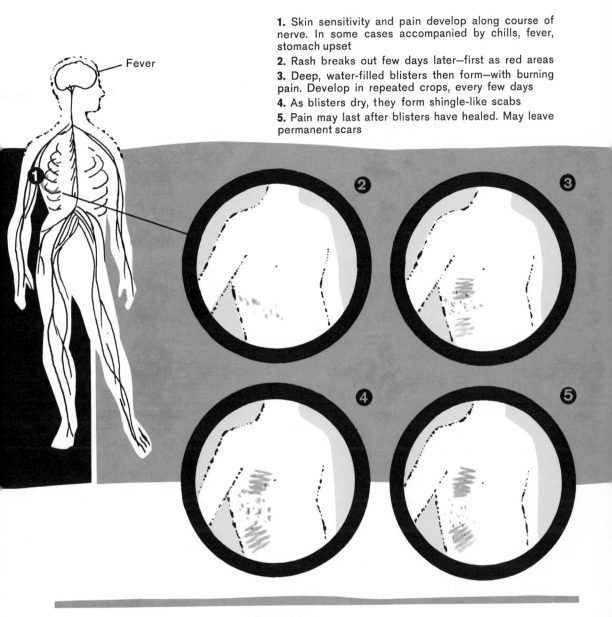

1. Skin sensitivity and pain develop along course of nerve. In some cases accompanied by chills, fever, stomach upset

2. Rash breaks out few days later—first as red areas

3. Deep, water-filled blisters then form—with burning pain. Develop in repeated crops, every few days

4. As blisters dry, they form shingle-like scabs

5. Pain may last after blisters have healed. May leave permanent scars

Fever

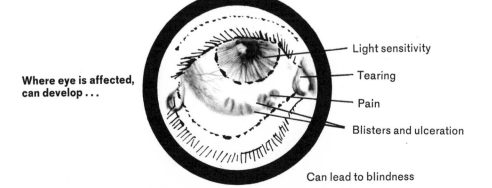

Where eye is affected, can develop . . .

Light sensitivity

Tearing

Pain

Blisters and ulceration

Can lead to blindness

the disease and its causes SICKLE CELL ANEMIA is an incurable, hereditary blood disorder that affects black people almost exclusively. One out of every 500 black Americans is estimated to have the disease in some state of severity.

Sickle cell anemia victims suffer from an abnormal form of *hemoglobin* —a substance in the blood that gives it its red color and has the vital job of conveying oxygen from the lungs to the other tissues of the body. The red blood cells of sufferers from the disease become sickle- or crescent-shaped and the hemoglobin does not carry enough oxygen to the tissues. Another result is that the sickle-shaped cells accumulate in a sludge or muddy form in the smaller blood vessels of the arms and legs. This tends to block circulation, cause pain in the extremities, and sometimes leads to strokes.

symptoms These are a result of the blood vessel blockage. The impairment of circulation to various parts of the body causes attacks of acute pain. The arms, legs and abdomen are the most frequent sites for this. The blocked circulation may also cause ulceration of the skin in the legs.

A lack of oxygen and blockage in circulation may also cause problems in the bones and joints, kidneys and lungs.

Since the sickle cells are fragile and easily destroyed, the victim also has such symptoms of general anemia (lack of red blood cells) as weakness, dizziness, and headache.

complications In severe cases of sickle cell anemia, the victim may develop an enlarged heart and suffer from heart failure. Blockage of circulation in the brain may lead to strokes. The bones may become deformed, and the poor circulation may leave the victim open to secondary infections. In cases that are severe and present since infancy, the children develop poorly—physically and mentally. Maturing of the sexual organs and other secondary sex characteristics are also retarded.

prevention (or lessening of impact) At present, there is no known cure or method of effectively treating this inherited illness. Mild forms occur that produce few or no symptoms. But in the severe cases of sickle cell anemia, death often occurs at an early age. The average lifespan of a baby born with a recognizable case of sickle cell anemia is 20 years—and he has only a 50% chance of surviving his first year of life.

However, promising research is going on at Rockefeller University that gives hope for the future.

Sickle Cell Anemia

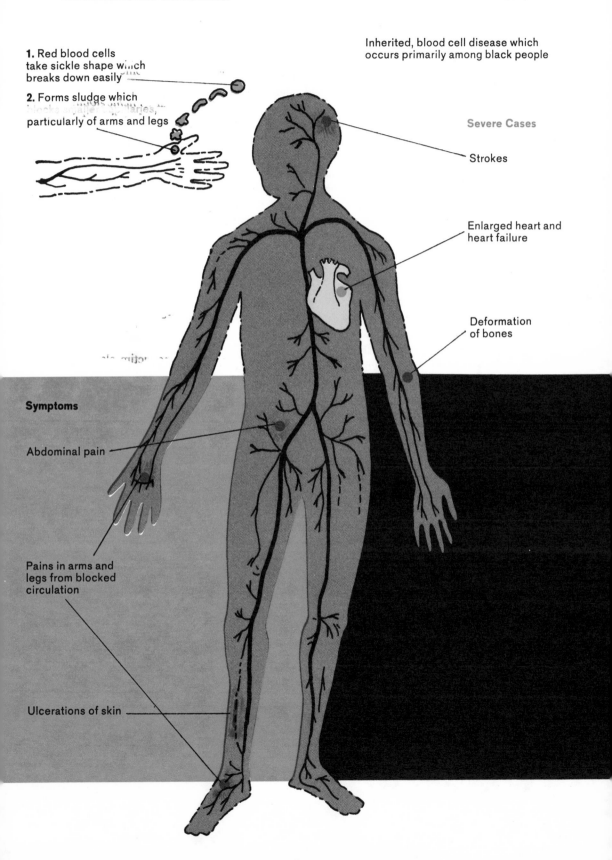

1. Red blood cells take sickle shape which breaks down easily

2. Forms sludge which blocks smaller capillaries, particularly of arms and legs

Inherited, blood cell disease which occurs primarily among black people

Severe Cases

Strokes

Enlarged heart and heart failure

Deformation of bones

Symptoms

Abdominal pain

Pains in arms and legs from blocked circulation

Ulcerations of skin

the disease and its cause   This is a disease of the lungs caused by prolonged inhalation of the fine particles of silica (quartz). It is an industrial disease among workers involved in mining, sand blasting, glass manufacture, tunneling, foundry work, and other rock cutting occupations.

Whether or not a worker develops silicosis depends on the amount of silica dust in the air at his job, the length of time he is exposed to it, and—to some degree—his individual makeup.

Under average working conditions, the disease may take a long time to develop—up to 20 years. With heavy exposure, it may occur sooner.

Silica dust attacks the lungs, causing fibrous tissues and nodules to form there and in nearby lymph glands. As a result, the lungs lose their elasticity. They no longer expand and contract easily, and breathing becomes difficult.

symptoms   Recognizable symptoms usually develop long after the disease has taken root in the lungs. These symptoms include shortness of breath, chest pain, cough and feelings of weakness.

Other characteristic symptoms of lung problems appear, including development of club-shaped fingers and a blueish tint to the skin.

Any exertion on the part of the silicosis victim causes an increase in the severity of the symptoms. Normal work, or even a mild exertion such as walking, cannot be undertaken.

complications   TB, emphysema, and advanced fibrosis of the lungs can develop if the worker is not taken out of the silica dust environment. Pulmonary heart disease, heart failure, and death are the eventual outcome.

prevention (or lessening of impact)   Carefully planned ventilation that removes the silica dust from the work area is the best way to prevent the development of silicosis. Protective masks are of some help and should be utilized. TB and other secondary infections should be treated when and if they develop. There is no specific treatment for silicosis itself.

Silicosis

Lung disease caused
by inhalation of
rock (silica) particles

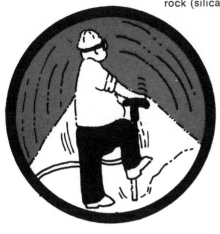

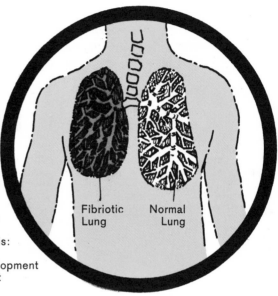

Rock particles
irritate lung,
causing fibrosis:
shrinking of
lung and development
of nodules in it

Fibriotic
Lung

Normal
Lung

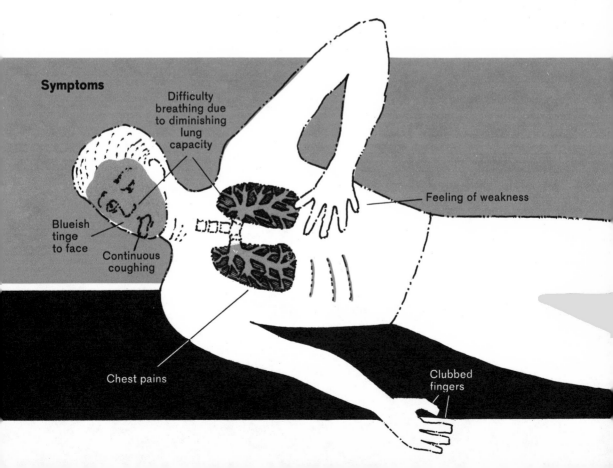

Symptoms

Difficulty
breathing due
to diminishing
lung
capacity

Feeling of weakness

Blueish
tinge
to face

Continuous
coughing

Chest pains

Clubbed
fingers

the disease and its causes   Sinusitis is an infection of the membranes lining the sinus cavities. It is caused by a variety of bacteria which live and grow there. Any obstruction in the nose, such as polyps, large adenoids, or a deviated septum, may interfere with normal sinus drainage and open the way for infection. Nasal allergies are often responsible because they frequently lead to secondary infections. Sinusitis may follow a simple cold or an abscessed upper molar rupturing into the maxillary sinus. Swimming and diving frequently cause it. It is a common disease, especially along the seaboard where there are sudden changes of temperature and humidity.

A patient is susceptible to repeated attacks once he is infected. Any sinus or combination of sinuses may be involved, but the frontal and maxillary sinuses are most often affected. Infection of the sphenoid sinus occurs less often but can be more serious.

symptoms   Sinusitis begins with low-grade fever, weakness, and pain over the particular sinus involved. The directions in which this pain radiates are shown on the accompanying diagram of sinuses. As a rule, there is a thick yellow or green discharge which increases and decreases as the position of the head changes. If the drainage is blocked, the infection may last beyond the few days it runs normally, and there is pain and a rise in temperature. Also, at this stage there may be swelling about the eyes and cheeks. Toothache may be the first sign of maxillary sinusitis.

complications   Without drainage an infection can become severe enough to involve the bone (osteomyelitis). Another complication is meningitis which is caused by direct invasion of the brain. This happens less often now with the proper use of antibiotics. The infection can also spread to the eye, throat, ear, and lungs.

prevention (or lessening of impact)   Since nasal obstructions are often specific causes of sinusitis, it is well to repair septal deviation, remove polyps and enlarged adenoid tissue, and make any other corrections necessary to permit discharge to drain freely from the nose. If a patient has an existing allergy, it should be treated. Nose clamps during swimming and diving are of help. Packaged cold vaccines relieve some people, while others benefit from a vaccine prepared from their own infected discharge.

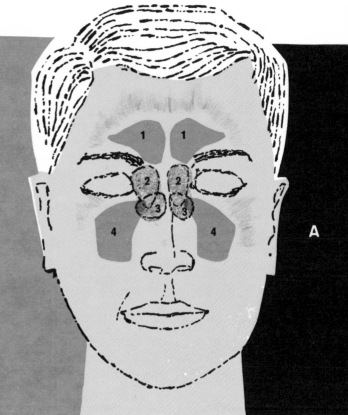

A. The Sinuses—and Where Pain from Them Strikes

1. Frontal Sinus — Directly outward to forehead.

2. Ethmoid Sinus—Back of the eyes and nose.

3. Sphenoid Sinus — Back of the head and neck.

4. Maxillary Sinus — Beneath eyes and up to forehead.

A

B. Cross-section View of Acute Sinusitis

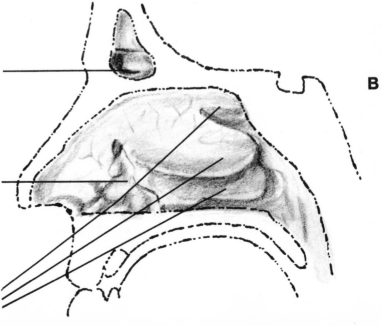

1. Infection creates pus in sinus.

B

2. Thick yellow or green discharge seeps down into nose and throat.

3. Infection blocks normal air passage through sinus, congests nasal lining, creates feeling of pressure, tenderness, pain in surrounding area.

the injury and its causes Between the vertebrae of the spine there are spinal discs made of cartilage which serve as shock absorbers. Acute injuries, congenital weakness, or chronic injuries which may have occurred years before the onset of pain, can cause weakening of the ligaments which bind the spine. At the weakest point these ligaments may tear, permitting the spinal disc to protrude, or herniate. Protrusion of the disc, with pressure on the nerve roots, is one of the commonest causes of low back pain, causing the kind of low back disorder which used to be described as lumbago, sciatica, sacro-iliac sprains, and low back sprains.

symptoms Low back pain or irritation of the involved nerve root is one of the earliest symptoms of a slipped disc. At this stage, rest will generally result in less pain because the disc works back to its more normal position. However, if it does not slip back completely, the nerve root irritation continues and causes pain down the back of the leg, sometimes numbness, and the kind of discomfort commonly called "sciatica." The continued pressure on the sciatic nerve causes intense pain which is aggravated by any back movements, sneezing, coughing, or other abrupt motion. The outer surface of the foot and toes may tingle or become numb. When the patient stands he tilts his back. When he raises his leg straight up, he gets a definite pain in the back. Continued nerve pressure causes weakness and atrophy of the muscles, and definite loss of sensation. Paralysis can result from this chronic pressure on the nerve, and the patient cannot use his bladder and bowel.
The sciatic pain from the buttock down the length of the affected leg can become so excruciating that motion becomes severely limited, if not impossible, and the patient is bedridden.

complications These depend on the extent of nerve damage caused by the pressure of the displaced disc. The paralysis and interference with bladder and bowel functions are serious problems. In addition to the further complications they may bring, they can prevent the patient from working or from carrying on other normal activities.

prevention (or lessening of impact) Any case of low back pain or sciatica should be thoroughly investigated to rule out the possibility of a herniated spinal disc. The diagnosis can generally be made from just a physical examination, but sometimes X ray or spinal canal studies are necessary. Bed rest and heat may prevent the development of the more serious effects of a slipped disc if they are used early enough. Many patients find orthopedic supports such as corsets or low back braces helpful. Heavy lifting, bending, pushing, and pulling should be avoided.
When there is no improvement after the simpler recommendations have been followed, back traction or surgery may be necessary.

Slipped Disc

Cross Section of Spine

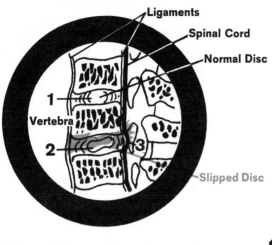

Ligaments
Spinal Cord
Normal Disc

1
Vertebra
2 3

Slipped Disc

1. Normal disc cushions impact along spine of walking, turning, other activities

2. Slipped disc is displaced by impact, exertion or congenital weakness

3. Slipped disc pinches spinal cord, causing back pain and other problems

4. Rest may speed slipped disc's return to normal position — eliminating pressure on spinal cord and ending backache

If slipped disc condition is not corrected . . .

Increased pain when walking, sneezing, coughing, any activity

Tilt to back when standing

Intense pain in back

Pain radiates down leg (frequent cause of "sciatica")

Prolonged pressure on nerves may bring paralysis

Possible loss of bladder and bowel control

Atrophy of muscles

Loss of reflexes

Numbness and tingling

the disease and its causes Smallpox is a highly contagious virus disease which can be very serious in unvaccinated people. It is spread by direct contact with an infected person or any article he has handled, or by a carrier. The virus is present in discharges from nose and throat, in skin blisters, in the scabs which later fall off, and in body excretions. There are no recognizable symptoms during the incubation period, which lasts from 10 to 14 days. A patient becomes permanently immune to smallpox after an attack.

symptoms The disease begins suddenly, with high fever accompanied by a rash. There may be vomiting, diarrhea, aches and pains. Convulsions and delirium may occur if the temperature climbs high enough.

In its early stages the rash may resemble measles. It starts on the face and forearms and spreads to the upper arms and body. By the third day the lower extremities are covered. About the fourth day it comes to look like a series of water blisters, as illustrated. These take on the appearance of pus blisters as the illness progresses. All of the rash on a person's body looks alike at any one time. This is different from the rash of chickenpox, where all the different stages of the rash may appear at one time. Throughout the development of the smallpox rash there is likely to be high fever.

A mild form of smallpox called variloid may occur in people who are *partially* protected by a vaccination they may have received years before.

complications In more severe forms of smallpox, bleeding occurs from the mouth and the rash may resemble blood blisters. In confluent smallpox, which is a severe form of the disease, the rash is so dense it appears to run together. Such cases are often fatal.

Complications include secondary infections of the skin, such as boils, abscesses, and erysipelas. Ear infections, pneumonia, and heart failure are also complicating features.

prevention (or lessening of impact) Everyone should be vaccinated because it is almost a guarantee that one will not get smallpox. This should be repeated every three years to maintain immunity. Anyone planning to spend time in a foreign country where smallpox is known to exist should be certain to get a revaccination.

Isolate the patient with this disease, and sterilize or destroy anything with which he has come in contact. Good care includes keeping the patient in bed, keeping him clean and comfortable, and seeing to it that he gets plenty of liquids.

Smallpox

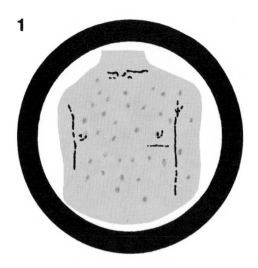

1. Rash
Sudden outbreak of fever is accompanied by rash. It starts on face and forearms, spreads to upper arms and rest of body by 3rd day. Rash turns from red spots to pimples.

2. Blisters
Around 4th day, blisters with grey pinpoint centers form over pimples.

3. Pus Globules
Blisters keep enlarging, and around 7th day fill with yellow pus.

4. Pockmarks
Around 10th day pus globules begin to dry up and form scabs. In more severe cases of smallpox, permanent pockmarks are left after scabs disappear.

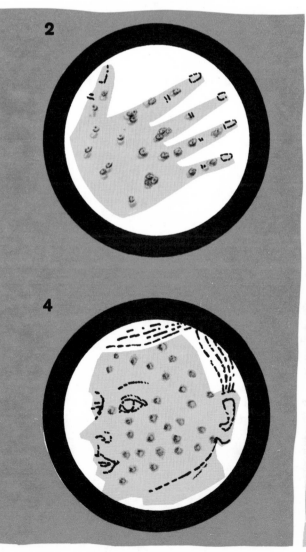

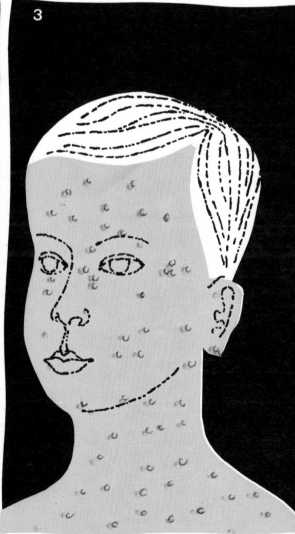

the condition and its cause The number of poisonous snakes found throughout the world is probably less than 250—about one-tenth of the total known types of snakes. In the U.S., there are four types of poisonous snakes: the coral snake, rattlesnake, copperhead, and water moccasin (cottonmouth). There are about 3000 reported cases of snake bites a year in the U.S.—but many more in parts of South America, Asia, and Africa. The rattlesnake, copperhead, and water moccasin are called "pit vipers" because of a small pit between the eye and the nostril. Their heads are triangular in shape. The rattlesnake has a horny tail which buzzes or rattles when the snake moves. This snake turns up in all sections of the country, with the diamondback being the most dangerous of the rattlesnake group.

The water moccasin is found in swampy areas—both in water and along the banks. It can bite under water. The copperhead is a related species with the least serious bite of the group.

The skin of the coral snake, found in the Southern states, bears alternating red and black bands followed by yellow rings. These snakes rarely bite man, but when they do, they inject a very toxic venom into multiple puncture wounds.

Snake bites on the face and neck are usually the most serious because of the closeness of the venom to the brain and central nervous system. The amount of venom injected also determines the seriousness of the bite— and young children, because of their small size, get the least help from their body in mobilizing to fight off the venom.

symptoms As the illustration shows, viper bites produce different types of symptoms from those produced by the coral snake or cobra. If unattended, viper bites can cause death within 8–48 hours. The bite of the coral snake can bring death even more quickly.

complications With prompt first aid and medical treatment, deaths from pit viper bites are rare and complications few.

However, impaired function of the hands and feet may sometimes occur. Secondary infections and gangrene occasionally develop. In the latter case, amputation of the involved limb may sometimes be necessary.

Of coral snake bite victims who developed symptoms, as many as one-third may die within 24 hours. The others can expect to recover without permanent effects.

prevention (or lessening of impact) By wearing long pants, boots and gloves in snake-infested areas, you help to ward off snake bites. If a snake bite is suffered, the steps shown in the bottom panel of the illustration should be followed. Though the disability and discomfort may be severe, the life can be saved with proper care.

Snake Bites (Poisonous Snakes)

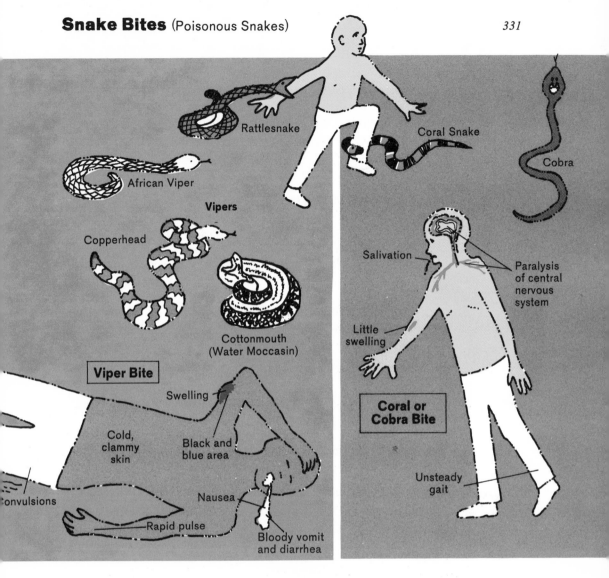

Rattlesnake

African Viper

Vipers

Copperhead

Cottonmouth
(Water Moccasin)

Coral Snake

Cobra

Salivation

Paralysis
of central
nervous
system

Little
swelling

**Coral or
Cobra Bite**

Unsteady
gait

Viper Bite

Swelling

Cold,
clammy
skin

Black and
blue area

Convulsions

Nausea

Rapid pulse

Bloody vomit
and diarrhea

1 Put tourniquet
above site of bite
to prevent spread
of infection

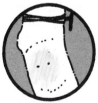

2 Make incision
crosswise thru
bite with
sterilized knife

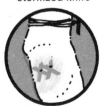

3 Use suction cup or
mouth to suck all
blood or venom in
wound

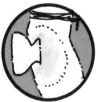

Quick Action Can Prevent Snake Bites from Becoming Fatal

4 Kill snake to
bring to doctor
for identification

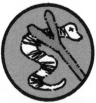

5 No exertion or
stimulants for
snakebite victim

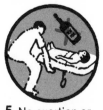

6 Rush victim to
doctor to administer
antivenom serum

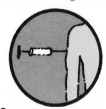

the injury and its causes SPRAIN   A sprain occurs when there is rupture of individual fibers or small groups of fibers of the *ligament* which holds a joint together. It is caused by the stretching of these ligaments in an injury. All joints can be involved in sprains. In areas where the ligaments surrounding a joint are very extensive, the involvement can extend over a considerable area. An example of this is the ankle, where discomfort from a sprain may extend to the top of the foot.

STRAIN   A strain is the parting or rupture of certain strands or fibers of a *muscle*. It is usually brought on by extreme muscle activity, particularly by heavy activity to which the muscle is not accustomed. Strains occur most commonly in the muscles of the back. However, the arms and legs are also subject to strains, especially in people involved in athletics or any activity in which these parts are used extensively.

symptoms   As shown in the Medi-Graph, the symptoms are pain and swelling which limit the use and motion of the joint or muscle involved. Pain increases when there is tension on the injured part, and decreases when the part is in a relaxed position. Black and blue marks discolor the skin, marking the spread of blood surrounding the injured area.

complications SPRAIN   There are no serious complications involved in sprains except the disability they cause.

STRAIN   Occasionally a complication of strain is the development of adhesions (an abnormal sticking together) between the torn muscle fibers. This results in prolonged pain and disability.

prevention (or lessening of impact) SPRAIN   Once it is established that there is no broken bone, the sprained area should be rested. For the first 24 hours cold should be applied to reduce the swelling. Follow with heat and general massage. In cases of severe swelling, it is best to strap the joint firmly so that the injured part is rested as much as possible. The physician will generally allow the patient to undertake modified activity, and suggest that the patient make progressive use of the injured part as he finds he can do so.

STRAIN   If the pain is very severe, the patient should be put to bed with the injured part raised up and at rest. Heat is usually very helpful, and gentle massage hastens recovery. It is advisable that the patient exercise the part in gradually increasing amounts as soon as he is able. If necessary, the part can be bandaged for support with a light splint or elastic type bandage.

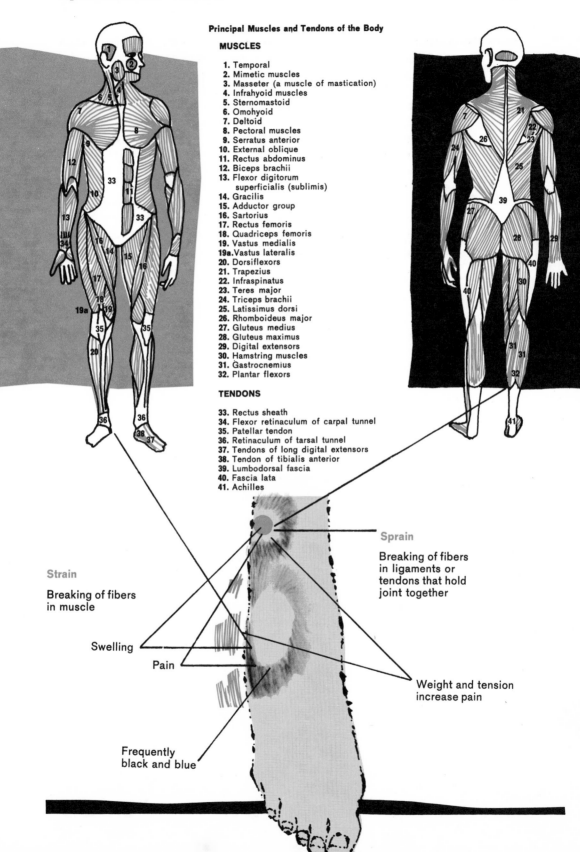

Principal Muscles and Tendons of the Body

MUSCLES

1. Temporal
2. Mimetic muscles
3. Masseter (a muscle of mastication)
4. Infrahyoid muscles
5. Sternomastoid
6. Omohyoid
7. Deltoid
8. Pectoral muscles
9. Serratus anterior
10. External oblique
11. Rectus abdominus
12. Biceps brachii
13. Flexor digitorum
   superficialis (sublimis)
14. Gracilis
15. Adductor group
16. Sartorius
17. Rectus femoris
18. Quadriceps femoris
19. Vastus medialis
19a. Vastus lateralis
20. Dorsiflexors
21. Trapezius
22. Infraspinatus
23. Teres major
24. Triceps brachii
25. Latissimus dorsi
26. Rhomboideus major
27. Gluteus medius
28. Gluteus maximus
29. Digital extensors
30. Hamstring muscles
31. Gastrocnemius
32. Plantar flexors

TENDONS

33. Rectus sheath
34. Flexor retinaculum of carpal tunnel
35. Patellar tendon
36. Retinaculum of tarsal tunnel
37. Tendons of long digital extensors
38. Tendon of tibialis anterior
39. Lumbodorsal fascia
40. Fascia lata
41. Achilles

Strain

Breaking of fibers
in muscle

Swelling

Pain

Frequently
black and blue

Sprain

Breaking of fibers
in ligaments or
tendons that hold
joint together

Weight and tension
increase pain

the condition and its causes Sterility—the inability of a couple to produce children —is a significant problem, affecting about 1 out of every 10 couples who want to have children. While it was formerly believed that a childless marriage was primarily the woman's fault, medical research now indicates that men are responsible for the sterility in 30%–40% of the cases. As the accompanying illustration shows, there are several places in the male's reproductive system where infection or injury may cut off production of the sperm cells. Or the sperm cells produced may be so weak or malformed that they cannot function properly in seeking out and fertilizing the female egg.

One cause of this is atrophy of the testicles—which can result from a birth defect, an infection such as mumps, an injury, exposure to X rays or other toxic substances, or endocrine disorders. Venereal diseases and other infections can also damage the testicles, the seminal vesicles, or the prostate gland, and cause sterility.

Birth defects or infections can take their toll of the female reproduction system too. Venereal disease or mumps may prevent the ovaries from producing healthy egg cells. This problem may also be caused by a lack of sex hormones produced by the endocrine glands or even by faulty diet. And birth defects in the uterus, vagina, or Fallopian tubes, or pelvic tumors, may block the normal route for sperm cell and egg cell to meet and mate.

Emotional problems may be a psychological bar to fertility for both male and female.

symptoms Of course, sterility is the symptom itself. However, medical tests will reveal if there are any underlying problems with the sperm or with the production of hormones by the endocrine glands. It will also show whether any anatomical problems and birth defects are present that must be corrected.

prevention (or lessening of impact) Among the measures that can be taken to counteract sterility are surgery for remediable defects, hormonal replacement drugs when needed, fertility drugs (although multiple births have been a problem with these), and timing of intercourse to take advantage of the most fertile time of the menstrual cycle. Advice on improvement of sexual intercourse techniques, psychotherapy, introduction of sperm high in the vagina, and artificial insemination are other possibilities. With patience and cooperation, fertility can replace sterility in 60% of the cases.

Sterility

Can have many causes ...

In the Male

1 Atrophy from disease or injury, harms production and delivery of normal sperm cells

2 Infection prevents passage of sperm cells to penis

Spermatic duct

Bladder

Prostate

Seminal vesicle

Penis

Epididymis

Testicles

Normal development and release route for male's sperm cells

3 Emotional problems prevent potency in male and receptivity in female

In the Female

4 Birth abnormality or infection blocks passage of sperm cell to meet egg

5 Birth abnormality or infection blocks egg from forming or passing to uterus to be fertilized

6 Lack of ovulation due to hormone problems

Ovary

Fallopian tube

Normal development and release route for female's egg cells

Uterus

Cervix

Vagina

Bladder

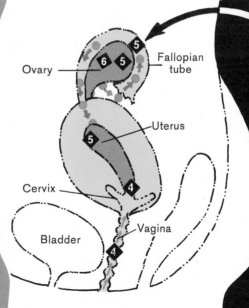

the disease and its causes   The term stroke is a broad descriptive word used to describe the effects of any interference with circulation within the brain. Strokes are properly called cerebral vascular accidents. They occur in a number of ways, as shown in the Medi-Graph. The blood supply to the brain is blocked by a thrombosis or clot which blocks the entrance to a narrowed and roughened section of artery; an embolus, which is a clot that is carried from another part of the body, usually the heart, blocks normal blood passage; a brain artery bursts and is unable to furnish brain cells with essential, nourishing blood; and, in rare instances, brain tumors or abscesses press on an artery and close it off.

A doctor cannot always be sure of the precise cause of a stroke, but he makes his diagnosis on the basis of the manner in which the attack occurred, the age of the patient, X ray studies, and the presence of possible contributing factors such as arteriosclerosis, high blood pressure, rheumatic or coronary heart disease, and diabetes. While the patient's condition seems to be the same regardless of the cause of the attack, the outlook and treatment differ.

Both men and women are affected, usually in the older age group.

symptoms   A stroke can occur without any warning and without any seeming relation to any event in the life of the patient or his physical condition. He can awake from sleep and show signs of paralysis affecting his extremities or his face. However, frequently there is warning—usually a period of numbness on one side, perhaps some headache, and often weakness of the face or an extremity which disappears after a time.

When the attack comes full force, there is paralysis of one side of the body, with all the symptoms noted in the Medi-Graph. Generally, strokes caused by a cerebral thrombosis are slower to develop than those caused by hemorrhage or emboli. In the case of emboli, there is immediate collapse and sometimes shock. Hemorrhage may cause severe headache and stiffness of the neck before the paralysis develops.

The areas of weakness or paralysis depend upon just where the accident occurs in the brain. Small blood vessel damage causes local areas of weakness or numbness; larger cerebral blood vessel damage causes larger areas of paralysis and weakness.

complications   These depend upon the severity of the attack. Severe brain destruction can cause death. Specific areas of brain damage can cause respiratory and cardiac failure. Patients who become paralyzed are subject to the complications of bed rest—pneumonia, kidney infections, bed sores, and blood clots.

prevention (or lessening of impact)   Anti-coagulants help patients with heart disease capable of forming emboli. Surgery is effective in cases with early signs of thrombosis in the neck arteries. Severe high blood pressure must be treated by a physician. When paralysis has occurred, the patient must be protected against secondary infection and started on physical therapy as soon as possible.

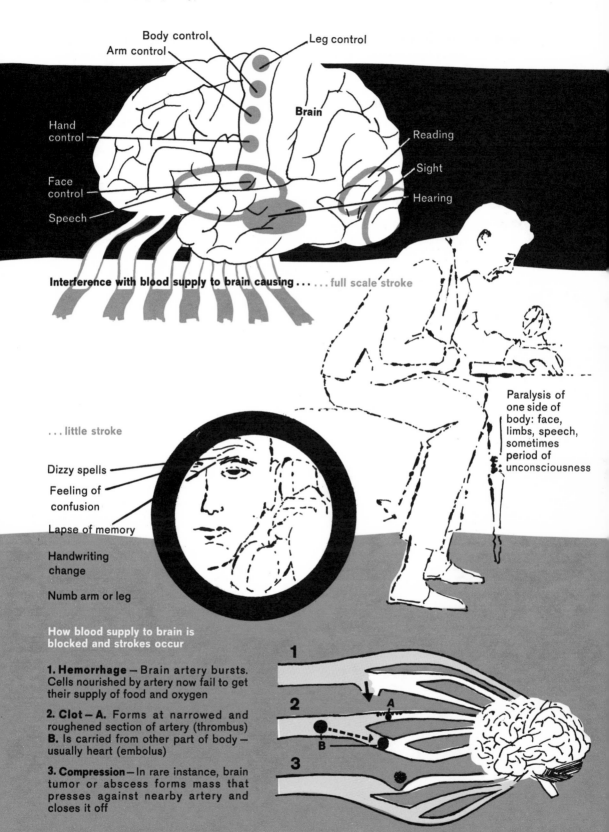

Body control
Arm control
Leg control

Hand control

Brain

Reading

Sight

Face control

Hearing

Speech

Interference with blood supply to brain causing . . . . full scale stroke

. . . little stroke

Dizzy spells

Feeling of confusion

Lapse of memory

Handwriting change

Numb arm or leg

Paralysis of one side of body: face, limbs, speech, sometimes period of unconsciousness

How blood supply to brain is blocked and strokes occur

1. Hemorrhage — Brain artery bursts. Cells nourished by artery now fail to get their supply of food and oxygen

2. Clot — A. Forms at narrowed and roughened section of artery (thrombus) **B.** Is carried from other part of body — usually heart (embolus)

3. Compression — In rare instance, brain tumor or abscess forms mass that presses against nearby artery and closes it off

the disease and its cause Styes develop as an inflammation of the glands at the edge of the eyelids—usually near hair follicles (the openings out of which hairs grow). The area becomes infected by bacteria—usually the Staphylococcus.

Styes occur at all ages—but commonly among children and young adults. They frequently occur in groups—several at one time; or in series—one after the other.

Styes are often associated with chronic eyelid irritations. Sometimes an uncorrected vision problem will cause eyestrain by weakening the eye and making it susceptible to styes. And any illness that lowers general resistance can precipitate the disease.

symptoms As the illustration shows, the stye behaves like a pimple or small boil. It starts as a red swelling, tender and painful. It grows in size—sometimes causing swelling of the entire lid.

A yellowish, pussy head develops on top of the red pimple. After a day or two, it softens and bursts. Yellowish pus is discharged.

complications Lack of cleanliness and sanitary precautions by the stye victim can spread the disease to others around him. The same failings can cause him to be afflicted with recurrent bouts of styes.

prevention (or lessening of impact) Hot compresses and antibiotics as prescribed by the doctor will usually suffice to clear up a case of styes. But, on occasion, a particularly troublesome one will have to be opened by the doctor.

Styes

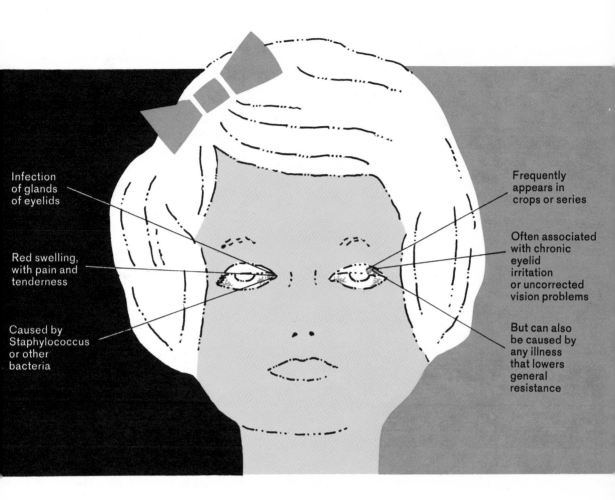

Infection
of glands
of eyelids

Red swelling,
with pain and
tenderness

Caused by
Staphylococcus
or other
bacteria

Frequently
appears in
crops or series

Often associated
with chronic
eyelid
irritation
or uncorrected
vision problems

But can also
be caused by
any illness
that lowers
general
resistance

Course of Development

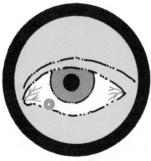

1 Starts as red
swelling with
pain and
tenderness

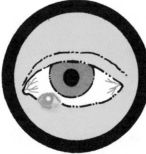

2 Grows in size,
comes to
yellowish head

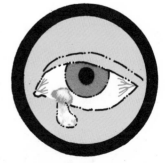

3 After day or two,
softens and bursts.
Yellowish pus
is discharged

the disease and its causes   Syphilis, the most serious of the venereal diseases, is caused by a spirochete. There are two ways people get this disease: It is acquired through intercourse with an infected person, by kissing, or on rare occasions by handling contaminated articles; or else it is transmitted via the blood from an infected mother to her unborn child. For that reason pregnant women should be examined carefully for syphilis and treated as soon as a diagnosis of syphilis is made. Along with the disease there are often extensive inflammatory reactions of the body in general and the central nervous system and heart in particular.

The disease is found throughout the world, experienced by every race and by both sexes. The incubation period varies from 10 to 50 days—usually it is about 3 weeks.

symptoms   First there may appear the characteristic chancre, which is an ulcerous sore about ½″ in diameter, as illustrated. It is painless and usually appears on the external genital organs, or occasionally on the lip, tongue, nipples, or fingers. The lymph glands enlarge but do not become painful. Without treatment the chancre heals slowly in from 4 to 6 weeks. It should be noted, however, that in this first stage neither the chancre nor other symptoms always appear. This is called the first stage of syphilis.

In the second stage, which begins as the chancre disappears, there may be weakness, chilliness, low-grade temperature, generalized aches and pains in glands and joints, and headache. Skin lesions in the form of raised red patches on the skin, or small patches in the mouth or reproductive organs, begin to appear. This rash may take different forms and can be confused with other skin diseases. There is no characteristic rash, many different parts of the body are involved, and the length of time it is present varies.

The third stage may occur at any time, from weeks to years after the initial infection. There are skin lesions of varying types, and there may be loss of hair. Serious effects can be involvement of the central nervous system, brain or heart, as well as the joints, bones, liver, and all organs of the body.

complications   These are related to the organ system involved. Late effects of the disease include heart disease, heart failure, rupture of the aorta (main artery of the body), brain damage, and destruction of the spinal cord.

prevention (or lessening of impact)   There is no sure preventive for this illness except abstinence from sexual intercourse with infected partners. Prophylactic care is of some benefit but offers no guarantee. Early recognition and prompt treatment are essential to prevent late destructive effects. Regardless of whether any symptoms appear, blood tests should be taken promptly in any cases where exposure to the disease is suspected.

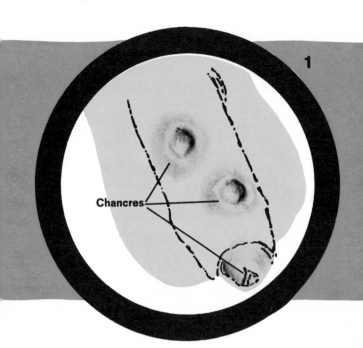

1

1. Primary Stage:
Chancre is characteristic symptom of primary stage of syphilis. Usually one but sometimes several chancres appear — generally in genital regions. Occasionally syphilis chancres emerge. on lip, tongue, nipples or finger.

1A. Frequently there is accompanying painless swelling of lymph glands near genitals. Chancres too are painless — and generally heal in 3-4 weeks without leaving scars.

1A

2. Secondary Stage:
Mild rash sometimes occurs after chancre disappears. May appear anywhere on body—and has no characteristic appearance.

Chancres

Swelling of Lymph Glands

Chancre

2

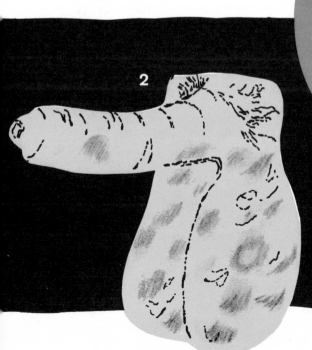

the disease and its causes   The tapeworm is a parasite that infects hogs, steers, and cows. When a person eats contaminated meat that is raw or under-cooked, the tapeworm larvae (young worms just out of the egg) that are present in the meat can pass into the person's small intestine. There, the tapeworms grow into mature worms from 6 to 20 feet long.

symptoms   As a rule, tapeworm infection causes no unusual disturbances. A patient may not know he has it until segments of the worm are dis-charged into his feces and he observes them. In occasional cases there can be some abdominal discomfort, nausea, vomiting, or a change in bowel habits. An outstanding characteristic of the infection is the patient's ravenous appetite. (Thus, there are good grounds for the folk saying "He eats so much and stays so thin—you'd think he had a tapeworm!")

complications   Generally there are no serious complications from beef tapeworm. The worm may live for years before it is detected, with no effect on the general health of the patient. Occasionally, a moderate anemia (loss of red blood cells) develops.
However, pork tapeworm larvae can cause serious complications by invading the muscles in general, the heart muscle, brain, eye, and ner-vous system.

prevention (and lessening of impact)   To prevent this infection it is essential that pork and beef be cooked thoroughly in order to destroy the larvae of the tapeworm. Once a patient is infected, the entire worm, including the head, must be removed, and this can be done medically. Removing the head is important because when it remains attached to the intestinal wall, it regenerates itself and the infection cycle starts all over again.

Tapeworm

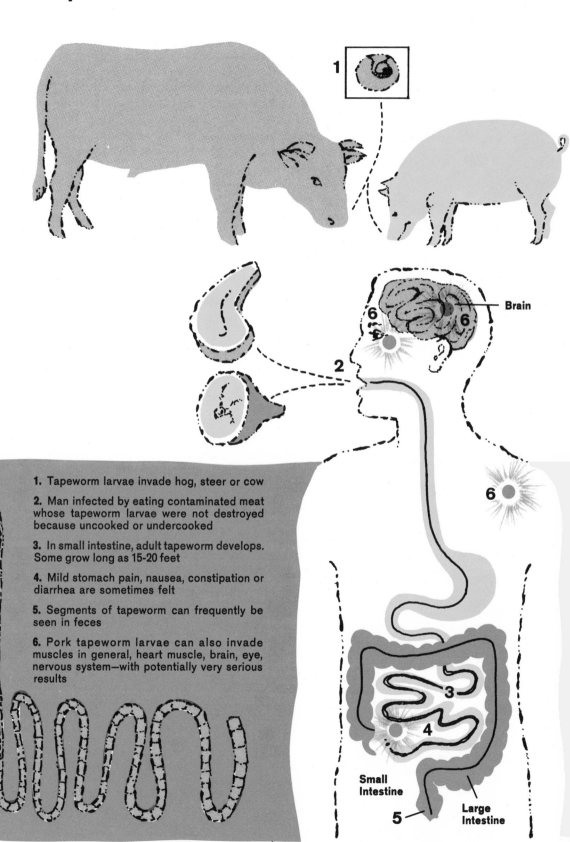

1. Tapeworm larvae invade hog, steer or cow

2. Man infected by eating contaminated meat whose tapeworm larvae were not destroyed because uncooked or undercooked

3. In small intestine, adult tapeworm develops. Some grow long as 15-20 feet

4. Mild stomach pain, nausea, constipation or diarrhea are sometimes felt

5. Segments of tapeworm can frequently be seen in feces

6. Pork tapeworm larvae can also invade muscles in general, heart muscle, brain, eye, nervous system—with potentially very serious results

Brain

Small Intestine

Large Intestine

the disease and its cause   This disease makes its appearance in the middle of the first year of life, and results in the death of the child in the next few years. It is caused by the accumulation of a fatty substance within the brain cells. In a normal person, the body manufactures an enzyme called hexosaminidase A (HEX A) which assists in the digestion of fatty substances. Medical research has recently discovered that in an infant suffering from Tay-Sachs disease this enzyme is absent. As a result, abnormal amounts of fatty material accumulate in the brain, eventually destroying the functioning of the brain and the central nervous system.

Infants inherit this disease from seemingly normal "carrier" parents. Tay-Sachs has gained a reputation as a "Jewish disease," because about 85% of the cases occur among Jews whose families are of East European origin.

symptoms   The affected child appears normal in the first few months of life. But sometime between 4–8 months, symptoms of the disease begin to appear. The child loses all of his physical skills—such as his ability to crawl or turn over. Mental retardation and deterioration also begin to set in.

Blindness develops due to degeneration of the retina. Convulsions usually occur, and death strikes by the time the child is 3–5 years old.

prevention (or lessening of impact)   Now that research has isolated the genetic cause of the disease, its prevention is within the grasp of prospective parents. Tay-Sachs is a recessive disease: both parents must be carriers in order for a Tay-Sachs child to be born—as shown in the illustration. If both parents are carriers, their chances are 1 out of 4 for a child with Tay-Sachs disease to be born from each pregnancy.

Fortunately, a simple blood test is available that detects whether seemingly normal people are carriers of the disease. It is particularly important that Jewish couples take this test. If it reveals that neither parent— or only one of the parents—is a carrier, then the couple know they will not produce an infant doomed with the disease. If both parents turn out to be carriers, a test of pregnant women is available which will detect the disease in the fetus as early as the 16th week.

Tay-Sachs Disease

345

Disease caused by abnormal accumulation of fatty substances in the Brain

Brain of

Normal Infant   **Tay-Sachs Victim**

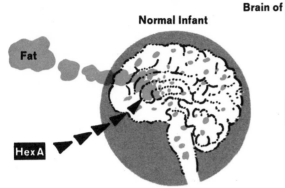

Fat

Fat

HexA

Enzyme HexA breaks up fatty substances so that they can be utilized by Brain and other organs

Lack of HexA enzyme means abnormal deposit of fatty substances in Brain—gradually stopping it from functioning

Course of Tay-Sachs Disease

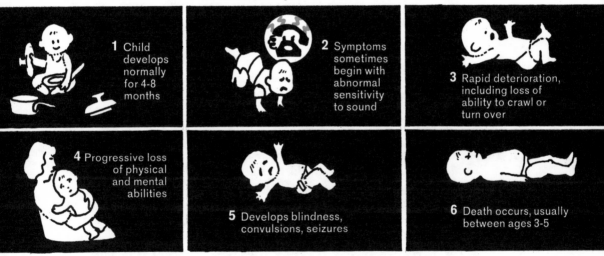

1 Child develops normally for 4-8 months

2 Symptoms sometimes begin with abnormal sensitivity to sound

3 Rapid deterioration, including loss of ability to crawl or turn over

4 Progressive loss of physical and mental abilities

5 Develops blindness, convulsions, seizures

6 Death occurs, usually between ages 3-5

Chance of Inheriting Tay-Sachs Disease if Parents are Carriers

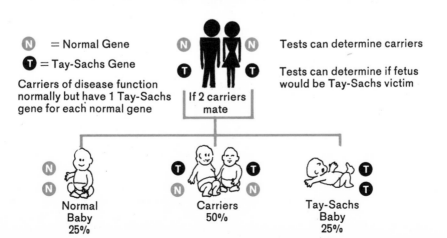

Ⓝ = Normal Gene

Ⓣ = Tay-Sachs Gene

Carriers of disease function normally but have 1 Tay-Sachs gene for each normal gene

If 2 carriers mate

Tests can determine carriers

Tests can determine if fetus would be Tay-Sachs victim

Normal Baby 25%

Carriers 50%

Tay-Sachs Baby 25%

the disease and its causes   Tetanus is an acute infection of the central nervous system caused by a specific type of bacteria and the poison they create. The bacteria are usually found in dust, dirt, and manure. The patient is infected through a puncture wound caused by anything sharp—such as a nail or splinter, or an insect or dog bite. Any skin opening is a port of entry, but deep wounds are dangerous because the tetanus germ thrives best without oxygen. It can occur in anyone . . . in any age group . . . at any time of the year. The incubation period is 3 days to 3 weeks.

symptoms   This disease is characterized by pain and stiffness of the muscles of any part of the body. This is usually preceded by headache, temperature, stiff neck, and then muscle spasm. The wound of entry shows all the signs of infection. The muscles of the jaw are particularly involved, and it becomes painful and difficult to open the mouth. It is from this that the name lockjaw comes.

Swallowing may be difficult. Breathing is labored and irregular. The entire back may go into such spasm that the victim arches until he is lying on just his head and heels. Convulsions occur. In severe cases the patient dies in as few as 3 days. In less severe instances, the course of the illness is 2 to 3 weeks.

complications   Secondary infections such as pneumonia are common. Heart failure can cause death. Patients who recover sometimes have deformed backs as a result of the severe muscle spasm. The disease is frequently fatal, although it need not be if properly diagnosed and treated early. When therapy is delayed, the poison or toxin invades the body disastrously.

prevention (or lessening of impact)   Since the tetanus vaccine available is highly effective, immunization should be started during the first year of life. It is a series of 3 injections. Booster shots should be given for any dirty, potentially infected wound. Patients who have not been immunized and require immediate protection can be given an antitoxin, but many people react adversely to it because it is made of horse serum. Highly specialized care is needed if there is to be any hope of saving the life of a patient ill with tetanus. Specific medications are available for the muscle spasms and for complications. Hospitalization is a "must." Often the patient must be fed intravenously and may require a respirator to help him breathe.

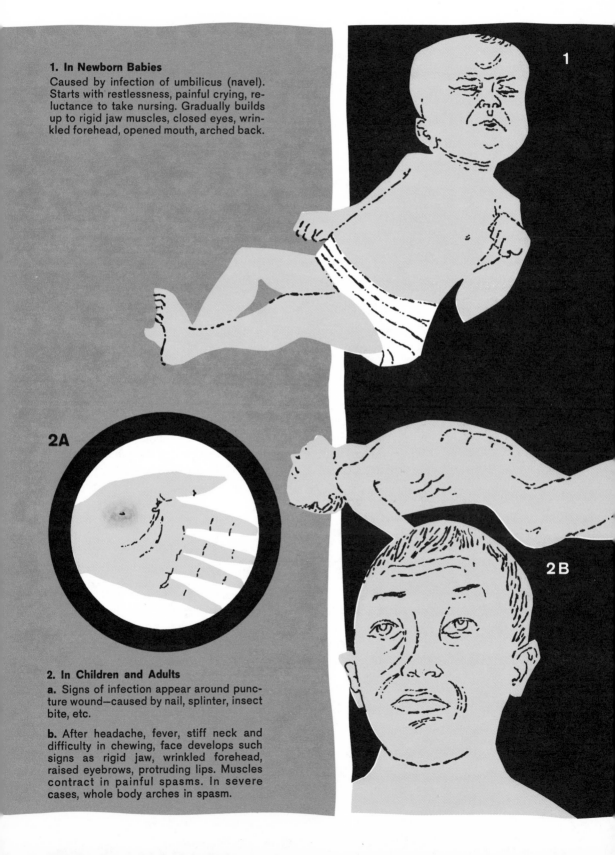

1. In Newborn Babies

Caused by infection of umbilicus (navel). Starts with restlessness, painful crying, reluctance to take nursing. Gradually builds up to rigid jaw muscles, closed eyes, wrinkled forehead, opened mouth, arched back.

2. In Children and Adults

a. Signs of infection appear around puncture wound—caused by nail, splinter, insect bite, etc.

b. After headache, fever, stiff neck and difficulty in chewing, face develops such signs as rigid jaw, wrinkled forehead, raised eyebrows, protruding lips. Muscles contract in painful spasms. In severe cases, whole body arches in spasm.

the disease and its causes   Many bacteria and viruses infect the tonsils, but it is the streptococcus which is the most common cause of tonsillitis—and from which it gets the alternate name of strep throat. The disease occurs most often in children, but affects every age group. Strep throat localizes on tonsils, stubs of tonsils, or in the pharynx. The incubation period can run from 1 to 10 days, but most generally lasts 2 to 4 days. The illness itself runs from 3 to 9 days without medication, and is shortened by treatment.

symptoms   Acute tonsillitis begins suddenly with chills, aches and pains, headache, and sore throat. The temperature rises quickly to 102°-104°, and it may go as high as 106°. Nausea and vomiting are frequent with children, diarrhea less so. The disease reaches its peak quickly, usually within 24 to 48 hours. The sore throat is severe and persists until the infection is brought under control. Pain is likely to spread to the ear and the neck. Here glands behind the angle of the jaw, below the ears, are most commonly affected. One out of 2 cases shows cold symptoms, with nasal discharge, cough, and loss of voice. As shown in the Medi-Graph, the mucous membrane of the pharynx, soft palate, and tonsils may be red and swollen and covered partially or entirely with a yellow, white or grayish membrane. The tongue is usually gray and coated.

complications   A frequent complication and disease to which tonsillitis is related is scarlet fever. It may appear 1 to 5 days after the onset of the infection and is identified by the rash. Other complications include sinusitis, ear infections, pneumonia, and a serious peritonsillar abscess called quinsy throat which occurs when the infection spreads about the tonsillar area. There is difficulty in swallowing, pain on opening the mouth, and very sore throat. Chronic tonsillitis can develop, with signs of the infection recurring in the same pattern every 2 or 3 weeks. Arthritis and meningitis are rare complications.

prevention (or lessening of impact)   There is no specific vaccine against the streptococcus bacteria. Since the greater number of people with this illness carry the organism in their respiratory discharge for as long as 3 months, preventing its spread is a problem. Good hygiene must be observed. Those who come in close contact with a patient should be treated promptly with antibiotics. Susceptible people can be given protection over long periods of time with drugs prescribed by the doctor. Good medical care during the illness helps to prevent the patient from becoming a carrier.

Acute Tonsillitis (Strep Throat)

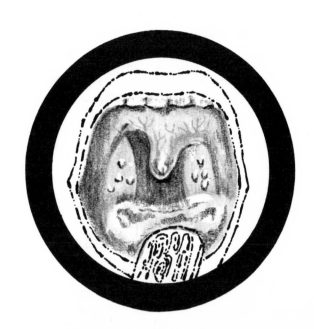

A. Red, swollen tonsils, pharynx, soft palate. Patches of yellow, gray or white membrane covers inflamed area. Tongue has heavy gray coating.

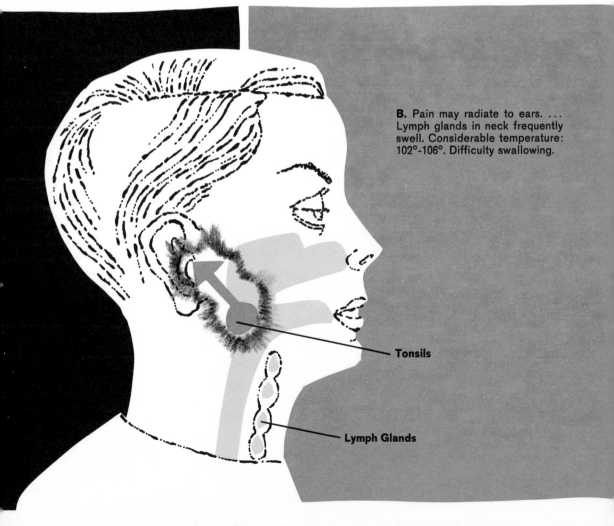

B. Pain may radiate to ears. ... Lymph glands in neck frequently swell. Considerable temperature: 102°-106°. Difficulty swallowing.

Tonsils

Lymph Glands

the disease and its causes   This is a common infection, transmitted by contact with the parasitic germ *Toxoplasmi gondii*. Recent research indicates that people contract toxoplasmosis in two main ways. The first is through eating raw or rare meat—since this parasitic germ finds a congenial home in the flesh of animals, even after they have been slaughtered for use as food.

The feline digestive system provides another favorable place for development of toxoplasmosis germs. Excreted into the cat's litter box or buried in the soil by the cat, the cyst in the feces becomes infective after a 2–4 day incubation period.

Toxoplasmosis' big threat is to the fetuses of pregnant women because, like German measles, it can cause birth defects.

symptoms   Toxoplasmosis may be fatal to as many as 10% of all babies born with the disease. If the baby is not stillborn, it can live on with brain damage, blindness, enlarged liver and spleen, fever, and jaundice. A majority of babies born with the disease show some permanent damage.

Many adults who contract the disease display no symptoms and apparently feel no ill effects. As the illustration shows, others may feel as if they have a cold or the flu, with the illness subsiding without serious problems or discomfort.

Your doctor diagnoses the disease by skin and blood tests.

complications   Among adults, complications are rare. Infants born with severe brain damage from the disease are prey to other infections that may prove fatal.

prevention (or lessening of impact)   Tests show that about one-fourth of U.S. adults have toxoplasmosis antibodies in their blood, developed from a previous bout with the disease. These antibodies are thought to make the person immune to further infection with the disease.

Pregnant women who are in the habit of eating raw meat (like steak tartare) or rare meat, or who have been in contact with cats, should be tested to see if they are protected by toxoplasmosis antibodies in their blood. If these antibodies are not present, the pregnant woman should avoid both hazards.

Toxoplasmosis can be controlled with a combination of drugs—but these may cause undesirable side effects. So treatment of pregnant women in this way must be guided by their individual reactions.

Toxoplasmosis

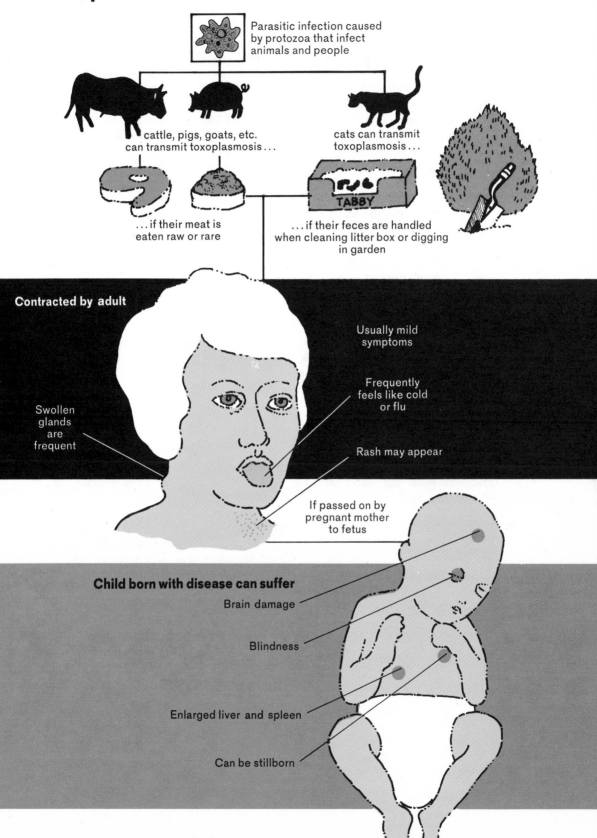

Parasitic infection caused by protozoa that infect animals and people

cattle, pigs, goats, etc. can transmit toxoplasmosis...

cats can transmit toxoplasmosis...

TABBY

...if their meat is eaten raw or rare

...if their feces are handled when cleaning litter box or digging in garden

Contracted by adult

Usually mild symptoms

Frequently feels like cold or flu

Swollen glands are frequent

Rash may appear

If passed on by pregnant mother to fetus

Child born with disease can suffer

Brain damage

Blindness

Enlarged liver and spleen

Can be stillborn

the disease and its causes Trench mouth is an infection of the mucous membrane of the mouth and throat, caused by two types of germs working together in individuals whose resistance has been lowered. It is very common in young adults. At one time it was assumed that the disease was transferred by direct contact, such as kissing. However, since the germs are present in the mouth of most individuals much of the time, it is now believed that the disease takes hold when resistance is lowered because of poor vitamin intake, intestinal disorders, blood diseases, poor oral hygiene, associated dental problems, emotional stress, or fatigue.

symptoms The disease usually begins with soreness of the mouth, a metallic taste, pain around the teeth, and bleeding gums. There may be sore throat, headache, earache, and weakness. The breath usually has a foul odor. If the throat is involved as well as the regional lymph glands, there is usually temperature up to 102°-103°. The tongue will usually swell and become furry.

In weak and elderly patients, trench mouth may be more acute. There are high temperature and marked generalized effects. The mouth may have punched-out, grayish ulcerations around the edge, near the teeth. On pressure these will bleed readily. There may be similar ulcerations on the inside of the cheeks and on the pharynx. Because there is a grayish membrane in the mouth and throat, this disease was at one time confused with diphtheria. In cases with throat or tonsil involvement, the infection may last 10 to 14 days with persistent temperature and pain.

complications Complications are rare, since the infection tends to be mild and responds to therapy. However, neglect can result in infection at the roots of the teeth, with eventual loosening and perhaps loss of the teeth.

prevention (or lessening of impact) Trench mouth may be avoided with proper dental hygiene and the correction of any dental abnormalities that make for poor mouth conditions. Since there is a possibility of contagion, it is wise to use separate dishes and silverware for an infected patient. An infected child need not be isolated at home, but he should not go to school. And since observation suggests that lowered resistance plays a role in the onset of this disease, it is important to maintain good dental and general health.

Trench Mouth (Vincent's Angina)

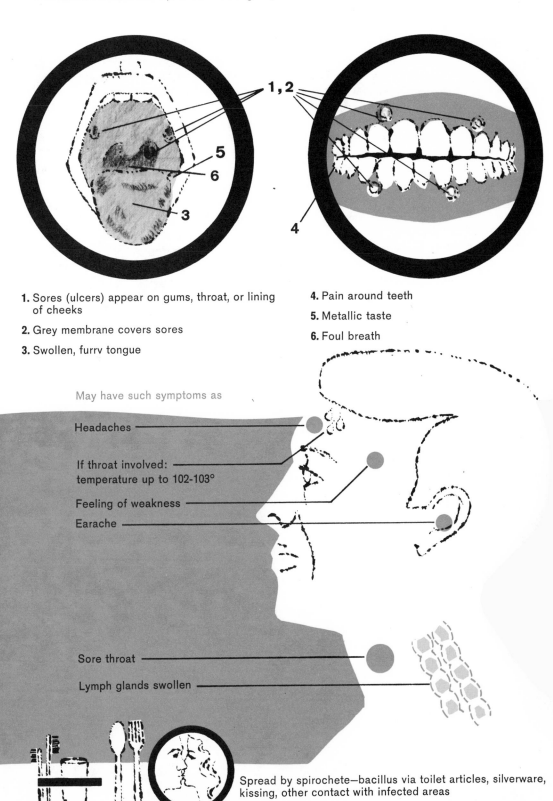

1. Sores (ulcers) appear on gums, throat, or lining of cheeks

2. Grey membrane covers sores

3. Swollen, furry tongue

4. Pain around teeth

5. Metallic taste

6. Foul breath

May have such symptoms as

Headaches

If throat involved: temperature up to 102-103°

Feeling of weakness

Earache

Sore throat

Lymph glands swollen

Spread by spirochete—bacillus via toilet articles, silverware, kissing, other contact with infected areas

the disease and its causes Trichinosis is a roundworm infection which man contracts when he eats infected pork. The life cycle of the roundworm is such that the larval stage (the stage of the young worm just after it comes out of its egg) exists in the infected pig. When man eats raw or partially cooked infected pork, these larvae are freed in the course of digestion and pass into the small intestine. There they attach themselves, develop into adult worms, and reproduce. Their eggs pass through the walls of the bowel and are carried via the bloodstream to the muscles, where they form cysts. In occasional cases, the roundworms may find their way to the heart muscle and eventually the brain. Trichinosis is a quite common ailment, especially among people who eat ham or pork in a raw or partially cooked state.

symptoms The number of roundworms eaten determines the symptoms. In many cases, there are no symptoms at all. But when a patient has eaten a good many of the worms, there is usually abdominal pain, nausea, vomiting, and occasionally diarrhea. This is followed by chills and fever up to 102°-104°. The muscles become very tender and are painful on motion. There may be respiratory signs such as shortness of breath and hoarseness. Swelling around the eyes is not unusual. There may be a red rash over the body. In severe cases, this stage can last as long as eight weeks.
As convalescence sets in, the larvae become locked into the muscles and the symptoms subside.

complications Complications can be severe. They include pneumonia, involvement of the heart, and phlebitis—which is a vein inflammation in which blood clots form.

prevention (or lessening of impact) Trichinosis can be prevented simply by cooking all pork and pork products thoroughly. This destroys any larvae in the meat to be eaten.

Trichinosis

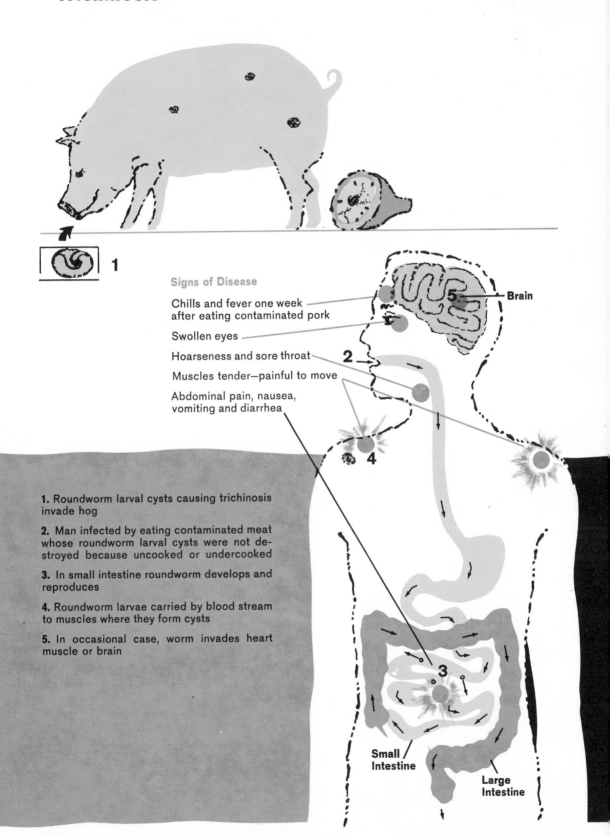

Signs of Disease

Chills and fever one week after eating contaminated pork

Swollen eyes

Hoarseness and sore throat

Muscles tender—painful to move

Abdominal pain, nausea, vomiting and diarrhea

Brain

2

4

5

3

1. Roundworm larval cysts causing trichinosis invade hog

2. Man infected by eating contaminated meat whose roundworm larval cysts were not destroyed because uncooked or undercooked

3. In small intestine roundworm develops and reproduces

4. Roundworm larvae carried by blood stream to muscles where they form cysts

5. In occasional case, worm invades heart muscle or brain

Small Intestine

Large Intestine

Trichomonas

Infectious disease of the genital organs, spread by protozoan parasite. Occurs much more commonly among women than men.

the disease and its causes   TRICHOMONAS is an infectious disease of the genital organs which is spread by a protozoan parasite. It occurs much more commonly among women than men—attacking the vagina and urethra in the former case and the penis and scrotum in the latter. Though not a serious infection, it can be a disabling and painful illness.

Trichomonas may be spread by the male through sexual intercourse.

symptoms   Among women, the typical symptoms of trichomonas are vaginal itching and burning, and a heavy, creamy, yellow discharge from the vagina. A burning sensation on urination is common as is irritation about the vulva—occasionally extending to the rectum. The doctor's examination reveals an inflammation of the vagina and occasionally ulceration or erosion of the vaginal wall. Sometimes small blood spots *(petechiae)* appear there.

In the male, trichomonas signals itself by itching and burning of the penis and scrotum, where a rash appears.

complications   Usually the disease is easily cured by the doctor without serious complications. But some patients, reacting to certain drugs used in treatment, have contracted fungi as a secondary infection.

prevention (or lessening of impact)   Strict personal hygiene—keeping the genital organs clean—will prevent attacks of trichomonas. The use of prophylactic douches is also helpful when the disease threatens. And if trichomonas is contracted, both husband and wife should present themselves to the doctor if the illness is persistent or recurrent. The doctor has a number of specific drugs at his disposal which are effective in eradicating the disease.

Trichomonas

Infectious disease of the genital organs, spread by protozoan parasite. Occurs much more commonly among women than men.

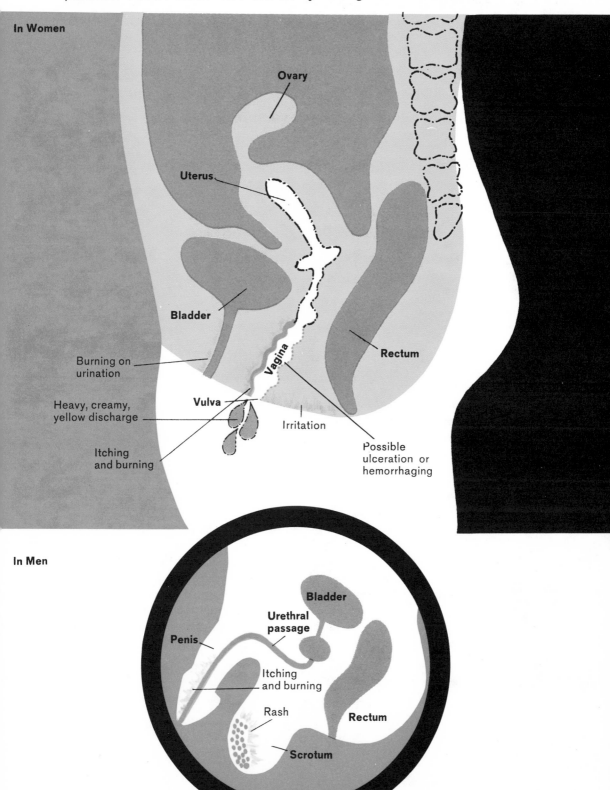

the disease and its causes   Tuberculosis is caused by the tubercle bacillus—found in humans, cows, and birds. These bacteria are spread by particles of dust or droplets which are expelled by a tubercular patient when he talks, coughs, laughs, or sneezes; or they are introduced into the intestinal tract by way of contaminated foods—such as milk from tubercular cows or objects placed in the mouth. Men and women between the ages of 20 and 40 are most susceptible. The exact incubation period is unknown and varies from days to many years.

symptoms   Tuberculosis is a generalized illness affecting all organ systems. Pulmonary tuberculosis, discussed here, and the most common form, affects the lungs. The onset is usually abrupt, and there may be no history of exposure to the disease. A main symptom is a cough which can be either dry or productive. There is some spitting which varies in quality. Blood spitting may occur, and there may be pain in the chest. Frequently the voice box is involved and hoarseness results. Shortness of breath may be noted, often an indication of long-standing or advanced disease. There is almost always fever in active pulmonary tuberculosis, generally accompanied by night sweats, loss of strength, and loss of weight. When the gastro-intestinal system is involved there may be marked loss of appetite and symptoms of indigestion. Occasionally there is diarrhea.

complications   The main complications are pleurisy, an involvement of the lining of the lung; pleural effusion, in which the chest fills with fluid; tuberculous laryngitis, the cause of the hoarseness; and pneumothorax, which is rupture of the lungs. A form of tuberculosis called miliary occurs when the infection is spread through the bloodstream to involve any part of the body, including the brain.

prevention (or lessening of impact)   As yet, there is no really effective vaccine for the prevention of tuberculosis, although one has been undergoing extensive clinical testing for many years. A tuberculin test is available which shows whether or not an individual has been exposed to tuberculosis, or has had a healed case.

High hygienic standards and good health are necessary to maintain resistance to the disease. All contact with infected people or foods from contaminated sources should be avoided. Anyone exposed should have routine chest X rays so that the infection can be detected early and treated promptly. Specific medical and surgical treatment is available once the diagnosis is established.

Pulmonary Tuberculosis

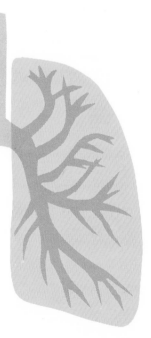

1. Symptoms that sometimes appear are coughing, spitting up of blood, pain in chest, hoarseness, fever, night sweats, loss of weight and strength.

2. Bacterial infection causes inflammation, abscess and scarring of lung. May heal and then reinfect. X rays reveal stage of infection, guide doctor in treatment.

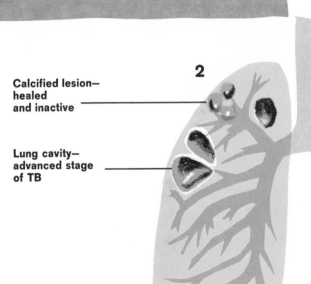

Calcified lesion—
healed
and inactive

Lung cavity—
advanced stage
of TB

the disease and its causes Typhoid fever is an acute, generalized infection caused by a specific type of bacteria. It is spread by infected water, milk, and other dairy products, other foods, or by direct contact with a typhoid carrier. It can occur at any season but appears most often in the fall. The incubation period is about 2 weeks. All age groups are involved, but the most frequent victims are young adults.

symptoms The disease usually begins as a mild, grippe-like infection, with head-ache and muscle aches. There may be nosebleeds, nausea, vomiting, constipation, or diarrhea. As the illness advances, the temperature goes higher, reaching levels of 104°-105°. The second week is marked by persistent high fever and an accompanying slow pulse. A rose-colored rash appears on the abdomen, back, and chest. The abdomen is dis-tended and uncomfortable. By the 3rd or 4th week there is gradual decrease in the temperature and rash, and disappearance of symptoms.

complications There may be hemorrhage or perforation of the intestinal tract. The liver may become infected, resulting in jaundice. The gallbladder may become infected and remain as a source of infection. As a result of this condition, a person may become a carrier. Pneumonia and meningitis are also possible complications.

prevention (or lessening of impact) There is a typhoid vaccine which is highly effective but not an assured preventive. It is given in three weekly doses and followed by a booster at regular intervals. Hygienic measures and proper sewage disposal are important factors in preventing illness. In areas known to have typhoid fever, all water should be sterilized properly and particular precautions should be taken with foods fertilized with human excrement.

Food handlers should have stool examinations to rule out the possibility that they are typhoid carriers.

A patient with typhoid fever requires good nursing care. He should be isolated and his bed linen and dishes sterilized. Toilet facilities in con-tact with the patient's stools and urine should be carefully disinfected. The patient should be kept clean throughout and bathed daily if pos-sible. His convalescent diet should include small amounts of low roughage-high calorie food at frequent intervals to maintain his strength and shorten his convalescence. Specific antibiotics are avail-able for treatment. Booster shots of vaccine may be given in cases of epidemics or if a person has been exposed.

1. First Week

Flushed face, glassy eyes, white or brownish coated tongue with reddened tip and edges. Chills, headache, other grippe-type symptoms. Fever mounting to 104-105°.

2. Second Week

Rash breaks out—usually on abdomen, sometimes on chest or back. 1-20 rose colored pimples appear in successive waves. Fade momentarily on pressure. Abdomen swells and is tender.

3. Third-Fourth Week

Rash disappears — leaving brownish stain. Fever declines and other symptoms gradually disappear.

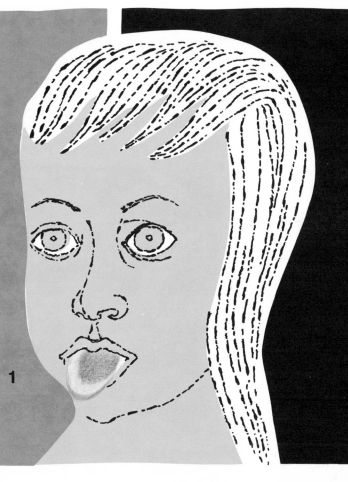

1

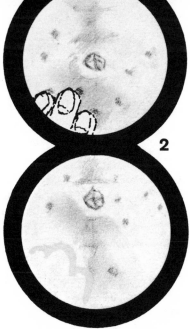

2

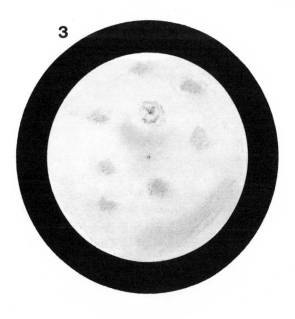

3

the disease and its causes Called stomach ulcers, gastric, peptic or duodenal ulcers, these are crater-like sores in the lining of the stomach and upper part of the small intestine (duodenum). Ulcers are believed to be caused by the stomach's producing an excess of digestive juices—pepsin and hydrochloric acid. In normal digestion, these juices break up food into forms that can be readily absorbed through the intestine. However, when the stomach produces too much hydrochloric acid, this may eat into the lining of the stomach or small intestine—causing ulcers. A majority of ulcers occur in the duodenum.

Tense, nervous people seem particularly prone to develop ulcers, as a result of a harmful cycle: emotional stress . . . leading to overproduction of stomach acid . . . leading to pain . . . leading to increased emotional stress . . . leading to ulcers.

symptoms During the digestive process food enters the stomach within several minutes after eating—but it takes a couple of hours to move on to the duodenum. Ulcer patients frequently have pain in the stomach area within minutes after eating (if they have stomach ulcers) or 2 to 3 hours after eating (if they have duodenal ulcers). This pain seems to be due to the effect on the ulcer of the digestive juices the stomach produces in response to the recently eaten food. The type of pain may vary from a mild upset stomach to a sharply gnawing or burning sensation. These ulcer pains are usually relieved if the patient takes an antacid, milk or other soft foods to neutralize the stomach acid. The pain is located high in the abdomen, as illustrated, and may radiate to the back.

However, some ulcer patients may experience no apparent pain or other symptoms for a long time after their ulcers have developed.

complications In the case of patients who are not warned by painful symptoms or who do not seek medical attention when these symptoms develop, an ulcer may eat all the way through (perforate) the wall of the stomach or duodenum. An ulcer may also break through the wall of a blood vessel, causing internal bleeding. Both these complications require immediate hospitalization and treatment.

If an ulcer patient finds his pain suddenly becoming much more intense than usual, and his usual medication doesn't relieve the pain, he can suspect perforation. Signs of possible internal bleeding would be vomiting of blood, or the passage of blood or black stool through the rectum. Stomach ulcers can become malignant.

prevention (or lessening of impact) Talking over emotional upsets and problems with a sympathetic or professional listener helps to get rid of the tensions which promote the formation of ulcers. Avoiding tobacco and other stimulants, developing relaxing hobbies, getting a good night's sleep regularly and following a doctor's advice regarding diet and medication help to prevent the formation of ulcers—or lessen the severity of attacks from ulcers, when they have developed.

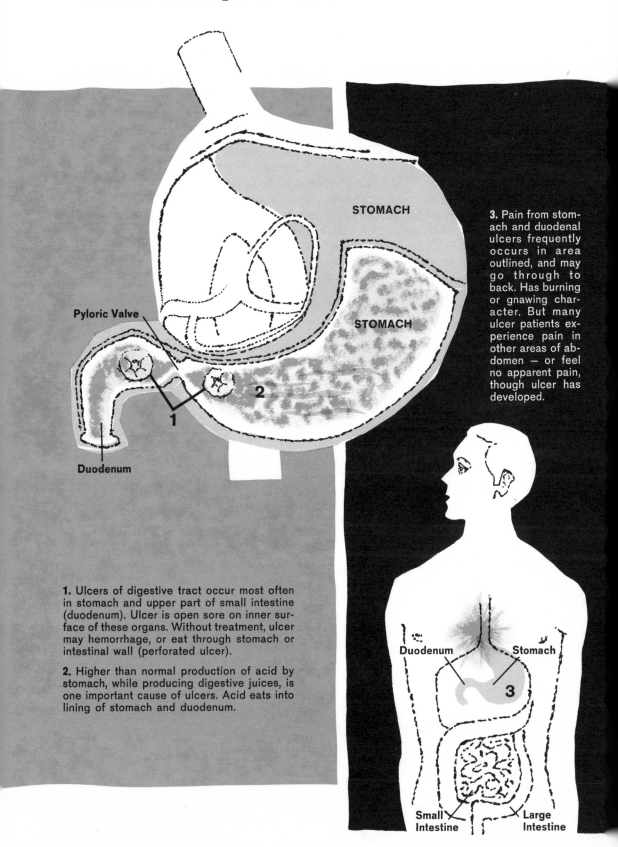

STOMACH

Pyloric Valve

STOMACH

2

1

Duodenum

3. Pain from stomach and duodenal ulcers frequently occurs in area outlined, and may go through to back. Has burning or gnawing character. But many ulcer patients experience pain in other areas of abdomen — or feel no apparent pain, though ulcer has developed.

1. Ulcers of digestive tract occur most often in stomach and upper part of small intestine (duodenum). Ulcer is open sore on inner surface of these organs. Without treatment, ulcer may hemorrhage, or eat through stomach or intestinal wall (perforated ulcer).

2. Higher than normal production of acid by stomach, while producing digestive juices, is one important cause of ulcers. Acid eats into lining of stomach and duodenum.

Duodenum   **Stomach**

3

Small   **Large**
Intestine   **Intestine**

the disease and its causes   To function normally, the testicles, which are egg-shaped glands, must operate in their natural environment—the scrotum (or sac). Normally, the testicles descend at birth from the abdominal cavity through the inguinal canal to the scrotum. When they do not descend, they are in an abnormal environment where there is interference with their production of sperm and the male sex hormone testosterone. Undescended testicles can be found anywhere between the abdomen and the scrotum—as shown in the Medi-Graph.

Undescended testicles are found in about 10% of boys at birth. There are a variety of causes that are thought to be responsible for this disease: failure of the hormone supply to provide its normal stimulation of the testes to descend at birth; a refusal of the testicles to respond to such hormone stimulation; mechanical blockage such as adhesions or anatomical obstacles that prevent the normal descent of the testicles from the abdominal cavity to the scrotum.

Fortunately, by the time a boy born with undescended testicles reaches puberty, the condition has frequently corrected itself without creating any other problems.

symptoms   When a testicle has not descended by the onset of puberty (the age when a boy matures sexually—usually between 12 and 15), it degenerates progressively. However, if the other testicle has descended, the only symptom observed as a rule is occasional pain over the undescended one—and even this symptom may not appear.

If both testicles do not descend and they fail to produce testosterone, the patient shows eunuchoid symptoms. The penis may fail to grow normally, the voice may remain high-pitched, and beard, armpit hair, and pubic hair may be absent. There is a tendency for the long bones to overgrow, and abnormal fat deposits may appear on the hips, buttocks, and breasts. This extreme picture appears only when there is a complete lack of hormone function. Very often an undescended testicle is capable of some hormone secretion.

complications   Testicles which do not descend not only result in hormonal defects but also can be painful and be the site of cancer. When the testicles remain in the abdomen, cancer occurs most often. The greater the distance they travel toward the scrotum, the less likely is cancer to develop.

Another complication, as noted above, is the possible development of eunuchoidism.

prevention (or lessening of impact)   If a diagnosis of the condition is made before a boy's puberty and the location of the undescended testicle established, it can be treated successfully. Testicles found in the inguinal canal usually descend by themselves. If not, they generally respond to specific hormone injections. When passage is blocked mechanically, surgery is used to relocate the testicle.

Undescended Testicles

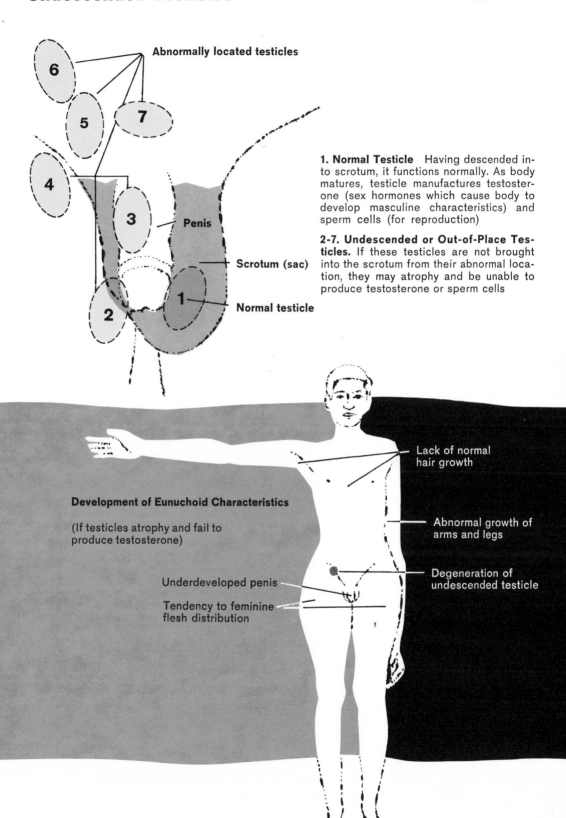

Abnormally located testicles

6

5

7

4

3

Penis

Scrotum (sac)

1

2

Normal testicle

1. Normal Testicle Having descended into scrotum, it functions normally. As body matures, testicle manufactures testosterone (sex hormones which cause body to develop masculine characteristics) and sperm cells (for reproduction)

2-7. Undescended or Out-of-Place Testicles. If these testicles are not brought into the scrotum from their abnormal location, they may atrophy and be unable to produce testosterone or sperm cells

Development of Eunuchoid Characteristics

(If testicles atrophy and fail to produce testosterone)

Underdeveloped penis

Tendency to feminine flesh distribution

Lack of normal hair growth

Abnormal growth of arms and legs

Degeneration of undescended testicle

the disease and its causes PYELITIS AND CYSTITIS Infections of the urinary tract are caused by a variety of bacteria. Common disorders which tend to recur, they may start in the urinary tract or as a secondary infection. Among the groups particularly subject to these infections are pregnant women, diabetics, patients subject to long periods of bed rest, and patients suffering from urinary tract problems such as kidney stones. Other sufferers are individuals with some neurological disorder that interferes with normal bladder function, and males in the older age groups who are subject to prostatic diseases which prevent free passage of urine.
TUMORS Malignant tumors of the kidney and bladder are fairly common. They are a source of concern because it is difficult to make early diagnosis. Except for one type which is seen in young children, kidney tumors occur most often after the age of 50, in both sexes, and in all races. The most common and most important sign that there may be a tumor present is the painless passage of blood in the urine. The amount may be microscopic or visible to the naked eye, and some time may pass before the blood appears again. On occasion there may be vague pains in the upper abdomen or flanks, and mild cramp.

symptoms PYELITIS AND CYSTITIS When the kidneys are infected, the disease is known as pyelitis. The onset is rapid, with the symptoms shown in the Medi-Graph. When the bladder is infected, the disease is called cystitis. In the latter disease the patient may have low-grade fever, chills, and aches and pains in addition to the symptoms noted in the accompanying Medi-Graph.
TUMORS Kidney tumor symptoms are somewhat similar—as shown in the Medi-Graph.

complications PYELITIS AND CYSTITIS Chronic urinary tract infection can lead to destructive changes in the kidneys. This in turn can lead to high blood pressure and, eventually, loss of ability of the kidneys to function, and uremia.
TUMORS Where there is a tumor, complications arise from infection and interference with urine flow. Severe pyelitis and the obstruction caused by a tumor can result in death. Spread of the tumor to other organ systems is a possible and serious complication.

prevention (or lessening of impact) PYELITIS AND CYSTITIS Pyelitis and cystitis require careful, prolonged treatment which should not be delayed. Fortunately, these urinary tract infections are usually highly responsive to proper care, if they are not neglected. The doctor will probably get urine cultures to identify the responsible bacteria, and will treat the patient with antibiotics or other specific drugs.
Infection in other parts of the body must be treated to prevent spread to the kidneys. Preventive measures are advisable for patients subject to long bed rest or catheterization.
TUMORS The only hope lies in early recognition and prompt surgery. Any neglect of any recognizable symptom can be calamitous.

Urinary Tract Tumors and Infections

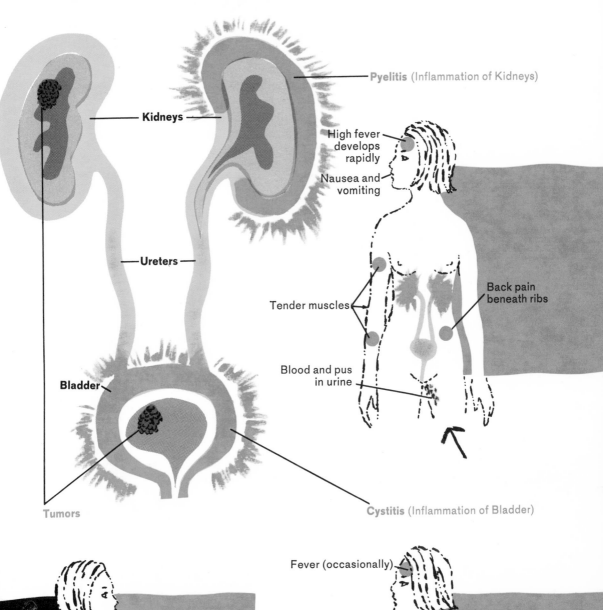

Pyelitis (Inflammation of Kidneys)

Kidneys

High fever develops rapidly

Nausea and vomiting

Ureters

Tender muscles

Back pain beneath ribs

Bladder

Blood and pus in urine

Tumors

Cystitis (Inflammation of Bladder)

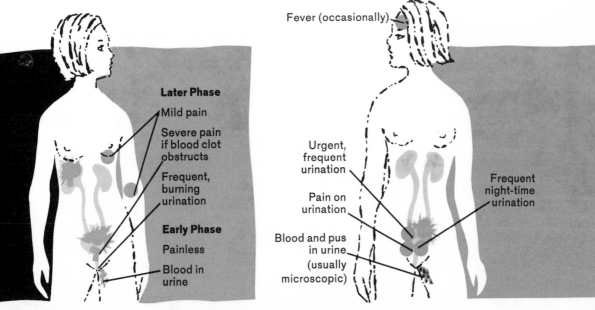

Later Phase

Mild pain

Severe pain if blood clot obstructs

Frequent, burning urination

Early Phase

Painless

Blood in urine

Fever (occasionally)

Urgent, frequent urination

Frequent night-time urination

Pain on urination

Blood and pus in urine (usually microscopic)

the disease and its causes   Varicose veins or varicosities are enlarged, twisted veins near the surface of the skin. They are caused by defective vein valves which can be present at birth; they can result from prolonged postural strain; or they can be the result of extra strain on the valves when the deep veins of the legs function ineffectively. Stagnation and back pressure on the vein result from these conditions, causing over-stretching, lengthening, and enlargement of the vein walls.

Varicosities are commonly seen in people whose work requires them to stand for long periods, and in women after pregnancy. Both men and women are subject to this disease, which usually appears in the legs and becomes more troublesome as age advances.

Sometimes only a short section of a single vein is involved; sometimes nearly all the veins in one or both legs are affected. Most cases involve the surface veins which lie just under the skin. If there are no other complications, these enlarged veins are not a serious threat to health. When varicose veins become severe, it may be the result of a disease or injury involving deep veins higher in the legs or in the body. In these cases, the underlying causes must be treated.

symptoms   In the early stages there is no discomfort and the patient is generally more concerned with the unsightly appearance of the swollen veins. The first symptom is usually a feeling of heaviness in the legs. As the disease progresses, the feet swell. Still later there is pain, explained by the fact that the veins are close to the nerves of sensation.

Skin changes commonly result, and there is deep pigmentation in some areas. Skin ulcerations can appear, with craters that become quite large and heal slowly. Other symptoms are shown in the Medi-Graph.

Because all of these are also symptoms of other diseases or conditions, they cannot always be blamed on varicose veins. Only a doctor can decide in each case.

Another kind of vein which makes an appearance is called the "spider burst" type. These are tiny, purple veins seen under the skin in spidery clusters. They do not have the same significance as varicose veins, and in most instances doctors say that no treatment is necessary. Sometimes treatment to improve their appearance is tried, but this is rarely successful.

complications   If varicose veins are not treated, eventually the enlarged veins, the ulcerated skin, and the swollen feet can disable the patient almost completely.

Phlebitis, which is an associated inflammation of the skin, and secondary infections related to the skin ulcers, are the complications of this disease. Rupture of the veins, with hemorrhage under the skin, is also seen frequently.

prevention (or lessening of impact)   Elastic stockings and raising up the feet during periods of rest can limit the further development of varicose veins. Injection therapy has been useful in limiting the disease. Surgery offers the best hope for cure once the varicosities are well established.

Varicose Veins

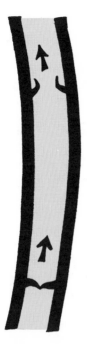

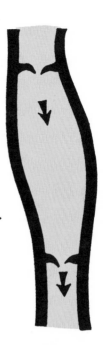

◄ **Operation of Normal Vein**
Valves along your veins channel flow of blood. When valve above opens to guide flow toward heart, valve below closes to prevent backward escape of blood.

Varicose Vein ▶

In varicose vein, walls swell out. Valves no longer close to prevent back flow of blood. Blood accumulates in vein.

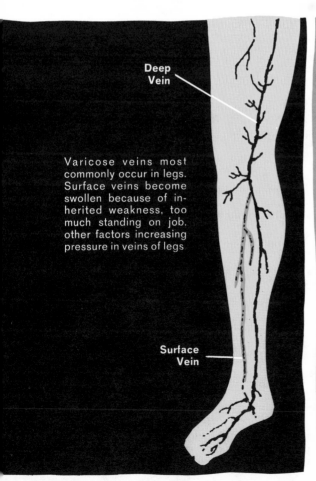

Deep Vein

Varicose veins most commonly occur in legs. Surface veins become swollen because of inherited weakness, too much standing on job. other factors increasing pressure in veins of legs

Surface Vein

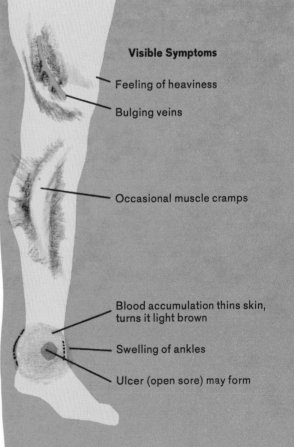

Visible Symptoms

Feeling of heaviness

Bulging veins

Occasional muscle cramps

Blood accumulation thins skin, turns it light brown

Swelling of ankles

Ulcer (open sore) may form

the disease and its causes   Vitamin A is a fat-soluble vitamin found in large amounts in liver, eggs, cream, butter, fish liver oil, and green and yellow vegetables. When a diet does not include enough of these foods, the result is a disease which affects principally the eyes and skin. The severest changes occur in young infants, but milder forms can appear in individuals of any age or race.

symptoms   The most serious effect is on the eyes of an infant. There is dryness and scaling of the cornea and the conjunctiva—which are the delicate membranes that line the eyelids and cover the eyeball. Vision is interfered with and there is extreme sensitivity to light. While adults with this disease show no positive signs when their eyes are examined, infants with severe cases develop some coloring or pigmentation of the eye membrane, and occasionally there are white spots around the cornea.
In the mild form there is night blindness or poor adaptation to the dark. The skin on the thighs, arms, and sometimes the face, thickens so that it resembles a permanent goose flesh. The hair tends to be dry and brittle. The tear ducts may waste away and dry out.

complications   If the cornea is extensively involved and there is some secondary infection, blindness can result. In young infants, bronchial pneumonia is often a complication.

prevention (or lessening of impact)   All that is necessary to prevent vitamin A deficiency is a diet that adequately includes the foods mentioned: liver, eggs, cream, butter, fish liver oil, and green and yellow vegetables. Supplementary doses of vitamin A can be bought commercially. For example, the simplest form is cod liver oil.
When the eyes of infants are involved, early recognition and treatment are important to prevent blindness.

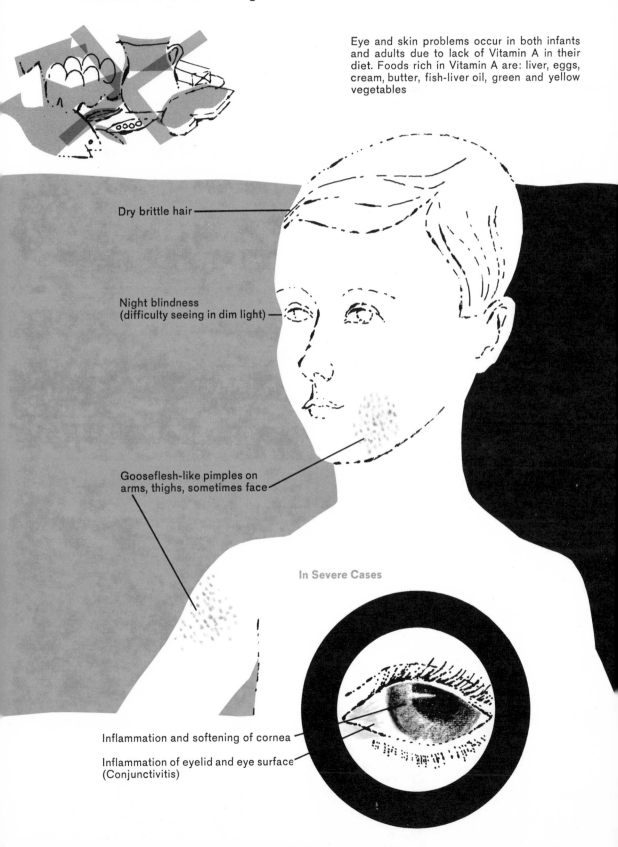

Eye and skin problems occur in both infants and adults due to lack of Vitamin A in their diet. Foods rich in Vitamin A are: liver, eggs, cream, butter, fish-liver oil, green and yellow vegetables

Dry brittle hair

Night blindness (difficulty seeing in dim light)

Gooseflesh-like pimples on arms, thighs, sometimes face

In Severe Cases

Inflammation and softening of cornea

Inflammation of eyelid and eye surface (Conjunctivitis)

the disease and its causes   Warts are elevations of the skin that can occur on any part of the body but occur most often on the fingers, face, and soles of the feet. They are caused by a virus and are moderately contagious, spreading from one area to another in the same person, or to several members of one family. They are extremely common in children. It is hard to say how long warts will last. Their response to medication is uncertain and, in fact, it is reported that cases of warts have been cured by suggestion or hypnosis! Often they disappear without any treatment at all.

symptoms   They appear at first as rather flat masses about the size of a pinhead. Rapidly they develop into raised, hard, rough-surfaced, horny bumps, usually grayish brown in color. It is not unusual to find a central large wart surrounded by a ring of small ones. There may be some local tenderness, but as a rule there is no real pain.
When warts occur on the feet (plantar warts) they are not usually raised because the constant pressure of walking flattens them and drives them under the skin. Because of this pressure, however, they can be quite painful and make walking difficult.

complications   There are no serious complications, and there is no relationship between warts and cancer. When they occur on the feet and attempts are made to root them out surgically, the healing can be slow and the patient can be somewhat handicapped during the healing process.

prevention (or lessening of impact)   There is no way to prevent warts from developing, nor is there a sure way to evaluate how effective treatment is. Plantar warts which are painful and disable the patient are treated by a variety of medical and surgical techniques. One method—where the doctor paints the affected area with acid as long as the wart is visible—is credited with some success without being painful to the patient.

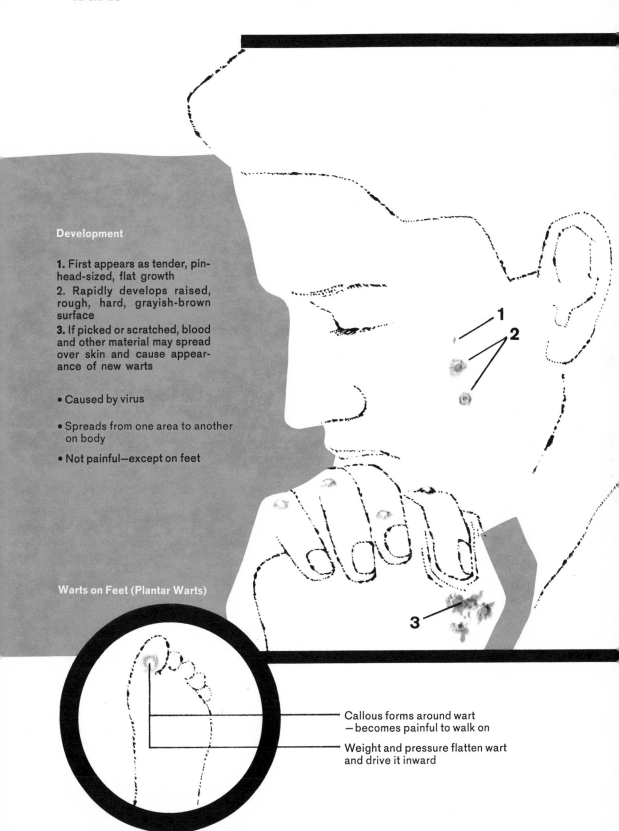

Development

1. First appears as tender, pinhead-sized, flat growth

2. Rapidly develops raised, rough, hard, grayish-brown surface

3. If picked or scratched, blood and other material may spread over skin and cause appearance of new warts

- Caused by virus

- Spreads from one area to another on body

- Not painful—except on feet

Warts on Feet (Plantar Warts)

Callous forms around wart —becomes painful to walk on

Weight and pressure flatten wart and drive it inward

the disease and its causes WENS Wens are cysts or sacs which form when the fatty material produced by the oil glands of the skin is unable to reach the surface of the skin.

MILIUM A milium is a nodule the size of a pinhead, which appears often on the face, especially in the region of the eyelids. The cause is unknown.

LIPOMA A lipoma is a tumor made up of an abnormal collection of fatty cells beneath the skin. It is quite common and may appear on any part of the body singly or in number. The growth is round, feels rubbery, and has a normal skin covering.

symptoms WENS They are found, as a rule, on the scalp, behind the ears, and on the back. Their size varies. Wens may appear singly or in combination with others.

MILIUM The nodules are yellowish white and usually hard.

LIPOMA Characteristically, they are soft masses that move freely. Usually they are painless, but they can be tender.

complications WENS Occasionally wens will become inflamed. Once open, they empty out a foul-smelling, cheesy material. However, they can be removed surgically and present no serious problems. They never become cancerous.

MILIUM The only complication is the unfavorable effect these have on one's appearance. However, milia are easily removed surgically and present no serious problems.

LIPOMA A lipoma never results in cancer and is easily removed surgically. Occasionally it becomes infected.

prevention (or lessening of impact) There is no way to prevent their development, but in cases where such growths have become infected, surgical removal is indicated to prevent further problems.

Wens, Milium and Lipoma (Non-malignant Skin Growths)

Cross-Section of Skin

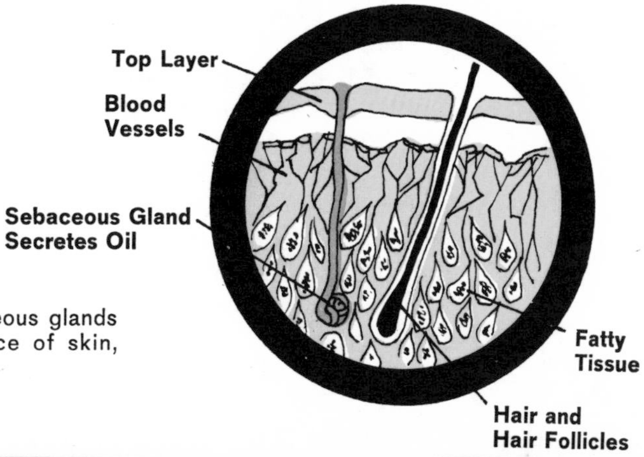

Top Layer

Blood Vessels

Sebaceous Gland Secretes Oil

Fatty Tissue

Hair and Hair Follicles

If fatty material produced by sebaceous glands is prevented from reaching surface of skin, resulting blockage can form...

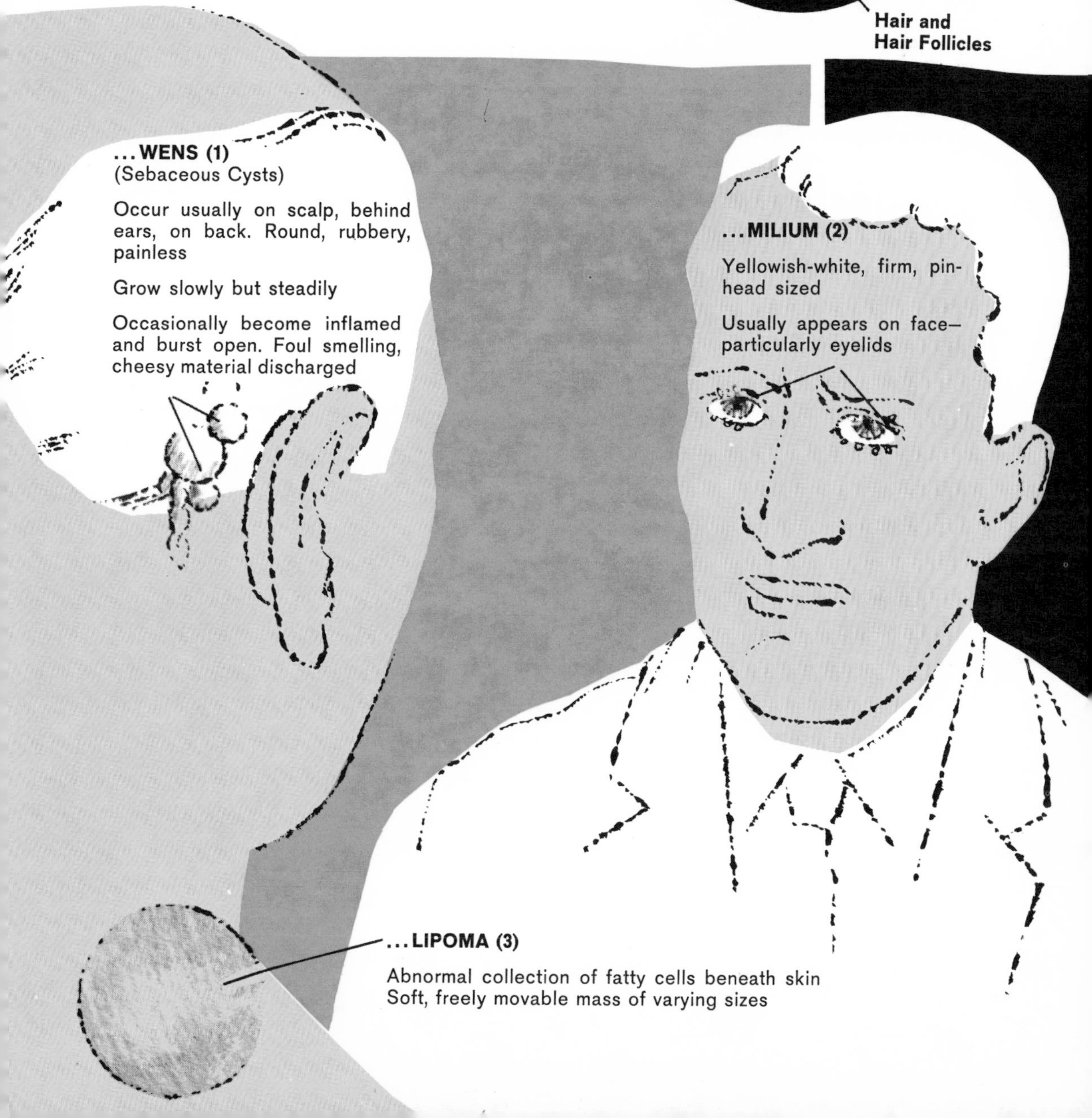

...WENS (1)
(Sebaceous Cysts)

Occur usually on scalp, behind ears, on back. Round, rubbery, painless

Grow slowly but steadily

Occasionally become inflamed and burst open. Foul smelling, cheesy material discharged

...MILIUM (2)

Yellowish-white, firm, pin-head sized

Usually appears on face—particularly eyelids

...LIPOMA (3)

Abnormal collection of fatty cells beneath skin
Soft, freely movable mass of varying sizes

the injury and its causes   Whiplash is seen more and more and has become a distressing medical and legal problem. It is generally the result of an automobile accident in which a car that is slowing down or completely stopped is hit forcibly from the rear. Studies show that in such cases the patient's head is first snapped back and then forward, with considerable force. A head-on collision with any object can also cause whiplash. The damage that results is something like a severe sprain that might be found about any joint. Damage is usually done to the ligaments supporting the vertebrae of the neck. There is stretching, some tearing, and sometimes internal bleeding around the injured area. The injury can take a very long time to heal, and during the recovery period the patient cannot do anything that would put strain on his arms, shoulders, and neck.

symptoms   At the time of the accident there may be only a few symptoms or none at all. The patient may complain of a slight neck pain or inability to move his head freely. After 24 hours the neck pain increases and the victim cannot move his head in any direction, particularly forward and backward, without pain. Muscles over the front or back of the neck can become very tight and tender to touch. The pain radiates into the shoulders or down to the fingertips. Weakness, numbness, or tingling in one or both arms is not unusual. Occasionally the patient complains that he has a headache and feels dizzy and nauseated when he changes his position.

complications   The accident causing whiplash can also cause a fracture or dislocation of a vertebra of the neck. Sometimes herniation of a cervical disc occurs. This means that one of the discs located between the neck's vertebrae has been pushed out of position. It may then press on the nerves emerging from the spinal column and cause severe pain.
This herniated disc or other severe nerve injury resulting from the whiplash can interfere with full use of the upper extremities and be a serious handicap to a working man or woman.

prevention (or lessening of impact)   The most logical preventive step is to drive carefully. Cars should be equipped with such safety equipment as seat belts and head rests and these should be used whenever the car is in use. Drug therapy, neck supports, and physiotherapy are available for the patient with a whiplash injury to the neck. Orthopedic and medical care can make him more comfortable and minimize his disability.

Whiplash Injury of the Neck

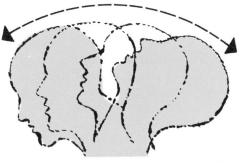

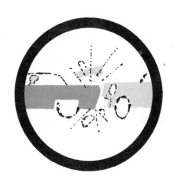

1. Accident As result of sharp impact, head snaps back and forth with great force

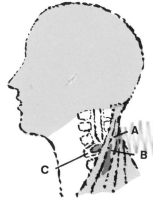

2. Damage
A. Stretching and tearing of ligaments
B. Bleeding around injured area
C. Occasionally goes on to severe nerve injury. Herniation of cervical disc, fracture or dislocation may be accompanying injuries

3. Initial Reaction
May be slight neck pain and limitation of head movement—or little noticeable pain

4. After 24 Hours

Weakness

Headache

Dizziness

Nausea

Front and back neck muscles tender to touch

Pain may radiate on position change

Increased pain— especially when moving head forward or backward

Numbness Tingling

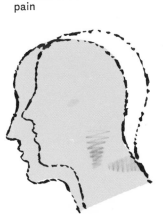

5. Next Several Weeks
Pain and weakness in neck, shoulders, arms during lifting or other strain producing activities

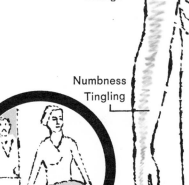

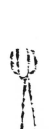

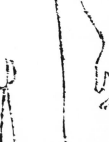

the disease and its causes   Whooping cough is a contagious disease involving the respiratory tract and is caused by a specific type of bacteria. It gets its name from the whooping sound produced by a patient taking a deep breath inward after a prolonged coughing seizure. It is a childhood disease primarily, and can be fatal to very young children if complications become severe. One attack gives lifelong immunity.

symptoms   It may begin with low-grade fever and mild cold-like symptoms. This is followed by a dry, hacking cough which becomes worse at night. By the 3rd week the typical explosive cough, followed by the long whoop, has developed. A coughing spell usually continues until the characteristic stringy mucus can be expelled. During this stage the child's face may become bluish, the eyes bloodshot, and he is most uncomfortable. This stage may go on for as long as a month. The final stage resembles an ordinary bronchitis and may continue another 3 or 4 weeks.

complications   Bronchopneumonia is a frequent complication because the thick mucus plugs block the bronchial tubes. Lung collapse and other destructive lung changes can also occur. Ear infections are another possibility. Sometimes intestinal problems are brought on by the repeated vomiting which follows severe coughing. The resulting loss of important chemicals in the blood can lead to serious problems. One is the development of a condition in which the muscles go into painful and prolonged spasms accompanied by tingling, numbness and sometimes twitching. This is called tetany. Meningitis and encephalitis are rare complications.

prevention (or lessening of impact)   Fortunately, a vaccine that prevents whooping cough is available and should be given to every child before he or she reaches school age. It consists of a series of three injections. Exposure to known cases of whooping cough should be avoided, but if a child does become exposed he should be given booster shots.
Antibiotics are used to prevent complications and control the long course of the illness. Sedation is used to control the cough and the distress of the patient. Oxygen is sometimes provided during severe, choking coughing.

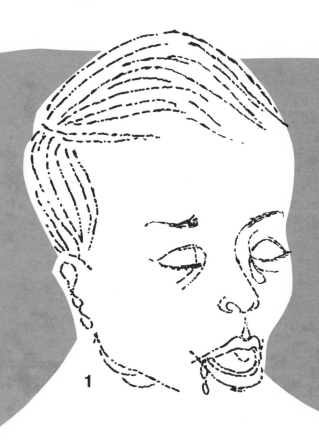

1. Puffy Face
3-4 days after heavy coughing stage starts, child's face becomes puffy and blueish in color. Eyes tear, tongue is pushed out and mucus is expelled during coughing spell.

2. Bloodshot Eyes
Around 5th day, heavy coughing causes bloodshot eyes because of breaking of some blood vessels in lining of eyes.

3. Sore Under Tongue
Rubbing of tongue against teeth during coughing spells usually produces sore under tongue by 6th day.

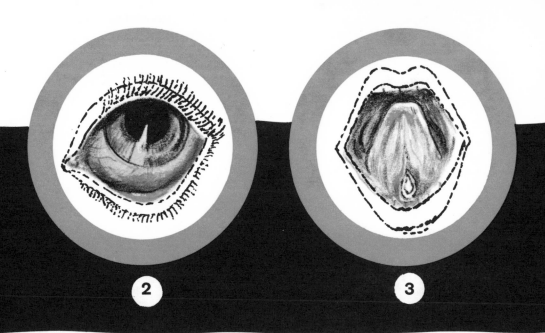

the disease and its causes   This disease is caused by a virus which is transmitted to man through the bite of an infected mosquito, *Aedes aegypti*. In the forests of Africa, South and Central America, where monkeys and possibly other animals carry the disease, another form of it is transmitted to man from monkeys by a "forest mosquito."

The incubation period for yellow fever is from 3–6 days following the bite of an infected mosquito. Once in the bloodstream, the virus is carried to the spleen, kidneys, lymph glands and bones.

symptoms   Yellow fever shows itself suddenly with chills, high fever, headache and backache. Nausea and vomiting are common—with a characteristic black vomit due to intestinal bleeding or blood from the gums. The patient's face becomes flushed and swollen, and his lips and tongue are bright red. The kidneys are frequently infected.

After 2 or 3 days, the patient's temperature frequently drops—and his pulse slows down—below normal. His skin grows cold and he takes on a jaundiced coloration. (This yellow coloration has given the disease its name: yellow fever.)

The chill-fever cycle may break in 3–4 days, only to recur again after a brief respite. But most patients start improving by the end of the first week.

The doctor diagnoses the disease by blood tests.

complications   About 5% of all yellow fever cases still end in death. This is due, in severe cases, to degeneration of the liver, kidneys and heart.

prevention (or lessening of impact)   Eradication of the mosquitoes that spread the disease is the weapon which has proved most effective against yellow fever. A vaccine has been developed which is also extemely effective— and should be taken if you have to enter an epidemic area.

No specific drugs have been found which can quickly cure the disease once it has taken hold. But one attack does give life-long immunity to yellow fever.

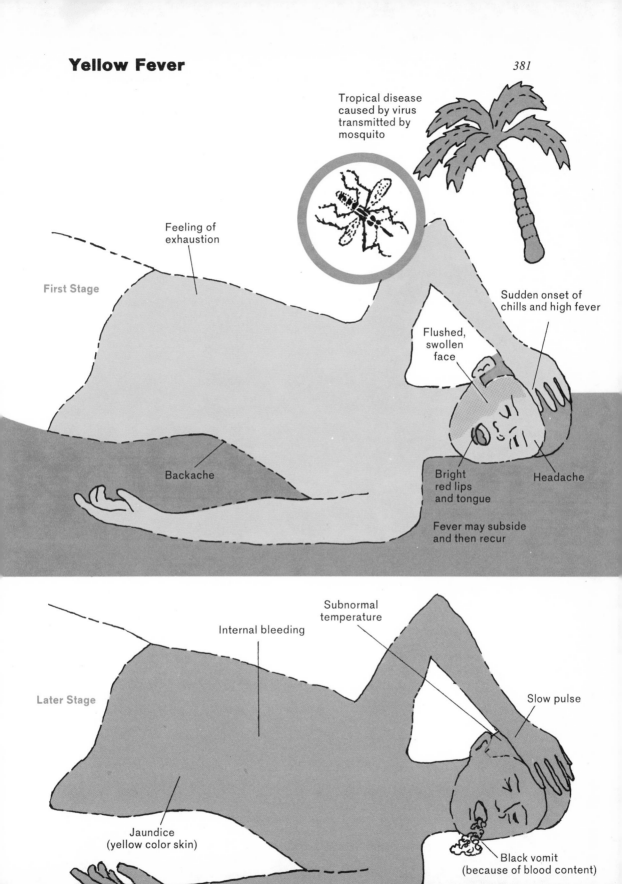

Yellow Fever

Tropical disease caused by virus transmitted by mosquito

First Stage

Feeling of exhaustion

Backache

Sudden onset of chills and high fever

Flushed, swollen face

Bright red lips and tongue

Headache

Fever may subside and then recur

Later Stage

Internal bleeding

Subnormal temperature

Slow pulse

Jaundice (yellow color skin)

Black vomit (because of blood content)

Index

A

abdomen, fluid in, 170, 172, 266
abdomen, swelling of, 64, 74, 84, 166, 206, 266, 268, 360
abdominal discomfort, 60, 68, 88, 306, 342
abdominal hernia, 184
abdominal pain, 16, 20, 28, 64, 112, 140, 146, 148, 154, 180, 182, 194, 206, 216, 254, 266, 268, 320, 354, 362
abscess, 12, 28, 226, 264, 280
abscess, lung, 226
aches and pains, 150, 218, 250, 310, 328, 348, 366
acne, 12
acromegaly, 14
Addison's disease, 16
adrenal cortex, underactive, 16
adrenal glands, overactive, 98
aerosols, sniffing of, 120
alcoholism, 18
allergy, 160, 190
amebiasis, 20
amebic dysentery, 20
amphetamines, drug abuse, 106
anal canal, tear in lining, 178
anemia, 58, 60, 188, 194, 198, 230, 254, 310
anemia, pernicious, 148, 276
anemia, sickle cell, 320
anesthetics, sniffing of, 120
aneurysms, 22
ankles, swelling of, 84, 98, 368
anthracosis, 24
anthrax, 26
anus area, itching and irritation of, 282
anxiety, 110, 118, 202, 258, 268
apathy, 42, 242
apoplexy, 336
appendicitis, 28
appetite, loss of, 16, 20, 64, 68, 74, 84, 88, 140, 148, 160, 180, 198, 220, 272, 276, 306, 314, 358
appetite, poor, 34, 288
arch pain, 52
armpit hair, absence of, 364
armpit hair, decrease in, 240
armpit pain, 56
arms, numbness, 376
arms, pains in, 320
arms, tingling, 376
arteries, hardening, 30, 102
arteries, narrowed, 32
arteriosclerosis, 22, 30, 202
arteriosclerosis obliterans, 32
arteriosclerosis, peripheral, 32
arthritis, 34, 312
asbestosis, 24
ascariasis, 306
asphyxia, 296
atherosclerosis, 30
athlete's foot, 144

B

backache, 98, 380
back, arched, 346
back, hunched, 14
back pain, 64, 136, 326, 366
bacterial endocarditis, subacute, 130
bacterial infections of skin, 70
balance, loss of, 236, 248
barbiturates, drug abuse, 108

beard, absence of, 364
behavior, drunken, 18, 108, 120
behavior, erratic, 18, 106, 110, 114, 116, 120, 132
belching, 146, 182
Bell's palsy, 36
beriberi, 38
bite(s), animal, 296
bite(s), snake, 330
bite, viper, 330
black and blue marks, 142, 176, 314, 330, 332
blackheads, 12
blackout, 19
blackwater fever, 230
bladder and bowel control, loss of, 132, 214, 248, 326
bladder pain, 58
Bleeder's disease, 176
bleeding, abnormal, 58, 176, 220
blindness, 344
blind spots, 42
blisters, 80, 86, 92, 144, 318, 328
blood pressure, high, 22, 98, 110, 122, 186, 254, 312
blood pressure, low, 16, 204
blood spitting, 22, 44, 62, 286, 306, 358
blood sugar, low, 16, 202, 204
blood vessels, broken, 84
blood vessel wall enlargement, 22
body hair, loss of, 204
body odor, 114
boils, 70
bones, easily broken, 74, 98, 198, 302
bone, infection of, 264
bone pain, 198, 220
botulism, 40
bowel habits, change in, 60, 342
bowel movement, painful, 178
bowel movements, interference with, 184
bowlegs, 302
brain, disease of, 132
brain tumors, 42
breastbone, pain beneath, 288
breast cancer, 56
breast, enlargement of, 124
breast, lump in, 56
breasts, atrophy of, 204
breasts, enlargement of male, 84
breath, gasping for, 46
breathing difficulty, 24, 38, 104, 126, 146, 160, 170, 172, 290, 322
breathlessness, 126, 174, 258
breath odor, 102, 104, 352
breath, shortness of, 24, 44, 46, 48, 50, 62, 94, 162, 164, 166, 170, 172, 182, 200, 220, 226, 228, 258, 274, 276, 322, 358
bronchial adenoma, 44
bronchial asthma, 46
bronchial tubes, inflammation of, 50
bronchiectasis, 48
bronchitis, 50
Buerger's disease, 52
bulbar polio, 290
bursitis, 54

C

calf pain, 32, 52, 278
cancer, blood, 220
cancer, breast, 56
cancer, cervix, 58
cancer, colon, 60
cancer, epidermoid, 66
cancer, lung, 62
cancer, lymph glands, 192
cancer, pancreas, 64
cancer, prostate, 292
cancer, rectum, 60
cancer, skin, 66
cancer, stomach, 68
cancer, uterus, 58
carbuncles, 70
cardiac neurosis, 258

cataracts, 72, 102
celiac disease, 74
central nervous system, disease of, 132, 248
cerebral palsy, 76
cervix, cancer of, 58
Chagas' disease, 78
chancre, 340
change of life, 240
chest, deformed, 22, 126, 302
chest discomfort, 94, 258
chest pain, 24, 48, 56, 62, 94, 122, 134, 140, 164, 166, 172, 188, 226, 258, 274, 276, 286, 322, 358
chewing difficulty, 252, 346
chickenpox, 80
chills, 26, 70, 112, 130, 140, 188, 218, 226, 230, 238, 260, 264, 288, 304, 310, 318, 340, 348, 354, 360, 366, 380
cholera, 82
circulation, blocked, 320
circulation, loss of, 312
cirrhosis, liver, 84
clitoris enlargement, 98
cocaine, drug abuse, 110
cold sores, 86
colic, 216
colitis, ulcerative, 88
collapse, 82
colon, cancer of, 60
coma, 18, 42, 46, 102, 118, 120, 122, 128, 186, 202, 216, 238, 254
confusion, 30, 98, 128, 202, 244, 272, 336
congenital heart disease, 162
conjunctiva, dryness and scaling of, 370
conjunctivitis, 90
constipation, 60, 64, 84, 88, 96, 136, 198, 206, 210, 268, 360
contact dermatitis, 92
convulsions, 78, 108, 110, 122, 128, 132, 174, 186, 202, 216, 238, 254, 296, 328, 330, 344, 346
coordination, impaired, 114, 276
coordination, loss of, 18, 116, 120
copperhead bite, 330
coral snake bite, 330
cornea, dryness and scaling of, 370
coronary artery disease, 94, 102
cottonmouth bite, 330
cough, 22, 24, 44, 100, 126, 162, 166, 170, 172, 188, 192, 194, 226, 234, 246, 274, 286, 296, 306, 322, 348, 358, 378
cough, dry, 46, 48, 50, 62
cough, hacking, 378
cough, persistent, 140
cretinism, 96
Cushing's syndrome, 98
cystitis, 366
cyst, pilonidal, 280
cyst, sebaceous, 374

D

deafness, 36, 42, 198, 236
dehydration, 82
delirium, 78, 108, 120, 128, 216, 238, 272, 296, 308, 328
delirium tremens, 18
depression, 74, 98, 106, 108, 118, 140, 240, 242, 244, 272, 276, 296
dermatitis, 92, 272, 316
deviated septum, 100
diabetes, 102
diaphragmatic hernia, 182
diarrhea, 20, 40, 60, 64, 74, 82, 84. 88, 112, 118, 140, 194, 238, 266, 272, 276, 306, 310, 328, 330, 354, 358, 360
diarrhea, bloody, 118, 206, 242
digestive tract, ulcers, 362
diphtheria, 104
disc, slipped, 326

dislocations, 142
dizziness, 30, 40, 42, 114, 120, 128, 162, 166, 174, 186, 236, 240, 258, 272, 320, 376
dizzy spells, 164, 336
drooling, 36, 76, 132, 270
drug abuse, 106-120
drug reactions, 92
duodenal ulcers, 362
dyspepsia, 68
dysentery, amebic, 20

E

earache, 352
ear, buzzing in, 236
ear lobes, elongated, 158
ear pain, 36, 348
ears, itching, 160
ears, ringing in, 36, 42, 236
ear, swelling behind, 232
eclampsia, 122
ectopic pregnancy, 124
effort syndrome, 258
emphysema, 126
encephalitis, 128
endocarditis, subacute bacterial, 130
enteritis, 206
epilepsy, 132
esophagus, diseases of, 134
eunuchoidism, development of, 364
exfoliative dermatitis, 92
exhaustion, 296, 380
exophthalmic goiter, 200
eyebrows, disappearance of, 158
eyebrows, raised, 346
eye, inability to close, 36
eye(s), itching, 90, 160
eyelid(s), drooping, 252
eyelid, inflammation of, 338
eyelid(s), swelling of, 90, 254, 338
eye muscle weakness, 128
eye pain, 152, 212, 318
eyes, blisters and ulcerations of, 318
eyes, bloodshot, 90, 152, 160, 378
eyes, crossed, 290
eye, sensitivity to light, 318
eyes, glassy, 360
eyes, protruding, 200
eyes, pus discharge from, 90
eyes, reddened, 150, 160, 234
eyes, spots before, 72
eyes, staring, 200, 270
eyes, swollen, 160, 324, 354, 318
eyes, tearing, 36, 160, 212, 318
eyes, uncontrolled movement of, 236
eyes, watery, 150, 234

F

face, blue, 166, 182, 226, 268, 378
face, flushed, 114, 174, 360, 380
face, puffy, 378
face, swelling of, 78, 254, 380
face, thickened skin of, 158
face, weakness of, 336
facial hair, increase in, 240
facial muscle weakness, 128
faintness, 162, 174, 258
Fallopian tube, obstruction of, 124
fatigue, 16, 40, 60, 160, 204, 242, 252, 276
feet, enlarged, 14
feet, itching, 194
feet, swelling of, 122, 164, 166, 170, 206, 368
feet, tingling, of 198, 242
fever, 20, 26, 34, 44, 48, 50, 70, 78, 80, 88, 92, 104, 128, 140, 156, 174, 188, 192, 194, 230, 232, 234, 238, 246, 254, 260, 264, 266, 272, 286, 290, 296, 300, 302, 304, 308, 310, 318, 346, 348, 350, 352, 354, 358, 360, 380
fever, absence of, 40
fever blisters, 86

fever, high, 210, 218, 220, 226, 232, 274, 328, 380
fever, irregular, 130
fever, low, 150, 154, 180, 206, 228, 250, 278, 288, 314, 324, 340, 366, 378
fibroid tumor, 136
fibromyositis, 138
finger joints, swelling of, 62
fingernails, blue, 170, 172, 268
fingers, clubbed, 48, 130, 162, 166, 322
fingers, knobby, 262
fingers, numb, 298
fingers, painful, 298
fissures, 178
flabbiness, 204
flashback, 114
flu, 140
folliculitis, 70
foot drop, 256
forehead, thickened skin, 158
forehead, wrinkled, 346
fractures, 142
fungus infections of the skin, 144
furuncles, 70

G

gait, abnormal, 76, 128, 242, 330
gallstones, 146
gangrene, 30, 52, 102
gassiness, 20, 60, 68, 206
gastric ulcers, 362
gastritis, 148
genital organs, disease of, 356
genital organs, ulcerous sore on, 340
German measles, 150
giantism, 14
glands, aches and pains in, 340
gland swelling, 36
glaucoma, 152
glue, sniffing of, 120
goiter, exophthalmic, 200
gonorrhea, 154
gout, 156
Graves' disease, 200
grippe, 140
groin, heaviness in, 196
groin pain, 184, 196
ground itch, 194
growth, excessive, 14
growth, poor, 302
growth, stunted, 74
gums, bleeding, 176, 314, 352
gums, lead line along, 216
gums, rough and grayish, 222
gums, ulceration of, 188

H

hair, coarsening, 96
hair, dry, brittle, 370
hair growth, abnormal, 98
hair, loss of, 84, 92, 96, 340
hair, standing on end, 114
hallucinations, 18, 106, 108, 110, 114, 116, 118, 120
hallucinogen, 114, 116, 118
hands, short, stubby, 96
hands, spade-like, 14
hands, tingling of 198, 242
hands, trembling, 106, 258
handwriting change, 336
Hansen's disease, 158
hashish, drug abuse, 116
hay fever, 160
headache, 14, 26, 42, 72, 98, 100, 104, 106, 122, 128, 132, 140, 148, 156, 164, 174, 186, 202, 218, 230, 238, 244, 246, 254, 272, 276, 288, 290, 296, 304, 310, 320, 336, 340, 346, 348, 352, 360, 376, 380
headache, migraine, 244
head noise, 236
head, pain on moving, 376
head pains, neuralgic, 100
head support, loss of, 290
head tremors, 270

hearing, defective, 100
hearing disturbances, 242
hearing impairment, 76
hearing loss, 232
heartbeat, rapid, 38
heartburn, 182
heart disease, congenital, 162
heart disease, hypertensive, 164
heart disease, pulmonary, 166
heart disease, rheumatic, 168
heart disease, thyroid, 170
heart, enlarged, 38, 166, 170, 172
heart failure, 168, 172
heart, irritable, 258
heart lesions, 312
heart, nervous, 258
heart palpitations, 38, 164, 170, 172, 186, 200, 240, 258, 276
heart rhythm, irregular, 168, 274
heart, soldier's, 258
heat stroke, 174
hematomas, 176
hemophilia, 176
hemorrhage, 22, 124, 130, 148, 236
hemorrhoids, 178
hepatitis, 180
hernia, abdominal, 184
hernia, hiatus (diaphragmatic), 182
hernia, inguinal, 184
heroin, drug abuse, 112
herpes simplex, 86
herpes zoster, 318
hiatus hernia, 182
hiccups, 16, 182
"high," 106, 108, 120
high blood pressure, 186
histoplasmosis, 188
hives, 190
hoarseness, 22, 38, 96, 104, 274, 354, 358
Hodgkin's disease, 192
hookworm, 194
hot flash, 240
hot flush, 240
hunger, 102, 202
hydrocele, 196
hydrophobia, 296
hyperparathyroidism, 198
hypertension, 186
hypertensive heart disease, 164
hyperthyroidism, 200
hypoglycemia, 202
hypogonadism, 204
hypothyroid diseases, 96

I

ileitis, 206
impetigo, 208
impotence, 14, 84, 102
indigestion, 182, 358
infantile paralysis, 290
infectious mononucleosis, 246
influenza, 140
inguinal hernia, 184
insomnia, 106, 272
intestinal obstruction, 210
intestine, inflammation of, 206
intoxication, 18, 108, 118, 120
iris, infection and inflammation of, 212
iritis, 212
irritability, 16, 42, 74, 98, 106, 116, 186, 200, 240, 244, 272, 290, 314
itching, 92, 102, 144, 190, 192, 224, 316

J

jaundice, 64, 84, 122, 180, 192, 218, 246, 268, 350, 380
jaw, protruding lower, 14
jaw, rigid, 346
jaws, clamped, 132
jaw, swelling of glands under, 250
jock itch, 144

joint aches and pains, 180, 262, 304, 340
joint deformity, 35
joint pain, 34, 130, 140, 156, 176, 228, 300, 314
joints, bony spurs on, 262
joints, grating of, 262
joints, fusion of, 34
joints, hemorrhage in, 314
joints, inflammation of, 34, 228
joints, stiffness of, 34, 262
joints, swelling of, 176, 300, 314

K

kidney area pain, 214, 254
kidney disease, 102, 122
kidney failure, 218, 230, 312
kidney stones, 214
knock knees, 302

L

labyrinthitis, 236
larynx, ulceration of, 188
lead poisoning, 216
legs, feeling of heaviness in, 368
legs, pain in, 314, 320
leg(s), swollen, 38, 278
leprosy, 158
leptospirosis, 218
lesions, 12, 144, 190, 208, 224, 272, 340
lethargy, 16, 18, 36, 84, 102, 108, 112, 202, 254, 276, 290
leukemia, 220
leukoplakia, 222
lice, 224
lion face, 158
lipoma, 374
lips, blue, 94, 170, 172, 268
lips, bright red, 380
lips, protruding, 346
liver, cirrhosis of, 18, 84
liver, enlarged, 64, 78, 102, 166, 172, 188, 192, 218, 246, 276, 310, 350
liver, inflammation of, 18, 180
lockjaw, 346
LSD, drug abuse, 114
lumbago, 138
lung abscess, 226
lung cancer, 62
lungs, calcification of, 188
lungs, disease of, 44, 48, 322
lungs, enlarged, 172
lungs, fibrosis of, 312
lungs, fluid in, 170, 172
lupus erythematosus, 228
lymph glands, enlarged, 246, 340
lymph glands, swelling of, 192, 220, 228, 348, 352

M

malaria, 230
malnutrition, 206
marijuana, drug abuse, 116
masculine characteristics, development of, 98
mastoiditis, 232
measles, 234
measles, German, 150
memory lapse, 336
memory, loss of, 30, 108, 128, 132, 272, 276
Ménière's disease, 236
meningitis, 238
menopause, 240
menstruation, abnormal, 58, 136, 240
menstruation, ceasing of, 14, 98, 200, 204
menstruation, delay in, 124
menstruation, recommencement of, 58
mental retardation, 76, 216, 344
mercury poisoning, 242
mescaline, drug abuse, 118
middle ear infection, 232
migraine headache, 244
milium, 374
mononucleosis, infectious, 246
moonface, 98

morning sickness, 124
mouth area, tingling of, 242
mouth, difficulty opening, 346
mouth, dry, 174
mouth, hemorrhage of, 220
mouth, painful, 242, 346
mouth, soreness of, 352
mouth, ulceration of, 188, 220
multiple sclerosis, 248
mumps, 250
muscle aches and pains, 34, 138, 140, 218, 230, 238, 304, 354, 360
muscle cramps, 82, 112, 368
muscle fatigue, 252
muscle rigidity, 35, 270
muscles, atrophied, 76, 252
muscles, inflammation of, 138
muscle spasms, 120, 270, 346
muscle twitching, 110, 112, 254, 290
muscle weakness, 16, 40, 98, 198, 200, 252, 272, 312
myasthenia gravis, 252
myocardial infarction, 94
myxedema, 96

N

nails, brittle, 32, 52
nails, concave, 200
nails, loss of, 92
nails, slow-growing, 32,
nasal allergies, 160
nasal congestion, 100
nasal discharge, 140, 160, 324, 348
nasal septum, 100
nausea, 16, 20, 26, 28, 64, 68, 84, 118, 128, 146, 148, 152, 198, 202, 206, 214, 218, 236, 238, 242, 244, 246, 254, 266, 268, 296, 318, 330, 342, 348, 354, 360, 366, 376, 380
nearsightedness, 72
neck pain, 348, 376
neck, stiff, 232, 238, 290, 346
neck, swelling of, 22
neck veins, swollen, 170, 172
neck, whiplash injury of, 376
nephritis, acute, 254
nervousness, 132, 170, 186, 200, 240, 258
neuritic pain, 22, 32, 216, 256, 318, 326
neuritis, 216, 256
neurocirculatory asthenia, 258
night blindness, 370
night sweats, 220, 358
nontropical sprue, 74
nosebleed, 104, 176, 186, 218, 300, 314, 360
nose, flat, 96
nose, itching, 160
nose, swelling of, 160
nose, thick, 96
numbness, 36, 132, 242, 256, 258, 276, 326, 336
nystagmus, 236

O

obstruction, intestinal, 210
obstruction, nasal, 100
orchitis, 260
osteoarthritis, 262
osteomyelitis, 264
ovarian infection, 266
overweight, 96

P

pain, radiating, 28, 54, 62, 94, 146, 182, 212, 232, 268, 286, 296, 324, 362, 376
pancreas, cancer of, 64
pancreatitis, acute, 268
paralysis, 30, 36, 40, 76, 128, 216, 256, 290, 296, 330, 336
paralysis agitans, 270

parasitic infestations of skin, 224
parathyroid glands, overactive, 198
Parkinson's disease, 270
pellagra, 272
pelvis, pain in, 292
penis, itching and burning, 154, 356
penis, pus discharge from, 154
penis, underdeveloped, 364
peptic ulcers, 362
perception, loss of, 42, 96, 108, 118, 158, 204, 242
pericarditis, 274
peripheral arteriosclerosis, 32
peritonitis, 28
pernicious anemia, 148, 276
peyote, drug abuse, 118
phlebitis, 52, 62, 64, 278
physical skills, loss of, 344
piles, 178
pilonidal cyst, 280
pimple(s), 13, 26, 70
pinkeye, 90
pinworm, 282
pituitary gland, overactive, 14
pituitary gland, underactive, 204
pityriasis rosea, 284
plantar warts, 372
pleurisy, 286
pleuritic pain, 228
pneumoconiosis, coal miner's, 24
pneumonia, 288
pneumonia, recurrent, 44, 62
poisoning, 40, 148, 216, 242
poisonous snakes, 330
poliomyelitis, 290
postnasal drip, 100
potbelly, 302
preeclampsia, 122
pregnancy, ectopic, 124
pregnancy, toxemia of, 122
prostate cancer, 292
prostate gland enlargement, 292
prostration, 174, 272
psoriasis, 294
psychic disturbances, 18, 38, 42, 78, 108, 110, 114, 116, 118, 120, 210, 272, 296, 344
pubic hair, absence of, 364
pubic hair, decrease in, 240
pulmonary heart disease, 166
pulmonary tuberculosis, 358
pulse, irregular, 170
pulse, rapid, 38, 170, 174, 202, 264, 276, 330
pulse, slow, 204, 360, 380
pupil, milky color, 72
pupils, dilated, 40, 106, 110, 118
pyelitis, 366

R

rabies, 296
rage, 242, 296
rash, 78, 80, 92, 102, 150, 224, 228, 234, 238, 246, 284, 300, 304, 308, 310, 328, 354, 356, 360
rattlesnake bite, 330
Raynaud's disease, 298
rectal pain, 20, 58, 60
rectum, cancer of, 60
rectum, varicose veins in, 178
red blood cells, lack of, 276
restlessness, 106, 202, 268, 296, 302
rheumatic fever, 300
rheumatic heart disease, 168
rheumatism, 138
rheumatoid arthritis, 34
rickets, 302
ringworm, 144
Rocky Mountain spotted fever, 304
rodent cancer, 66
roundworm, 306
rubeola, 234
rupture, 184

S

St. Vitus' dance, 300
salivary glands, swelling of, 250
salivation, 270, 330
scabies, 224
scarlatina, 308
scarlet fever, 308
schistosomiasis, 310
sciatica, 326
scleroderma, 312
scrotum, enlarged, 184
scrotum, itching and burning, 356
scrotum, swelling of, 196
scurvy, 314
seborrheic dermatitis, 316
sensitivity to cold, 96, 204
sensitivity to light, 370
sensitivity to sound, 36
sex drive, decreased, 16
sex organs, atrophy of, 204
sexual organs, undeveloped, 96
sex urge, decrease in, 204
shingles, 318
shock, 94, 210, 238
sickle cell anemia, 320
sighing, frequent deep, 258
silicosis, 322
Simmonds' disease, 204
sinusitis, 324
skin, blood spots under, 74, 130, 218, 220, 238, 304, 314
skin, blue tint to, 46, 82, 162, 230, 322
skin cancer, 66
skin, clammy, 200, 330
skin, cold, 230, 330, 380
skin, discoloration of, 16, 34, 52, 54
skin, dry, 96, 174
skin, flaky, 92, 308, 316
skin, fungus infections of, 144
skin growths, 374
skin, pallid, 106, 204, 216, 244, 276, 314
skin, parasitic infestations of, 224
skin, patches on, 158, 284, 294
skin, reddened, 92, 200, 264, 316
skin, scaly, 294, 316
skin, thickening of, 312, 370
skin, thin and shiny, 32
skin ulceration, 66, 320, 368
skull, deformity of, 302
slipped disc, 326
smallpox, 328
snake bites, 330
sneezing, 160
solvents, sniffing of, 120
speaking difficulty, 40, 202, 248, 290, 296
speech, abnormal, 18, 76, 106, 114, 118, 132
spine, pain in, 22, 280
spine, rigid, 290
spleen, enlarged, 78, 130, 188, 192, 220, 230, 246, 276, 310, 350
sprains, 332
sputum, blood in, 48, 62, 218, 226
sputum, foul smelling, 48, 226
sterility, 334
stomach, cancer of, 68
stomach cramps, 16, 74
stomach lining, inflammation and irritation, 148
stomach ulcers, 362
stool, pencil-shaped, 60
stools, blood in, 20, 60, 88, 206, 218, 310, 314
stools, blood on, 178
stools, light colored, 180
stools, mucus in, 60, 88, 206
strains, 332
strength, loss of, 14, 38, 68, 102, 220, 358
strep throat, 348
stroke, 174, 336
stupor, 18, 112, 128, 132, 202
styes, 338

subacute bacterial endocarditis, 130
sunstroke, 174
swallowing difficulty, 22, 40, 62, 104, 134, 274, 290, 296, 312, 346, 348
sweating, 112, 130, 192, 202, 214, 258, 268, 302
sweating, decrease in, 174
sweating, excessive, 34, 106, 170, 200, 230, 240, 244, 300
swelling, 22, 54, 56, 62, 86, 92, 142, 150, 232
syphilis, 340

T

tapeworm, 342
taste, loss of, 36
taste, metallic, 352
Tay-Sachs disease, 344
teething, delayed, 302
teeth, loosening of, 314
teeth, pain around, 352
testicle(s), infection and inflammation of, 260
testicle(s), pain in, 260
testicle(s), swelling of, 260
testicles, undescended, 364
tetanus, 346
thiamine deficiency, 38
thigh bones, pain in, 292
thirst, excessive, 82, 102, 198
throat, gray membrane in, 104
throat, inflamed, 140
throat, itching, 160
throat muscles, spasms of, 296
throat, scratchy, 188, 288
throat, severe pain in, 242
throat, sore, 104, 150, 246, 308, 348, 352, 354
throat, strep, 348
thrombo-angiitis obliterans, 52
thyroid gland enlargement, 200
thyroid gland, underactive, 96
thyroid heart disease, 170
tics, 270
tingling, 114, 132, 256, 276, 326
tinnitus, 236
toes, clubbed, 162
toes, numb, 298
toes, painful, 298
toes, ulceration of, 52
tongue, bright red, 276, 308, 380
tongue, coated, 348, 352, 360
tongue, protruding, 76, 96
tongue, ulceration of, 188, 276, 378
tonsillitis, acute, 348
tonsils, inflamed, 140
toothache, 324
toxemia of pregnancy, 122
toxoplasmosis, 350
trench mouth, 352
trichinosis, 354
trichomonas, 356
tuberculosis, pulmonary, 358
tumor, brain, 42
tumor, fibroid, 136
tumors, urinary tract, 366
typhoid fever, 360

U

ulcerative colitis, 88
ulcers of digestive tract, 362
ulcers, gray membrane on, 352
unconsciousness, 118, 120, 132, 174, 336
uremia, 242
urinary tract infections, 366
urinary tract stones, 214
urinary tract tumors, 366
urinating, discomfort on, 154, 292, 356, 366
urination, decrease in, 254
urination, difficulty starting, 292
urination, excessive, 102, 198

urination, frequent, 136, 154, 198, 214, 266, 292, 366
urine, black, 230
urine, blood in, 214, 292, 314, 366
urine, cloudy, 154, 254
urine, dark, 180
urine, decrease in output, 122
urine, inability to pass, 122, 292
urine, protein in, 122
urticaria, 190
uterus, cancer of, 58

V

vaginal bleeding, 124
vaginal discharge, 58, 356
vaginal itching and burning, 356
varicocele, 196
varicose veins, 368
vein inflammation, 26
vein, pain along, 278
veins, bulging, 368
veins, needlemark tracks over, 112
venereal disease, 334
Vincent's angina, 352
vision, blurred, 40, 42, 72, 114, 122, 152, 212, 248
vision difficulty, 102, 202
vision, double, 42, 72, 248, 252
vision, progressive loss of, 72
visual disturbances, 132, 186, 242, 244
vitamin A deficiency, 370
vitamin B₁ deficiency, 38
vitamin K deficiency, 74
voice, change in, 98, 192
voice, high-pitched, 364
voice, loss of, 38, 128, 348
voice, nasalized, 100, 252
voice, weakened, 16, 252
vomiting, 16, 20, 28, 38, 40, 42, 68, 82, 84, 112, 118, 128, 134, 140, 146, 148, 152, 180, 182, 186, 194, 210, 214, 218, 236, 238, 242, 244, 246, 254, 266, 272, 296, 308, 328, 342, 348, 354, 360, 366
vomiting, black, 380
vomiting, bloody, 314, 330
vulva, irritation, 356

W

walking, delayed, 302
walking difficulty, 248, 256, 270
walking, painful, 278
warts, 372
warty growth, 66
water moccasin bite, 330
water retention, 122
weakness, 14, 20, 26, 34, 42, 48, 56, 60, 62, 70, 84, 88, 92, 114, 124, 130, 140, 156, 166, 170, 186, 194, 202, 204, 228, 240, 242, 246, 248, 254, 258, 260, 264, 266, 268, 272, 274, 276, 288, 290, 292, 302, 314, 318, 320, 322, 324, 340, 352, 376
weight gain, lack of, 314
weight, increase in, 98
weight loss, 16, 20, 34, 38, 48, 56, 62, 64, 68, 74, 88, 102, 120, 170, 188, 192, 198, 200, 206, 220, 228, 272, 314, 358
Weil's disease, 218
wens, 374
wheezing, 44, 46, 62, 126
whiplash injury of neck, 376
whooping cough, 378
windpipe, inflammation of, 50
worm infection, 194, 282, 306, 310, 342, 354
wrist drop, 216, 256
writing difficulty, 242

Y

yellow fever, 380

Male and Female

THE HUMAN BODY
in
Anatomical Transparencies

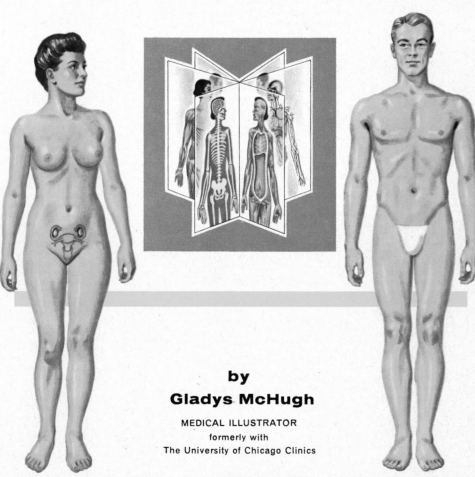

by
Gladys McHugh

MEDICAL ILLUSTRATOR
formerly with
The University of Chicago Clinics

NUMERICAL INDEX

1. Clavicle
2. Sternum
3. Rib
4. Rib cartilage
5. Sterno-mastoid muscle, moves head sideways
6. Trapezius muscle, raises shoulder
7. Deltoid, raises upper arm
8. Major pectoral, moves arm across chest
9. Latissimus dorsi, pulls arm backward
10. External oblique muscle of abdomen
11. Rectus abdominis in fascial sheath
12. Sartorius, "tailor's muscle," used in crossing leg (Beside it is the saphenous vein)
13. Rectus femoris, flexes thigh, extends leg
14. Transverse muscle of abdomen
15. Diaphragm, breathing muscle
16. Intercostals, breathing muscles
17. Skull
18. Temporal, chewing muscle
19. Parotid salivary gland
20. Masseter, chewing muscle
21. Thyroid cartilage
22. Thyroid gland
23. Lung
24. Liver
25. Gall bladder
26. Stomach
27. Small intestine
28. Ascending colon
29. Transverse colon
30. Descending colon
31. Cerebral septum
32. Brain stem
33. Cerebellum
34. Nasal septum
35. Tongue
36. Larynx
37. Superior vena cava
38. Pancreas
39. Duodenum
40. Appendix
41. Trachea
42. Aorta
43. Pulmonary artery
44. Heart
45. Esophagus
46. Inferior vena cava
47. Renal veins
48. Kidney
49. Adrenal gland
50. Spleen
51. Bladder
52. Femoral artery and vein
53. Renal arteries
54. Iliac artery and vein
55. Cerebrum
56. Nasal cavity
57. Brachial nerve plexus
58. Spinal column
59. Scapula
60. Humerus
61. Radius
62. Ulna
63. Hipbone of pelvis
64. Femoral nerve
65. Pelvic plexus
66. Rectum
67. Femur
68. Biceps, flexes arm
69. Extensors of hand
70. Flexors of hand
71. Muscles that pull trunk forward or flex thigh
72. Vastus, flexes thigh, extends leg
73. Muscles that move legs together
74. Triceps, extends arm
75. Greater gluteal, extends thigh, holds trunk upright
76. Tensor fascia lata, counteracts back pull of gluteus
77. Hamstrings, flex leg at knee joint
78. Lumbo-sacral joint
79. Sacrum
80. Sciatic nerve

DESCRIPTION OF PLATES

Plate 1

Front view of male figure with muscles on the right side and bony framework on the left, seen in relation to the vital organs of the body. On this plate is the rib cage, and external muscles of the neck, shoulder, chest, abdomen, hip, and leg. Over the center of the body the abdominal muscles fuse into a heavy sheet of white fascia (connective tissue).

Plate 2

Inside view of structures on first page, showing the attachments of some of the muscles to the bones. Between the ribs are the intercostal muscles that act in breathing. Note defect in lower part of abdominal wall where the spermatic duct pierces it. This is a common site of hernia in men. In the leg, the saphenous vein is seen passing through a hole in the fascia, beside the muscles. This vein and its branches are the site of varicosities when they occur.

Plate 3

The head, lungs, and digestive organs are the main structures here. Part of the skin is removed from the face to show the chewing muscles and the salivary glands. One gland has a duct piercing the cheek muscle; the other gland, visible beneath the jawbone, has ducts entering mouth beneath the tongue. The lungs (and heart) rest upon the diaphragm, a sheet of muscle which divides the chest and abdominal cavities. It acts with the intercostals to expand and contract the rib cage. Beneath the diaphragm is the liver, largest organ in the body, and the stomach. Filling the rest of the abdomen are the intestines.

Plate 4

On this plate is a midplane section through the head, neck, and lungs; in the abdomen, a back view of the digestive organs with their blood supply—the digestive circulation. In this view the bile and pancreatic ducts can be seen entering the duodenum (first part of small intestine).

Plate 5

The circulatory and urogenital systems. The latter is described on Plate 9. In the center of the chest is the heart with the aorta arching above it. Behind the aorta is the trachea. Its branches can be seen in the sectioned lungs with the pulmonary vessels. In the heart-lung circulation the arteries carry stale blood to the lungs and are shown in blue; the veins return oxygenated blood to the heart and are shown in red. This is the reverse of the general body circulation where arteries carry the fresh blood. Except in lungs all arteries are shown in red and veins in blue. The spleen, beneath the diaphragm, lies behind the stomach but is related to the circulatory system.

ALPHABETIC

NAME	NO.	PLATES
Adrenal gland	49	5, 6
Aorta	42	5, 6
Appendix	40	4
Biceps, flexes arm	68	7
Bladder	51	5, 6
Brachial nerve plexus	57	7
Brain stem	32	4
Cerebellum	33	4
Cerebral septum	31	4
Cerebrum	55	7
Clavicle	1	1, 2, 7, 8
Colon, ascending	28	3, 4
Colon, descending	30	3, 4
Colon, transverse	29	3
Deltoid, raises upper arm	7	1, 2, 8
Diaphragm, breathing muscle	15	2, 3, 5, 6, 7
Duodenum	39	4
Esophagus	45	5, 6
Extensors of hand	69	7, 8
External oblique muscle of abdomen	10	1
Femoral artery and vein	52	5, 6
Femoral nerve	64	7
Femur	67	7, 8
Flexors of hand	70	7, 8
Gall bladder	25	3, 4
Gluteal, greater, extends thigh, holds trunk upright	75	8
Hamstrings, flex leg at knee joint	77	8
Heart	44	5
Hipbone of pelvis	63	7, 8
Humerus	60	7, 8
Iliac artery and vein	54	6
Inferior vena cava	46	5, 6
Intercostals, breathing muscles	16	2, 7
Kidney	48	5, 6
Larynx	36	4
Latissimus dorsi, pulls arm backward	9	1, 8
Liver	24	3, 4
Lumbo-sacral joint	78	8
Lung	23	3, 4, 6
Masseter, chewing muscle	20	3
Muscles that move legs together	73	7

ON THE HUMAN BODY

Plate 6

Back view of lungs, trachea, esophagus, great vessels, and urogenital organs. Atop the kidneys are the adrenal glands which secrete cortisone and other hormones. Descending from the kidneys to enter the bladder are the ureters. Near them, at back of bladder, are genital glands. The lower one at base of bladder is the prostate. The pubic bone has been cut from front of pelvis—see matching cut on Plate 7— and with it the inguinal ligaments which were attached to the hipbones.

Plate 7

Midplane section of head and neck and deep structures of chest and abdomen. With the viscera removed we see here the back walls of the chest and abdominal cavities. Only the rectum, down in the pelvis, remains. On the figure's right side are muscles of the arm, leg, and torso; on the left are the bones. Note the cartilage (shown in blue) that covers the bones at the joints — shoulder, elbow, and hip. The head, sectioned in the midplane, reveals the nose, mouth, and throat cavities and the vocal cleft in the larynx. In the cerebrum is the left half of the brain, beneath it the spinal cord and nerve roots. At base of neck they form the brachial plexus. Emerging from the lower end of the spinal canal are nerves to the legs.

Plate 8

Back view of figure, with skeleton on the left, in relation to the vital organs, and muscles of the back on the right. The skull is seen in side view. From the bony pelvis the sacral nerve plexus emerges, giving off branches to muscles of the back. The largest branch, the sciatic nerve, passes over the hip joint to supply the muscles of the back of the leg.

Plate 9

Front and back views of the male urogenital system are shown, with the structures fully labeled and described. These include the urinary organs and the male reproductive or genital organs.

Plate 10

The structures of the female reproductive system are explained on this plate with front and side views of these organs in the pelvis.

Plate 11

The female organs in pregnancy are depicted here with a mid-section through the body of a pregnant woman. A comparative view of a twin pregnancy is also shown and an illustration of the milk structures in the breast.

INDEX

NAME	NO.	PLATES
Muscles that pull trunk forward or flex thigh	71	7
Nasal cavity	56	7
Nasal septum	34	4
Pancreas	38	4
Parotid salivary gland	19	3
Pectoral, major, moves arm across chest	8	1, 2
Pelvic plexus	65	7
Pulmonary artery	43	5
Radius	61	7, 8
Rectum	66	7, 8
Rectus abdominis in fascial sheath	11	1, 2
Rectus femoris, flexes thigh, extends leg	13	1, 2
Renal arteries	53	6
Renal veins	47	5
Rib	3	1, 2
Rib cartilage	4	1, 2
Sacrum	79	8
Sartorius, "tailor's muscle," used in crossing leg (Beside it is the saphenous vein)	12	1, 2
Scapula	59	7, 8
Sciatic nerve	80	8
Skull	17	3, 8
Small intestine	27	3, 4
Spinal column	58	7, 8
Spleen	50	5, 6
Sterno-mastoid muscle, moves head sideways	5	1, 2
Sternum	2	1, 2
Stomach	26	3, 4
Superior vena cava	37	4
Temporal, chewing muscle	18	3
Tensor fascia lata, counteracts back pull of gluteus	76	8
Thyroid cartilage	21	3, 8
Thyroid gland	22	3, 4
Tongue	35	4
Trachea	41	5, 6
Transverse muscle of abdomen	14	2
Trapezius muscle, raises shoulder	6	1, 2, 8
Triceps, extends arm	74	8
Ulna	62	7, 8
Vastus, flexes thigh, extends leg	72	7

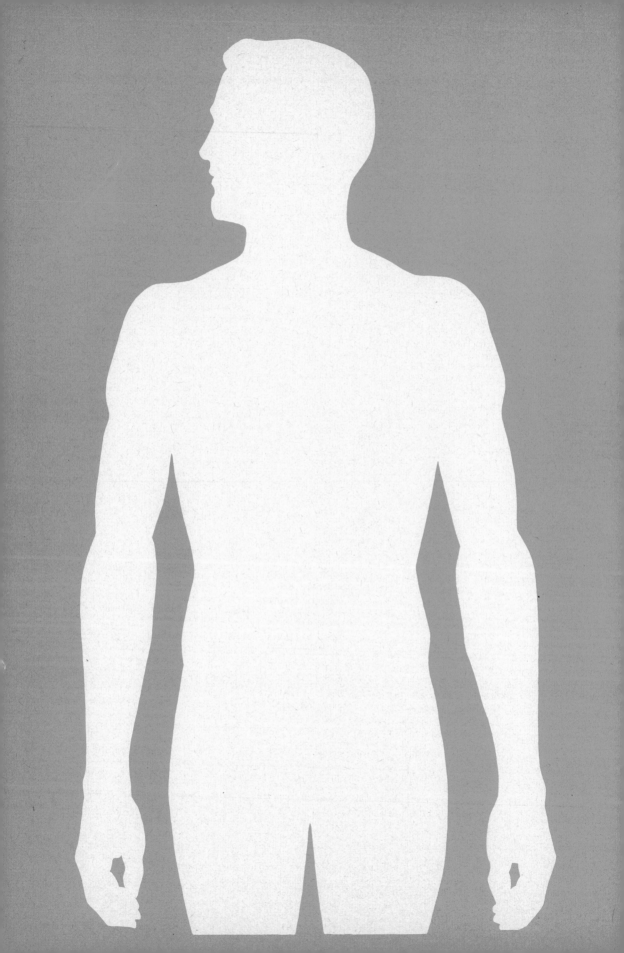

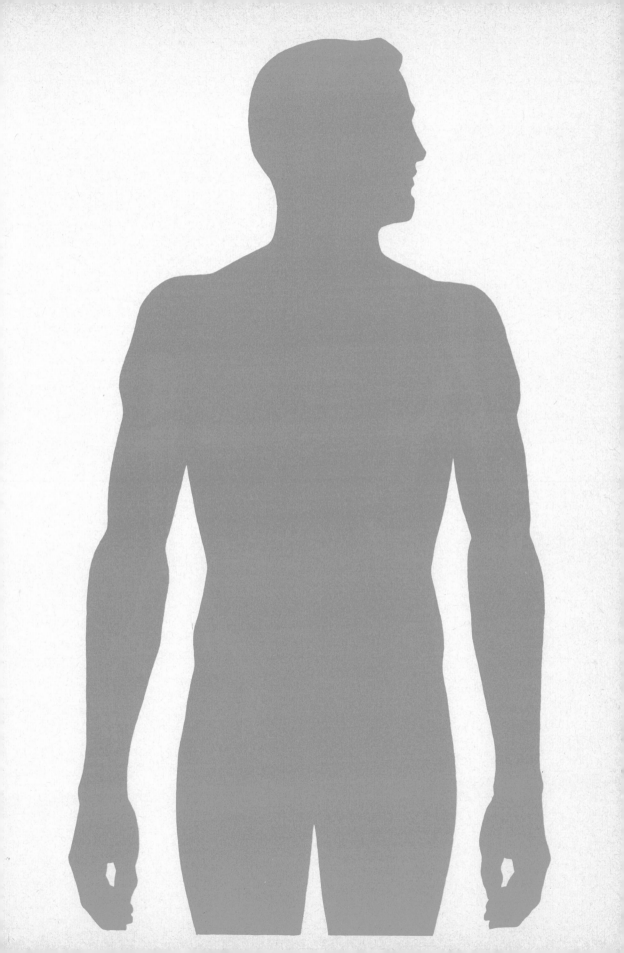

THE MALE UROGENITAL SYSTEM

The male reproductive organs are closely associated with the urinary organs. The sperm produced in the testicles have to pass through the urethra in the penis to leave the body.

THE URINARY ORGANS are the **kidneys,** where blood is filtered and urine is made, the **ureters,** which convey urine to the bladder, the **bladder,** where urine is collected, and the **urethra,** the channel through which it is voided.

THE MALE GENITAL ORGANS are the **testicles** in the scrotum, the **spermatic ducts** (vas deferens) from testicles to urethra, the **seminal vesicles** joining the spermatic ducts, the **prostate gland** surrounding the urethra where the ducts enter it, and the **penis.**

FRONT VIEW

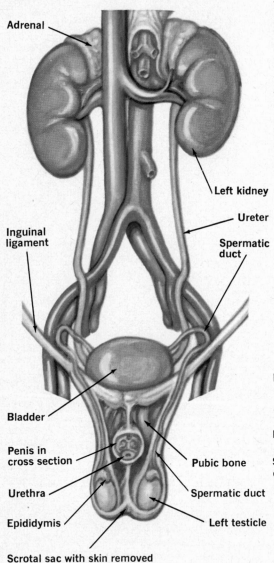

Adrenal

Left kidney

Ureter

Inguinal
ligament

Spermatic
duct

Bladder

Penis in
cross section

Pubic bone

Urethra

Spermatic duct

Epididymis

Left testicle

Scrotal sac with skin removed

BACK VIEW

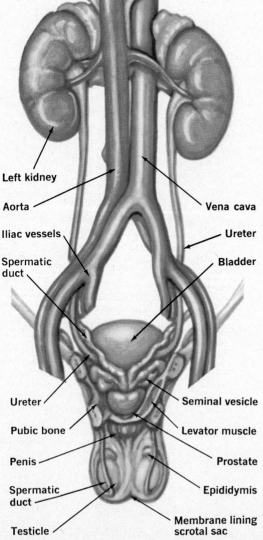

Left kidney

Aorta

Vena cava

Iliac vessels

Ureter

Spermatic
duct

Bladder

Ureter

Seminal vesicle

Pubic bone

Levator muscle

Penis

Prostate

Spermatic
duct

Epididymis

Testicle

Membrane lining
scrotal sac

The testicles manufacture sperm cells, the epididymis stores them for ripening. The latter, a mass of tubules arising from each testicle, continue into the spermatic ducts. The ducts transport the sperm, passing upward, into the abdomen, behind the bladder and through the prostate to reach the urethra. The seminal vesicles and prostate gland secrete fluids which are ejaculated with the sperm to increase their motility.

THE FEMALE REPRODUCTIVE SYSTEM

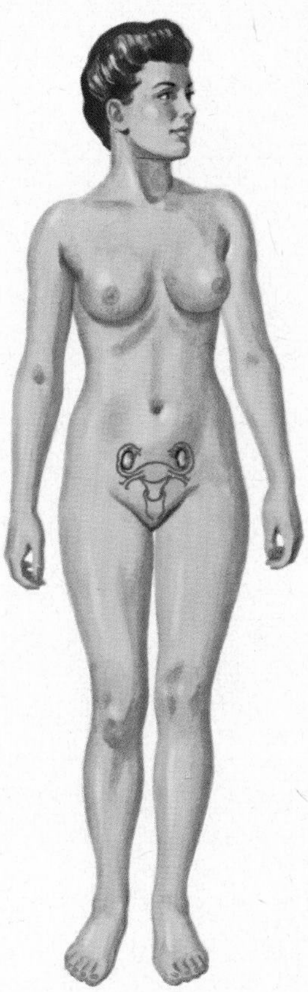

The primary reproductive organs of the female are located in the pelvic part of the abdominal cavity. They are the **ovaries,** which produce the eggs or ova, the **Fallopian tubes,** which transport the eggs to the uterus, and the **uterus,** which houses the baby in pregnancy. The top of the uterus, leaning forward over the bladder, is the fundus, the lower end is the cervix. It projects into the **vagina,** a tube leading to the outside and encircled by the labia, minor and major, of the external genitalia. The Fallopian tubes have open, fimbriated ends. During ovulation, rhythmic movements of the fimbria draw the ovum into the tube and toward the uterus. Accessory reproductive organs are the female breasts.

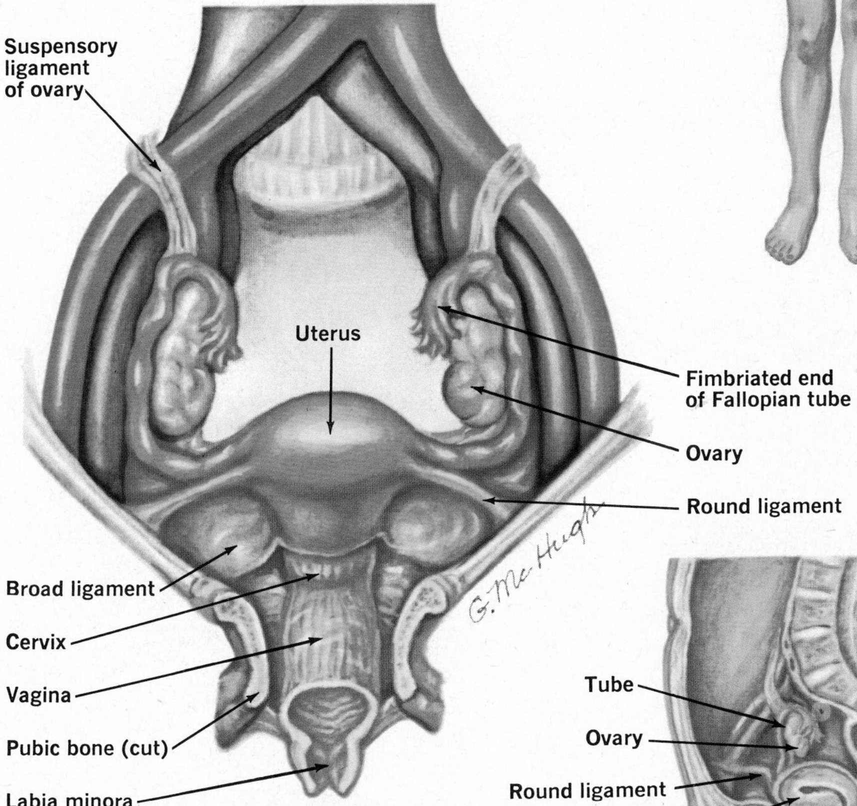

Suspensory ligament of ovary

Uterus

Fimbriated end of Fallopian tube

Ovary

Round ligament

Broad ligament

Cervix

Vagina

Pubic bone (cut)

Labia minora

Front view of Uterus, Tubes and Ovaries. The Bladder and part of the Pubic Bones have been removed.

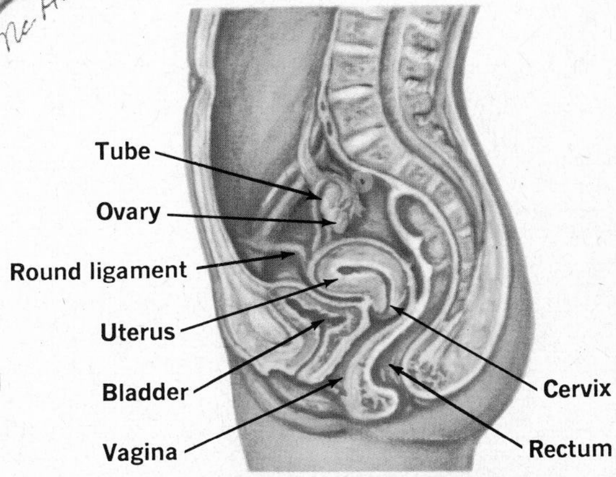

Tube

Ovary

Round ligament

Uterus

Bladder

Vagina

Cervix

Rectum

Side view of Pelvic Organs in Midplane Section.

THE FEMALE ORGANS IN PREGNANCY

During pregnancy the breasts—mammary glands — enlarge as the milk structures grow, but milk is not secreted until after the child is born. The uterus, normally the size of a small pear, undergoes phenomenal enlargement.

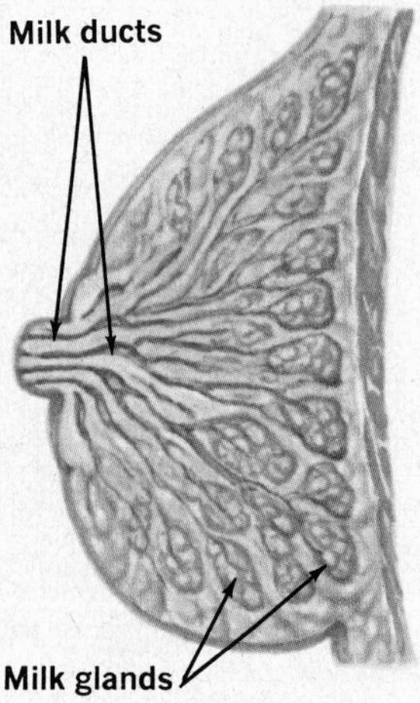

Heart

Liver

Stomach

Placenta

Spine

Milk ducts

Milk glands

Section through a Breast

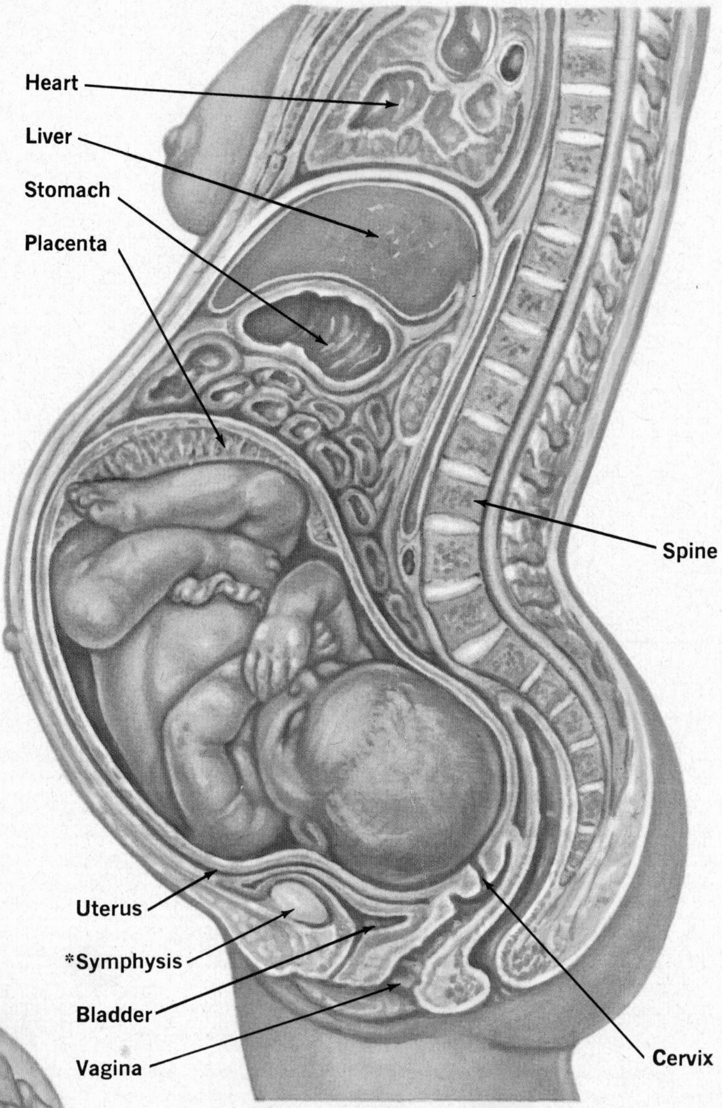

Uterus

*Symphysis

Bladder

Vagina

Cervix

*Cartilage between pubic bones

G. McHugh

Full Term Pregnancy

In this figure the baby's head has dropped down into the pelvis (lightening). This puts pressure on the bladder, cervix and rectum. Note also the adjustment of the abdominal organs to the enlarged uterus.

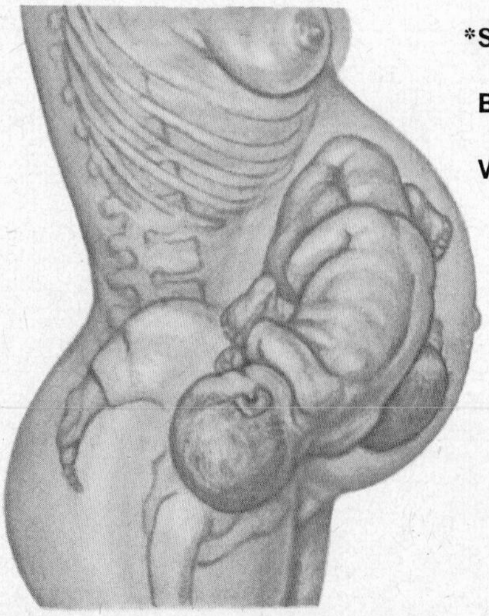

Twin Pregnancy drawn from an X-ray

Printed in Germany